Psychopharmacology Supplementum 2

Dyskinesia

Research and Treatment

Editors:
D. E. Casey T. N. Chase A.V. Christensen J. Gerlach

With 55 Figures

Springer-Verlag
Berlin Heidelberg New York Tokyo

Daniel E. Casey, MD
Clinical Investigator, Medical Research, Psychiatry and Neurology Services at the Veterans Administration Medical Center, and
Associate Professor, Departments of Psychiatry and Neurology at the Oregon Health Sciences University, Portland, OR 97207, and
Collaborative Scientist, Oregon Regional Primate Research Center, Beaverton, OR 97006, USA

Thomas N. Chase, MD
Director, Intramural Research Program, National Institute of Neurological and Communicative Disorders and Stroke, Department of Health and Human Services, National Institute of Health, Bethesda, MD 20205, USA

Anne Vibeke Christensen, MSc Pharm, DSc
Vice-President, Director of Research, H. Lundbeck A/S, Ottiliavej 7–9, DK-2500 Copenhagen-Valby, Denmark

Jes Gerlach, MD
Sct. Hans Mental Hospital, Department AEH, DK-4000 Roskilde, Denmark

---

The figure on the cover has been reproduced in part from L. Uhrbrand, A. Faurbye (1960) Psychopharmacologia I, fasc. 5, Fig. 1, p. 409

ISBN-13: 978-3-642-70142-9 e-ISBN-13: 978-3-642-70140-5
DOI: 10.1007/978-3-642-70140-5

Library of Congress Cataloging in Publication Data
Main entry under title:
Dyskinesia : research and treatment.
(Psychopharmacology. Supplementum ; 2)
Papers presented at an international symposium held in 1984 at Kollekolle, Denmark, and sponsored by the Lundbeck Foundation. Includes bibliographies and index. 1. Tardive dyskinesia–Congresses. I. Casey, Daniel E., 1947–. II. Lundbeck Foundation. III. Series. [DNLM: 1. Dyskinesia, Drug-Induced–congresses. W1 PS774 no. 2 / WL 390 D998 1984] RC394.T37D97 1985 616.8′3 85-2810
ISBN-13: 978-3-642-70142-9 (U.S.)

Typesetting: Daten- und Lichtsatz-Service, 8700 Würzburg

2125/3140-543210

Preface

More than a quarter century has passed since the initial descriptions of tardive dyskinesia (Schonecker, 1957; Sigwald et al., 1959). The earliest epidemiologic study of this disorder was carried out in Roskilde, Denmark, by Uhrbrand and Faurbye (1960); the term tardive dyskinesia was first used a few years later in a subsequent paper (Faurbye et al., 1964). Despite 25 years of intensive investigative scrutiny, the syndrome persists, and approaches to its prevention and treatment continue to have limited efficacy. It is thus fitting to evaluate what has already been learned and consider future directions for research.

Tardive dyskinesia is generally defined as an involuntary movement disorder, mainly involving the mouth, which attends long-term neuroleptic exposure. Beyond these simple facts, however, there has been relatively little consensus about this disorder. A desire to address the controversies associated with tardive dyskinesia prompted the organization of an international symposium at Kollekolle, just outside Copenhagen. This publication comprises all 26 presentations.

The following chapters focus on pathogenetic mechanisms, especially as this knowledge may contribute to the prevention of tardive dyskinesia. Topics include a review of clinical phenomenology and epidemiology; special attention is devoted to an examination of risk factors, particularly in relation to how advancing age or antecedent brain dysfunction might influence individual susceptibility. The contribution of striatal dopamine receptor hypersensitivity to the pathogenesis of tardive dyskinesia is extensively considered; the established hypothesis that this hypersensitivity is responsible for all known characteristics of the disorder can no longer be accepted. While no generally acceptable alternatives have emerged, the presence of GABA system dysfunction receives comprehensive elaboration. The central pharmacological actions of neuroleptics, especially their differential effects on portions of the dopamine system, are critically examined; evidence is presented suggesting that neuroleptics can no longer be considered either necessary or sufficient to produce tardive dyskinesia. Observations deriving from the recent development of suitable animal models for this disorder also receive special attention. Novel approaches to the symptomatic relief of tardive dyskinesia are

---

References:

Faurbye A, Rasch PJ, Bender Peterson P, et al. (1964) Acta Psychiatr Scand 40:10–26
Schonecker M (1957) Nervenarzt 28:35
Sigwald J, Bouttier D, Raymondeaud C (1959) Rev Neurol 100:751–755
Uhrbrand L, Faurbye A (1960) Psychopharmacologia 1:408–418

critically reviewed. Finally, data about antiparkinson drug-induced dyskinesias, as well as idiopathic dystonia and other dyskinesias, contribute additional perspectives to questions surrounding tardive dyskinesia.

We gratefully acknowledge the support provided by the Lundbeck Foundation, which organized and sponsored this Symposium.

Kollekolle, Denmark
January 1985

Daniel E. Casey
Thomas N. Chase
Anne Vibeke Christensen
Jes Gerlach

Contents

Preclinical Aspects

Brain Dopamine Receptors in Schizophrenia and Tardive Dyskinesia
P. Seeman 2

Receptor-Binding Profiles of Neuroleptics
J. Hyttel, J.-J. Larsen, A.V. Christensen, and J. Arnt 9

Functional Classification of Different Dopamine Receptors
U. Ungerstedt, M. Herrera-Marschitz, L. Ståhle, U. Tossman, and T. Zetterström 19

Pharmacological Properties of Presynaptic Dopamine Receptor Agonists
A. Carlsson 31

Influence of GABA Mimetics and Lithium on Biochemical Manifestations of Striatal Dopamine Target Cell Hypersensitivity
B. Scatton, D. Fage, A. Oblin, B. Zivkovic, S. Arbilla, S. Z. Langer, and G. Bartholini 39

New Aspects on the Role of Dopamine, Acetylcholine, and GABA in the Development of Tardive Dyskinesia
J. Scheel-Krüger and J. Arnt 46

Discussion Section

Differential Effects of Dopamine D-1 and D-2 Agonists and Antagonists in 6-Hydroxydopamine-Lesioned Rats
J. Arnt 60

Clinical Aspects

Is Tardive Dyskinesia a Unique Disorder?
C. D. Marsden 64

Tardive Dyskinesia: Prevalence, Incidence, and Risk Factors
J. M. Kane, M. Woerner, and J. Lieberman 72

Involuntary Disorders of Movement in Chronic Schizophrenia
The Role of the Illness and Its Treatment
D. G. Cunningham Owens 79

Tardive Dyskinesia: Reversible and Irreversible
D. E. Casey 88

Pathophysiological Mechanisms Underlying Tardive Dyskinesia
J. Gerlach 98

Chemical and Structural Changes in the Brain in Patients with Movement Disorder
A. J. Cross, T. J. Crow, I. N. Ferrier, J. A. Johnson, E. C. Johnstone, F. Owen, D. G. C. Owens, and M. Poulter 104

Medical Treatment of Dystonia
H. Pakkenberg and B. Pedersen 111

The Effect of Dopamine Antagonists in Spontaneous and Tardive Dyskinesia
R. Fog 118

GABA Dysfunction in the Pathophysiology of Tardive Dyskinesia
C. A. Tamminga, G. K. Thaker, and T. N. Chase 122

Clinical Activity of GABA Agonists in Neuroleptic- and L-Dopa-Induced Dyskinesia
P. L. Morselli, V. Fournier, L. Bossi, and B. Musch 128

Tardive Dyskinesia: Nondopaminergic Treatment Approaches
D. E. Casey 137

Pathophysiology of L-Dopa-Induced Abnormal Involuntary Movements
Y. Agid, A.-M. Bonnet, M. Ruberg, and F. Javoy-Agid 145

Discussion Section

Prevalence of Tardive Dyskinesia in a Clinic Population
J. Fleischhauer, R. Kocher, V. Hobi, and U. Gilsdorf 162

Animal Models

Differential Alteration of Striatal D-1 and D-2 Receptors Induced by the Long-Term Administration of Haloperidol, Sulpiride or Clozapine to Rats
P. Jenner, N. M. J. Rupniak, and C. D. Marsden 174

Pharmacological Differentiation of Dopamine D-1 and D-2 Antagonists After Single and Repeated Administration
A. V. Christensen, J. Arnt, and O. Svendsen 182

Pathophysiology of Tardive Dyskinesia
L. M. Gunne and J.-E. Häggström 191

Intermittent Treatment with Droperidol, a Short-Acting Neuroleptic, Increases Behavioral Dopamine Receptor Sensitivity
R. H. Belmaker, A. Elami, and J. Bannet 194

Induction and Reversal of Dopamine Dyskinesia in Rat, Cat, and Monkey
K. G. Lloyd, M. T. Willigens, and M. Goldstein 200

Behavioral Effects of Long-Term Neuroleptic Treatment in Cebus Monkeys
D. E. Casey 211

Induction of Tardive Dyskinesia in *Cebus apella* and *Macaca speciosa* Monkeys: A Review
E. F. Domino 217

List of Contributors 225

Subject Index 226

Preclinical Aspects

Brain Dopamine Receptors in Schizophrenia and Tardive Dyskinesia [1]

P. Seeman [2]

Contents

Abstract 2
1 The D_1 and the D_2 Dopaminergic Sites 2
2 The D_2 Dopamine Receptor 3
3 Conversion of State of the D_2 Dopamine Receptor from D_2^{high} into D_2^{low} 3
4 Functional Significance of the D_2^{high} and D_2^{low} States 4
5 Brain Dopamine Receptors in Schizophrenia 5
6 Brain Dopamine Receptors and Tardive Dyskinesia 6
References 6

Abstract

Brain dopamine receptors (type D_2) mediate the psychomotor effects of dopamine. The D_2 dopamine receptor can exist in either a high-affinity state for dopamine (nanomolar dissociation constant) or in a low-affinity state (micromolar dissociation constant). Both states of the receptor, however, have high affinity for neuroleptics (60 p*M* for spiperone). The postsynaptic receptor probably operates mainly in the D_2^{low} state. The presynaptic dopamine receptor, and also the dopamine receptors in the pituitary gland and the area postrema, probably function in the D_2^{high} state. The density of brain D_2 dopamine receptors is elevated in schizophrenia. The control densities were 10.5 pmol per g tissue. Half of the schizophrenic tissues (putamen, caudate nucleus, and nucleus accumbens) revealed densities of about 11.9 pmol per g, while the other half of the tissues revealed a density mode of 23.8 pmol per g. The bimodal distribution may support the concept of two types of schizophrenia. Future work must decide which group has more tardive dyskinesia.

1 The D_1 and the D_2 Dopaminergic Sites

A dopamine receptor is defined as a receptor which is more sensitive to dopamine than to any other endogenous neurotransmitter and which has a correlate with the biological potencies of dopaminergic drugs.

The D_1 site is dopamine-stimulated adenylate cyclase (Kebabian and Calne 1979). Since the D_1 site results in stimulation of the enzyme, the D_1 site may be considered as a receptor. At present, however, a major objective is to identify a functional role for D_1 in the nervous system.

1 The work described in this paper was supported by the Ontario Mental Health Foundation, the Medical Research Council of Canada, the Canadian Friends of Schizophrenics and the Rotary Club of Toronto

2 Department of Pharmacology, Faculty of Medicine, University of Toronto, Toronto, Ontario M5S 1A8, Canada

Dyskinesia – Research and Treatment
(Psychopharmacology Supplementum 2)
Editors: Casey, Chase, Christensen, Gerlach

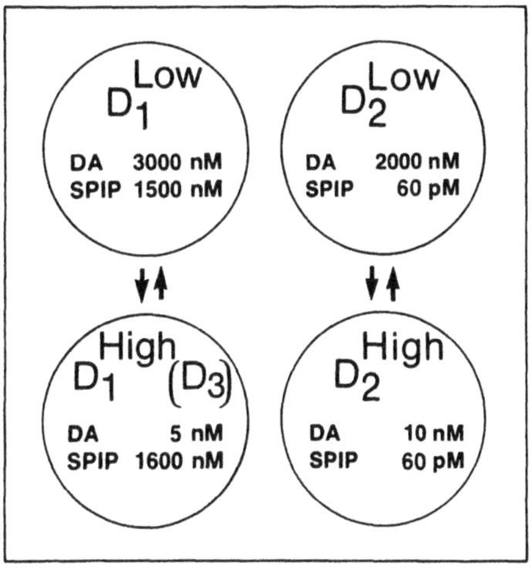

Fig. 1. Nomenclature of brain dopamine receptors and their states. D_1 is dopamine-inhibited adenylate cyclase, while D_2 inhibits adenylate cyclase (pituitary tissue) or interferes with the release of cyclic AMP from brain tissue slices (Stoof and Kebabian 1982). Both D_1 and D_2 can exist in either a high-affinity state for dopamine or a low-affinity state for dopamine. The concentrations shown for *DA* (dopamine) and *SPIP* (spiperone) are the approximate dissociation constants which define D_1, D_2, D_3 and their high- and low-affinity states. The D_3 site may be identical with D_1^{high}. The D_2^{high} state was formerly designated D_4 (Seeman 1980, 1982)

There is increasing evidence that, whatever its role, the D_1 protein may exist in a high- and a low-affinity state for dopamine (Hamblin and Creese 1982; Leff and Creese 1983), as shown in Fig. 1. The D_1^{high} state may be identical with a site previously identified as D_3 (List et al. 1980; List and Seeman 1982), as noted in Fig. 1.

2 The D_2 Dopamine Receptor

The D_2 dopamine receptor inhibits adenylate cyclase in the anterior pituitary gland (De Camilli et al. 1979) and in the intermediate lobe of the pituitary (Meunier et al. 1980; Cote et al. 1981). There is good (but indirect) evidence for a similar type of inhibition in the brain striatum (Stoof and Kebabian 1981).

The D_2 receptor mediates psychomotor dopaminergic behaviors (rotation, locomotion, anti-Parkinson action, psychotomimetic action, emesis and stereotypy) and a prolactin-lowering action, since the in vitro concentrations of agonists and antagonists (which inhibit ^{3}H-spiperone binding to the receptor) correlate very well with the doses eliciting the dopaminergic actions (Seeman 1980).

3 Conversion of State of the D_2 Dopamine Receptor from D_2^{high} into D_2^{low}

D_2 dopamine receptors in the anterior pituitary tissue can be readily converted from their state of high affinity for dopamine to their state of low affinity for dopamine and related agonists (Sibley et al. 1982; Sibley and Creese 1983; George et al. 1983a, b; Watanabe et al. 1983; De Lean et al. 1982).

In brain tissue, however, such complete conversion had not been obtained until recently (Grigoriadis and Seeman 1984). Previous work had indicated, for

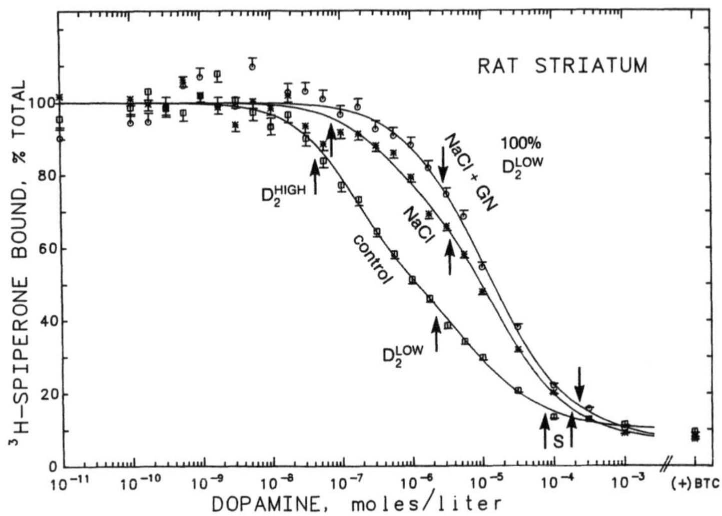

Fig. 2. Complete conversion of rat brain D_2^{high} dopamine receptors into their D_2^{low} state by guanine nucleotide and NaCl, calculated by iteration (program LIGAND; Munson and Rodbard 1980) to three ^{3}H-spiperone-binding sites (D_2^{high}, D_2^{low}, and serotonergic). (Adapted from Grigoriadis and Seeman 1984)

example, that approximately 22% of the ^{3}H-spiperone binding sites remained apparently resistant to conversion into D_2^{low} by guanine nucleotide (Huff and Molinoff 1982; Wreggett and Seeman 1984). It is now clear that these "resistant" ^{3}H-spiperone sites were serotonergic. Thus, if appropriate allowance is made in the computer-assisted analysis of the ^{3}H-spiperone/agonist competition data for this serotonergic component, it is possible to demonstrate complete conversion of D_2^{high} into D_2^{low} in rat brain striatum (Fig. 2).

4 Functional Significance of the D_2^{high} and D_2^{low} States

Presynaptic D_2 dopamine receptors (dopamine autoreceptors) appear to operate in the high-affinity state, D_2^{high}, since the dissociation constants (K) for agonists at D_2^{high} are approximately identical with the concentrations of them that inhibit the release of ^{3}H-dopamine from striatal slices (Seeman et al. 1984c).

The pituitary D_2 dopamine receptors also function in the D_2^{high} state, since the agonist K values are similar to those which inhibit the release of prolactin (George et al. 1984; Seeman et al. 1984c).

Postsynaptic D_2 dopamine receptors, however, appear to function in the D_2^{low} state, since the agonist K values at D_2^{low} are similar to the agonist concentrations which act postsynaptically to inhibit the release of ^{3}H-acetylcholine from striatal slices (Seeman et al. 1984c).

A diagram of the functional states of D_2 is shown in Fig. 3, where the presynaptic D_2 dopamine receptor is illustrated as being in the high-affinity form (i.e.,

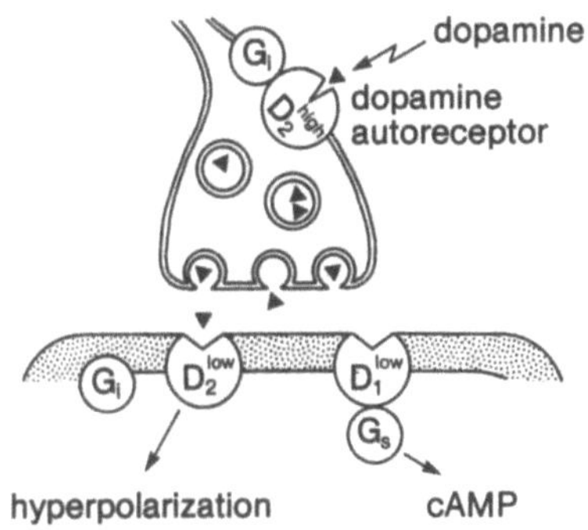

Fig. 3. The postsynaptic D_2 dopamine receptor may operate in the D_2^{low} state, as indicated by the loose fit between the receptor and the micromolar concentration of dopamine in the synaptic cleft. The highly sensitive presynaptic D_2 dopamine receptor appears to function in the D_2^{high} state, as indicated by the tight fit between D_2^{high} and the nanomolar concentration of dopamine expected on the edge of the synaptic terminal. D_1 is dopamine-stimulated adenylate cyclase. G_i and G_s are the nucleotide-sensitive regulatory proteins. Note that D_2^{high} is tightly coupled to G_i, while D_2^{low} is not coupled to the G_i protein

tight fit at nanomolar concentrations of dopamine), while the postsynaptic D_2 receptor is in the low-affinity state (i.e., loose fit at micromolar concentrations of dopamine).

5 Brain Dopamine Receptors in Schizophrenia

A consistent biological finding in schizophrenia has been that of an increased density of D_2 dopamine receptors in post-mortem brain tissue from schizophrenic patients (Lee and Seeman 1977, 1980; Seeman and Lee 1977; Lee et al. 1978; Seeman 1981; Owen et al. 1978). No changes have been detected in the D_1 or D_3 dopaminergic sites or other neurotransmitter receptors (Cross et al. 1981; Seeman and Lee 1982). While neuroleptic treatment appears to elevate the D_2 receptor density (Reynolds et al. 1980; MacKay et al. 1980, 1982), it is known that

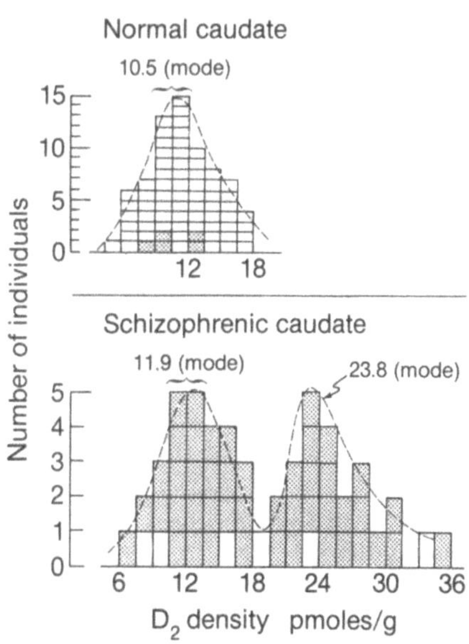

Fig. 4. Bimodal distribution of D_2 dopamine receptor densities in schizophrenic caudate nucleus. Each *small rectangle* indicates one brain tissue. The *dark rectangles* indicate that the patients had taken neuroleptics during their lifetime; the *white rectangles* indicate that the subjects either never had neuroleptics or had not taken neuroleptics for at least 6 months before death. (Adapted from Seeman et al. 1984b)

neuroleptic-free schizophrenic tissues also exhibit markedly elevated densities (Lee and Seeman 1980; Seeman 1981; Crow 1982).

Using improved experimental conditions (Seeman et al. 1982, 1984 a), we have now studied a new series of tissues (Seeman et al. 1984 b). Some of these recent data recorded in normal and schizophrenic caudate nucleus are shown in Fig. 4. The control mode was 10.5 pmol D_2 receptors per g wet original tissue. The schizophrenic tissues revealed one mode at 11.9 pmol/g (an increase of 13% over control) and a second mode at 23.8 pmol/g, representing a 2.3-fold increase over control. A similar pattern was obtained in the putamen and the nucleus accumbens.

The two subgroups of schizophrenic brain dopamine receptors (Fig. 4) are compatible with, but not necessarily synonymous with, the two-syndrome concept of schizophrenia suggested by Crow (1980). For example, the high-density mode of 23.8 pmol/g might represent Crow's type I syndrome of hallucinations and delusions associated with acute schizophrenia.

6 Brain Dopamine Receptors and Tardive Dyskinesia

One interpretation of the data in Fig. 4 is that there are two categories of schizophrenia, biologically resolved by the bimodal pattern of D_2 receptor densities.

A second interpretation is that the high-density mode with the 2.3-fold increase over control is associated with a history of high neuroleptic dosage and possibly tardive dyskinesia. The clinical records available to us, however, were not sufficiently detailed for us to ascertain this. It should be noted, however, that the ^{3}H-spiperone dissociation constants for the two modes of schizophrenic tissues (Fig. 4) were not significantly different from each other (between 110 and 150 p*M*). This suggests that the residual amount of neuroleptic remaining in the two populations of tissues was not significantly different, and thus, their lifetime neuroleptic doses during may have been about the same.

A third possible interpretation of the data in Fig. 4 is that although both modes of schizophrenic patients might have received about the same neuroleptic dosage, the high-density group might be a subset of patients in whom the brain responded with a more vigorous synthesis of D_2 receptors. These patients could be the ones who develop tardive dyskinesia.

Acknowledgements. I thank C. Ulpian, D. Grigoriadis, Dr. Susan R. George and Dr. M. Watanabe for their advice and assistance.

References

Cote TE, Greve CW, Kebabian JW (1981) Stimulation of a D-2 dopamine receptor in the intermediate lobe of the rat pituitary gland decreases the responsiveness of the beta-adrenoceptor: biochemical mechanism. Endocrinology 108:420–426

Cross AJ, Crow TJ, Owen F (1981) ^{3}H-Flupenthixol binding in post-mortem brains of schizophrenics: evidence for a selective increase in dopamine D_2 receptors. Psychopharmacology 74:122–124

Crow TJ (1980) Molecular pathology of schizophrenia: more than one disease process? Br Med J 280:66
Crow TJ (1982) The biology of schizophrenia. Experientia 38:1275–1282
DeCamilli P, Macconi D, Spada A (1979) Dopamine inhibits adenylate cyclase in human prolactin-secreting pituitary adenomas. Nature 278:252–254
DeLean A, Kilpatrick BF, Caron MG (1982) Dopamine receptor of porcine anterior pituitary gland. Evidence for two affinity states discriminated by both agonists and antagonists. Mol Pharmacol 22:290–297
George SR, Watanabe M, Seeman P (1983a) Commentary: the dopamine receptor of the anterior pituitary gland. In: Kaiser C, Kebabian JW (eds) Dopamine receptors. Am Chem Soc, Washington
George SR, Binkley K, Seeman P (1983b) Dopamine receptor sites and states in human brain. J Neural Transm [Suppl] 18:149–156
George SR, Watanabe M, Di Paolo T, Labrie F, Seeman P (1984) The functional state of the dopamine receptor in the anterior pituitary is in the high-affinity form. Endocrinology (to be published)
Grigoriadis D, Seeman P (1984) Complete conversion of brain D_2 dopamine receptors from the high- to the low-affinity state for dopamine agonists, using sodium ions and guanine nucleotide. J Neurochem (to be published)
Hamblin MW, Creese I (1982) ^{3}H-Dopamine binding to rat striatal D-2 and D-3 sites: enhancement by magnesium and inhibition by guanine nucleotides and sodium. Life Sci 30:1587–1595
Huff RM, Molinoff PB (1982) Quantitative determination of dopamine receptor subtypes not linked to activation of adenylate cyclase in rat striatum. Proc Natl Acad Sci USA 79:7561–7565
Kebabian JW, Calne DB (1979) Multiple receptors for dopamine. Nature 277:93–96
Lee T, Seeman P (1977) Dopamine receptors in normal and schizophrenic human brains. Abstracts of the Society for Neuroscience 3:443
Lee T, Seeman P (1980) Elevation of brain neuroleptic/dopamine receptors in schizophrenia. Am J Psychiatry 137:191–197
Lee T, Seeman P, Tourtellote WW, Farley IJ, Hornykiewicz O (1978) Binding of ^{3}H-neuroleptics and ^{3}H-apomorphine in schizophrenic brains. Nature 274:897–900
Leff SE, Creese I (1983) Dopamine receptors re-explained. Trends in Pharmacological Science 4:463–467
List S, Seeman P (1982) ^{3}H-Dopamine labelling of D_3 dopaminergic sites in human, rat and calf brain. J Neurochem 39:1363–1373
List S, Titeler M, Seeman P (1980) High-affinity ^{3}H-dopamine receptors (D_3 sites) in human and rat brain. Biochem Pharmacol 29:1621–1622
MacKay AVP, Bird ED, Spokes EG, Rossor M, Iversen LL, Creese I, Snyder SH (1980) Dopamine receptors and schizophrenia: drug effect or illness? Lancet II:915–916
MacKay AVP, Iversen LL, Rossor M, Spokes E, Bird E, Arregui A, Creese I, Snyder SH (1982) Increased brain dopamine and dopamine receptors in schizophrenia. Arch Gen Psychiatry 39:991–997
Meunier H, Giguere V, Labrie F (1980) Dopamine receptors are negatively coupled to adenylate cyclase in rat intermediate pituitary cells. Proceedings of the 4th international conference on cyclic nucleotides, July 1980, Abstr. THA9
Munson P, Rodbard D (1980) "Ligand": a versatile computerized approach for characterization of ligand-binding systems. Anal Biochem 107:220–239
Owen F, Crow TJ, Poulter M, Cross AJ, Longden A, Riley GJ (1978) Increased dopamine-receptor sensitivity in schizophrenia. Lancet II:223–226
Reynolds GP, Reynolds LM, Riederer P, Jellinger K, Gabriel E (1980) Dopamine receptors and schizophrenia: drug effect or illness. Lancet II:1251
Seeman P (1980) Brain dopamine receptors. Pharmacol Rev 32:229–313
Seeman P (1981) Dopamine receptors in post-mortem schizophrenic brains. Lancet I:1103
Seeman P (1982) Nomenclature of central and peripheral dopaminergic sites and receptors. Biochem Pharmacol 31:2563–2568

Seeman P, Lee T (1977) In: Timnick L (ed) Scientists find 'sites of craziness'. Los Angeles Times 200:1
Seeman P, Lee T (1982) Dopamine receptors in the schizophrenic brain. In: Namba M, Kaiya H (eds) Psychobiology of schizophrenia. Pergamon, Oxford, pp 241–247
Seeman P, Ulpian C, Wells J (1982) Dopamine receptor parameters (detected by ^{3}H-spiperone) depend on tissue concentration. Abstracts of the Society for Neuroscience 8:718
Seeman P, Ulpian C, Wreggett KA, Wells J (1984a) Dopamine receptor parameters detected by ^{3}H-spiperone depend on tissue concentration: analysis and examples. J Neurochem (to be published)
Seeman P, Ulpian C, Bergeron C, Riederer P, Jellinger K, Gabriel E, Reynolds GP, Tourtellotte WW (1984b) Bimodal distribution of schizophrenic brain dopamine receptor densities (to be published)
Seeman P, Grigoriadis D, George SR, Watanabe M (1984c) Functional states of dopamine receptors. In: Woodruff GN, Creese I, Gessa GL, Hornykiewicz O, Poat JA, Roberts PJ (eds) Dopaminergic systems and their regulation. Macmillan, London (to be published)
Sibley DR, Creese I (1983) Regulation of ligand binding to pituitary D-2 dopaminergic receptors. Effects of divalent cations and functional group modification. J Biol Chem 258:4957–4965
Sibley DR, DeLean A, Creese I (1982) Anterior pituitary dopamine receptors. Demonstration of interconvertible high and low affinity states of the D_2 dopamine receptor. J Biol Chem 257:6351–6361
Stoof JC, Kebabian JW (1981) Opposing roles for D-1 and D-2 dopamine receptors in efflux of cyclic AMP from rat neostriatum. Nature 294:366–368
Stoof JC, Kebabian JW (1982) Independent in vitro regulation by the D-2 dopamine receptor of dopamine-stimulated efflux of cyclic AMP and K-stimulated release of acetylcholine from rat neostriatum. Brain Res 250:263–270
Watanabe M, George SR, Seeman P (1983) The proportion of D_2 dopamine receptors in high and low affinity states depends on the agonist, cations, guanine nucleotides and temperature. Abstracts of the Society for Neuroscience 9:994
Wreggett KA, Seeman P (1984) Agonist high- and low-affinity states of the D_2 dopamine receptor in calf brain: partial conversion by guanine nucleotide. Mol Pharmacol (to be published)

Receptor-Binding Profiles of Neuroleptics

J. Hyttel, J.-J. Larsen, A. V. Christensen, and J. Arnt[1]

Contents

Abstract 9
1 Introduction 9
2 Dopamine D-1 and D-2 Receptors 10
3 Other Receptors 14
4 Concluding Remarks 16
References 17

Abstract

Dopamine-receptor blockade seems to be a prominent effect of neuroleptics. Blockade of other receptors might, however, contribute to the therapeutic effect. A series of neuroleptics have been tested for affinity to DA D-1 and D-2 receptors, serotonin receptors (S_2), α-adrenoceptors (α_1), histamine receptors (H_1), and muscarinic cholinergic receptors.

According to the affinity to DA D-1 and D-2 receptors, neuroleptics can be divided into different groups. Thioxanthenes have affinity for both D-1 and D-2 receptors; phenothiazines have affinity for D-2 receptors and considerably lower affinity for D-1 receptors; and butyrophenones, diphenylbutylpiperidines, and benzamides have affinity only for D-2 receptors.

Concerning affinity to other receptors the only consistent finding is affinity for S_2 receptors.

The clinical significance of these findings is speculative. In several behavioral tests the D-1/D-2 classification is also observed, and it is suggested that D-1-receptor activation is responsible for dyskinesia, and that thioxanthenes – due to their D-1 receptor blocking effect – induce less dyskinesia than other neuroleptics.

1 Introduction

It is well known that the antipsychotic potency of neuroleptics is closely correlated with their dopamine (DA) receptor blocking potency (Creese et al. 1976). In this respect only DA D-2 receptor blockade seems of interest.

The fact that neuroleptics constitute a group of drugs whose neurochemical profile varies widely, i.e., different neurotransmitter receptors are blocked to varying degrees, has been extensively described by many authors. Peroutka and Snyder (1980) examined 22 neuroleptics for affinity to DA receptors, serotonin (5-HT) receptors, α-adrenoceptors, and histamine receptors in rat brain membranes. They concluded that "... the average antipsychotic clinical potency correlates closely only with the drug affinity for DA receptors labelled by ^{3}H-spiroperidol... the substantial occupancy of 5-HT receptors, α-adreno-

1 H. Lundbeck A/S, Ottiliavej 7–9, DK-2500 Copenhagen-Valby, Denmark

Dyskinesia – Research and Treatment
(Psychopharmacology Supplementum 2)
Editors: Casey, Chase, Christensen, Gerlach

ceptors, and histamine receptors often occurs and may account for some of the auxiliary actions of neuroleptics." A similar conclusion was reached by Leysen (1982), who refers sedation and hypotension to blockade of $histamine_1$ and α_1-adrenoceptors, respectively. She also underlines the relation of antipsychotic effect to blockade of DA D-2 receptors and states that "since D_1, D_3 and D_4 sites cannot be related to a known pharmacological or physiological effect of DA, these sites cannot be considered receptors."

We think that these points of view are too narrow. Although no correlation can be found between clinical potency and affinities for receptors other than D-2 one cannot exclude the possibility that these affinities may have beneficial as well as undesirable influences and thereby contribute to the therapeutic differences which are indeed found between the neuroleptics. Furthermore, affinity for DA D-1 receptors can be related to several pharmacological effects exerted via DA or DA agonists (Christensen et al. 1979; Christensen and Hyttel 1982; Rosengarten et al. 1983; Christensen et al. this volume; Arnt and Hyttel 1984; Molloy and Waddington 1984). Surely these discoveries will lead to speculations as to a therapeutic relevance.

2 Dopamine D-1 and D-2 Receptors

Classification of DA-receptors into two types, D-1 and D-2, is well accepted (Kebabian and Calne 1979). The D-1 receptors are coupled to a DA-dependent adenylate cyclase (AC) in a stimulatory manner, whereas the D-2 receptors are independent of AC or coupled in an inhibitory manner (Stoof and Kebabian 1982). We have characterized D-1 receptors by AC experiments and by a receptor-binding technique using thioxanthene ligands, ^{3}H-*cis*(Z)-flupentixol (^{3}H-FPT) and ^{3}H-piflutixol (^{3}H-PIF) (Hyttel 1983; Hyttel et al. 1983). D-2 receptors were characterized by butyrophenone ligands, ^{3}H-haloperidol (^{3}H-HAL) or ^{3}H-spiroperidol (^{3}H-SPI) (Hyttel 1983; Hyttel et al. 1983).

The conclusion that thioxanthene and butyrophenone ligands differentiate D-1 and D-2 receptors is based on the observations that they are bound with a different distribution in the brain (Hyttel 1978), differ in neuronal localization (Leff et al. 1981), number (Hyttel 1978) and molecular size (Nielsen et al. 1984), and are changed differently by age (O'Boyle and Waddington 1984), prolonged neuroleptic treatment (Fleminger et al. 1983), or 6-OHDA lesions (Hyttel et al. 1983). Finally, the affinities of neuroleptics for thioxanthene-binding sites correlates closely with their inhibitory potency on DA-stimulated AC, whereas no such correlation is found for the affinity to butyrophenone-binding sites and their inhibitory potency on DA-stimulated AC (Hyttel 1978, 1981, 1982). According to their affinity for D-1 and D-2 sites, DA antagonists can be divided into three different groups (Hyttel 1978; Hyttel and Christensen 1983; Hyttel et al. 1983).

1. The experimental substance SCH 23390 shows selective affinity for D-1 receptors (Hyttel 1983).
2. Thioxanthenes show high affinity for both D-1 and D-2 receptors. Phenothiazines belong to this group, although the affinity to D-1 receptors is much lower than that to D-2 receptors.

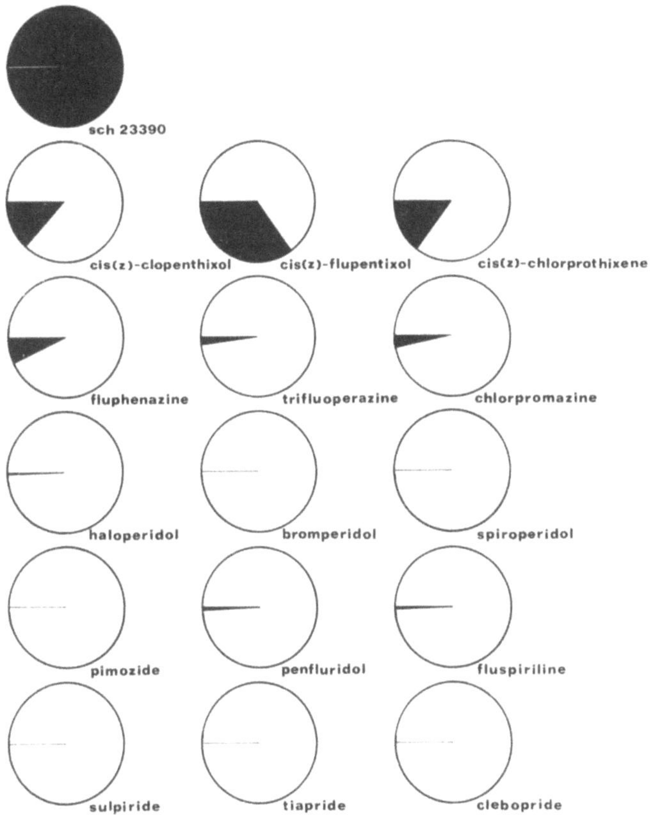

Fig. 1. Pie charts of the dopamine receptor profiles of neuroleptics and SCH 23390. The binding affinities to D-1 and D-2 receptors are shown as percentages of the total binding calculated from (1/D-1) + (1/D-2) = 100%. D-1 (*black area*) and D-2 (*white area*) receptor affinities were measured as ^{3}H-piflutixol and ^{3}H-spiperone binding, respectively

3. Butyrophenones, diphenylbutylpiperidines, and substituted benzamides show selective affinity for D-2 receptors.

This division can be schematically shown in pie charts (Fig. 1).

It has been shown that D-2 receptor affinities of neuroleptics correlate closely with antistereotypic and antiemetic potencies of neuroleptics (Creese et al. 1976). We also find such a correlation, e.g., antagonism of ^{3}H-SPI binding versus methylphenidate-induced compulsive gnawing in mice and amphetamine-induced stereotypy in rats. No such correlation can be found when ^{3}H-PIF binding substitutes ^{3}H-SPI binding (Fig. 2).

The lack of correlation with these DA-dependent behaviors has led to the erroneous interpretation that either these receptors are artifacts (or simply unspecific binding sites) or they have no significance for DA-mediated behavior.

However, many experiments have now been published showing the involvement of DA D-1 receptors in behavior. These behaviors are inhibited only by

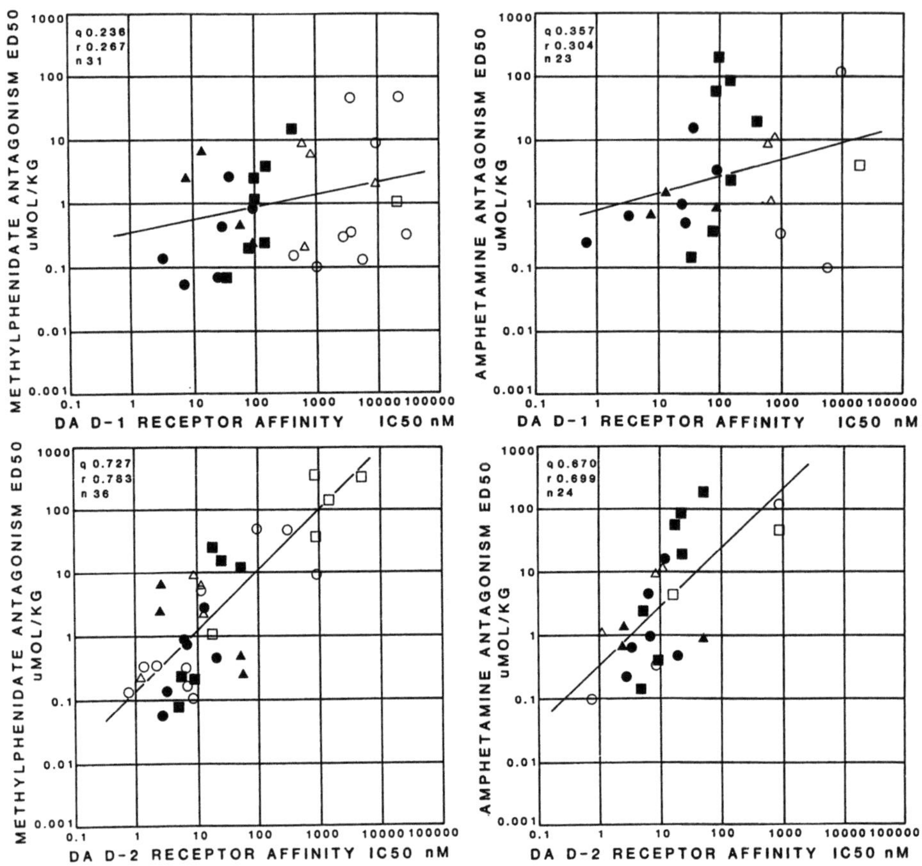

Fig. 2. Correlation between the antistereotypic potencies of neuroleptics and their D-1 and D-2 receptor affinities. D-1 and D-2 receptor affinities are represented by IC50 values (n*M*) in ^{3}H-piflutixol and ^{3}H-spiperone binding, respectively. Antistereotypic effects are represented by inhibition (ED50, μmol/kg IP) of methylphenidate-induced gnawing in mice and amphetamine-induced stereotypy in rats. ●, thioxanthenes; ■, phenothiazines; ○, butyrophenones; △, diphenylbutylpiperidines; □, benzamides; ▲, miscellaneous; *r* and *ϱ*, parametric and nonparametric correlation coefficients, respectively, *n*, number of neuroleptics included

neuroleptics possessing D-1 receptor affinity. Although this behavioral differentiation is the topic treated by Christensen et al. (this volume) it will be mentioned briefly here.

The methylphenidate antagonistic effect of neuroleptics is attenuated by concomitant treatment with scopolamine (Christensen et al. 1979, 1980). The attenuation becomes less pronounced with increasing affinity for D-1 receptors. The same differentiation is found in other behavioral tests after combination with scopolamine, e.g., amphetamine stereotypy, 6,7-ADTN-induced hyperactivity, conditioned avoidance response, and catalepsy in rats (Arnt and Christensen 1981; Arnt et al. 1981). These experiments are complemented by those of Ungerstedt et al. (1983). They found that in unilaterally 6-OHDA-lesioned rats the ability of *cis*(Z)-flupentixol and sulpiride to antagonize the rotational behavior after apomorphine and pergolide differed markedly. *cis*(Z)-Flupentixol was considerably more potent than sulpiride in antagonizing apomorphine (mixed D-1/ D-2 agonist) rotation, whereas the two neuroleptics were equipotent in antagonizing pergolide (D-2 agonist) rotation.

Prolonged treatment with neuroleptics leads to the development of tolerance. This tolerance becomes less pronounced with increasing D-1-receptor affinity (Christensen 1981; Christensen and Hyttel 1982; Hyttel et al. 1983). In Fig. 3 the correlations between D-1 and D-2 receptor affinity and the potencies in two of these behavioral tests are shown. It is evident that D-1 receptors play a central role in these DA-mediated behaviors.

More direct evidence for involvement of D-1 receptors in behavioral effects has been given by Arnt and Hyttel (1984), who showed that the D-1 agonist SK&F 38393 induced contralateral circling in unilaterally 6-OHDA-lesioned rats. This circling was selectively inhibited by neuroleptics possessing D-1 receptor affinity. Molloy and Waddington (1984) induced grooming and stereotypy in rats with SK&F 38393. This behavior was inhibited by SCH 23390 but not by metoclopramide. Finally, Rosengarten et al. (1983) showed that perioral movements in rats was dependent on D-1 receptor stimulation.

In brains removed from schizophrenic patients post mortem, increased number of D-2 receptors has been found (Lee et al. 1978; Lee and Seeman 1980a, b; Owen et al. 1978), whereas no changes were seen in the number of D-1 receptors (Cross et al. 1981; Crow et al. 1982). A recent investigation by Memo et al. (1983) suggests a link between schizophrenia and DA D-1 receptor function. These authors found that NaF, guanylimidodiphosphate (GppNHp), and SK&F 38393 elicited a greater activation of AC in homogenates of caudate nucleus in schizophrenic than in nonschizophrenic subjects. The findings suggest that the coupling of DA D-1 recognition sites with AC is more efficient in the brains of schizophrenic subjects, presumably because of an increased affinity for guanosine-5′-triphosphate (GTP).

To conclude, D-2-receptor affinity is of major importance for DA-mediated behavior and clinical effects. D-1-receptor affinity, however, has a crucial role in combination with other agents and in long-term treatment.

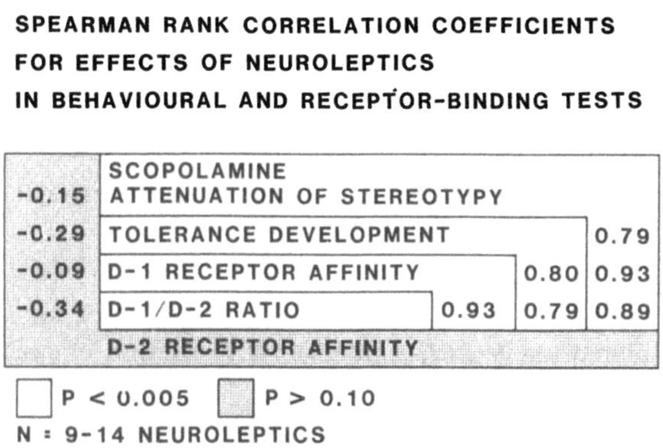

Fig. 3. Spearman rank correlation coefficients for effects of neuroleptics ($n = 9-14$) in behavioral and receptor-binding tests

3 Other Receptors

As pointed out above, neuroleptics possess high affinity for receptors other than DA receptors. This is probably best illustrated by pie charts, as shown in Figs. 4–6. The affinity for D-1 receptors, D-2 receptors, α_1-adrenoceptors, 5-HT_2 (S_2) receptors, and muscarinic (Ach) receptors is measured by the receptor-binding technique, whereas histamine (H_1) receptor affinity is determined by the guinea-pig ileum method.

First of all, only very few neuroleptics (pimozide, penfluridol, sulpiride, sultopride and clebopride) can be classified as selective DA antagonists.

Among the thioxanthenes varying degrees of S_2 and α_1 receptor affinity are apparent, whereas H_1 and Ach affinity is low. The high-dose phenothiazines, levomepromazine, chlorpromazine, and thioridazine, resemble chlorprothixene in that they possess high S_2 and α_1 affinity. Some H_1 affinity is also apparent. The low-dose phenothiazines, fluphenazine, perphenazine, and trifluoperazine, are more selective for DA receptors and resemble the low-dose thioxanthenes, *cis*(Z)-clopenthixol and *cis*(Z)-flupentixol.

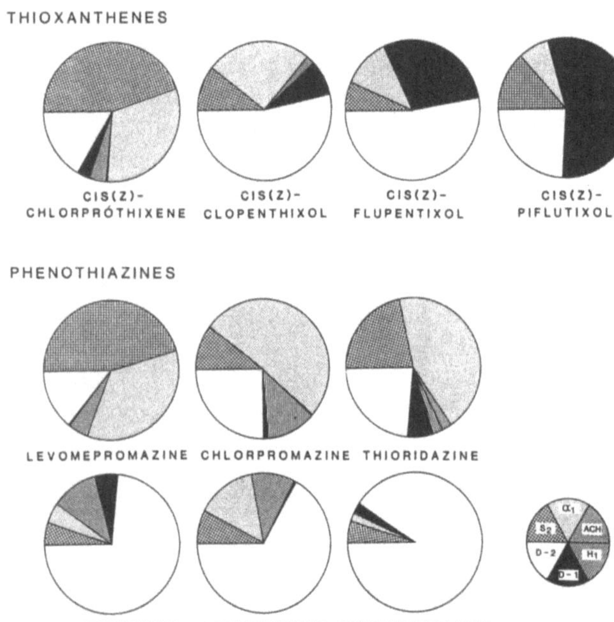

Fig. 4. Pie charts of receptor profiles of thioxanthenes and phenothiazines. The affinities, for the receptors are shown as percentages of the total binding calculated from:

$$\frac{1}{D-1}+\frac{1}{D-2}+\frac{1}{H_1}+\frac{1}{Ach}+\frac{1}{\alpha_1}+\frac{1}{S_2}=100\%$$

D-1, D-2, Ach, α_1, and S_2 receptor affinity was determined from receptor-binding experiments with ^{3}H-piflutixol, ^{3}H-spiroperidol, ^{3}H-PrBCM, ^{3}H-prazosin, and ^{3}H-spiroperidol, respectively. H_1 receptor affinity was determined from inhibition of histamine-induced contractions of guinea-pig ileum in in vitro experiments

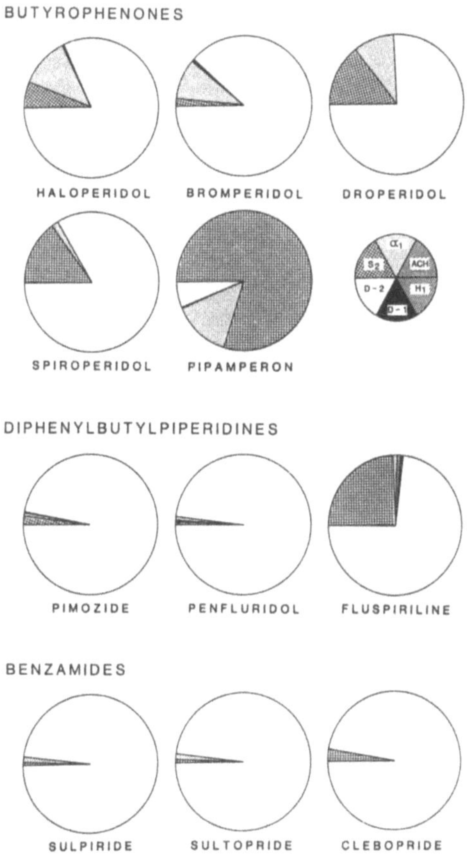

Fig. 5. Pie charts of receptor profiles of butyrophenones, diphenylbutylpiperidines and benzamides. For explanation see legend to Fig. 4

Butyrophenones, often referred to as selective DA antagonists, possess some S_2 and α_1 affinity. For pipamperon these effects seem to dominate. Some of the diphenylbutylpiperidines, pimozide and penfluridol, are indeed DA selective, whereas fluspirilene possesses a large S_2 component. The benzamides are also selective DA antagonists.

Some of the neuroleptics in Fig. 6 have a mixed profile. For clozapine, S_2 and α_1 affinity dominate and some Ach affinity is also apparent. Clothiapine and loxapine have affinity for all receptors examined. In fluperlapine the DA affinity is negligible compared with the affinity for other receptors. (+) Butaclamol has high affinity for D-1, D-2, and S_2 receptors. The new neuroleptic tefludazine has equal affinity for D-2 and S_2 receptors, some affinity for α_1 receptors, and slight affinity for D-1 receptors. The D-1 selectivity of SCH 23390 has been commented on above. Otherwise the substance possesses only weak S_2 affinity. In a larger series of neuroleptics than those in Figs. 4–6 the antagonistic potencies of methylphenidate-induced compulsive gnawing in mice and amphetamine-induced stereotypy in rats have been compared with the affinity for the different receptors (D-1, D-2, S_2, α_1, Ach, H_1) and with the ratios between some of these affinities (D-1/D-2 and S_2/D-2). Affinity to D-2 receptors was the only parameter

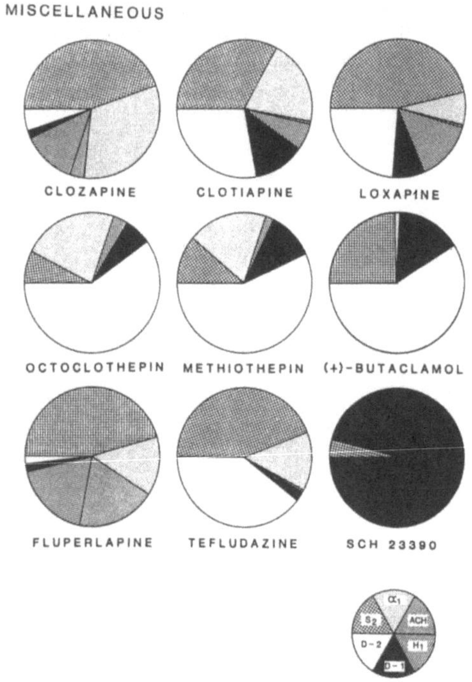

Fig. 6. Pie charts of receptor profiles of miscellaneous neuroleptics. For explanation see legend to Fig. 4

which correlated to inhibition of methylphenidate and amphetamine stereotypies [Spearman rank correlation coefficients (ϱ) were 0.727 and 0.670, respectively] (Fig. 2). Affinity for Ach receptors had a low negative correlation to these two tests ($\varrho = -0.447$ and -0.528). Correlation coefficients for D-1 receptor affinity versus antagonism of methylphenidate and amphetamine were 0.236 and 0.357, respectively (Fig. 2).

It is difficult to draw any conclusions from these pie charts and the correlation analysis. However, all neuroleptics possess affinity for DA (D-1, D-2, or both) and S_2 receptors. It would therefore be erroneous to state that only DA receptor blockade is responsible for neuroleptic activity. Although there is a high correlation between DA receptor blockade and neuroleptic activity this correlation does not imply a causal relationship.

4 Concluding Remarks

DA receptor blockade is certainly a prominent effect of neuroleptics and no doubt this blockade contributes to the antipsychotic effect, as stated above. Affinity to certain receptors other than DA receptors is often implicated in side-effects. The α_1-adrenoceptor blocking effect is claimed to be responsible for cardiovascular side-effects such as orthostatic hypotension and tachycardia. An antihistaminic effect is considered responsible for sedation and drowsiness, and an anticholinergic effect for dry mouth, obstipation, urine retention, and visual disturbances. However, one cannot exclude the possibility that affinity for these receptors – in some parts of the brain – may have a beneficial effect. The observation that noradrenaline and 5-HT levels were significantly increased in the putamen in schizophrenics (Crow et al. 1979) indicates a possible role for these transmitters in the disease.

Since the blockade of S_2 receptors seems to be common to all neuroleptics it is tempting to relate this effect also to the antipsychotic effect. It is claimed that hallucinations caused by hallucinogenic drugs are mediated by 5-HT. The similarity of these hallucinations and those experienced by some schizophrenic patients supports the idea of an involvement of 5-HT in certain schizophrenic symptoms. Thus, 5-HT receptor blockade could be expected to be of value in controlling these symptoms.

Finally, the D-1 receptor blockade effected by certain neuroleptics has attracted a great deal of attention. The experiments by Rosengarten et al. (1983) showing that perioral movements in rats were dependent on D-1 receptor stimulation may lead to the suggestion that D-1 receptor activation is responsible for similar effects in man, i.e., dyskinesias.

Since tardive dyskinesia is often claimed to develop upon long-term treatment with neuroleptics, blockade of D-1 receptors should therefore be advantageous. Furthermore, if tardive dyskinesia is caused by the development of DA receptor hypersensitivity, the neuroleptics least capable of inducing this should be used. The neuroleptics inducing the least tolerance and hypersensitivity are thioxanthenes, which should therefore be regarded as the drugs of choice for long-term maintenance therapy.

References

Arnt J, Christensen AV (1981) Differential reversal by scopolamine and THIP of the antistereotypic and cataleptic effects of neuroleptics. Eur J Pharmacol 69:107–111

Arnt J, Christensen AV, Hyttel J (1981) Differential reversal by scopolamine of effects of neuroleptics in rats. Relevance for evaluation of therapeutic and extrapyramidal side-effect potential. Neuropharmacology 20:1331–1334

Arnt J, Hyttel J (1984) Differential inhibition by dopamine D-1 and D-2 antagonists of circling behaviour induced by dopamine agonists in rats with unilateral 6-hydroxydopamine lesions. Eur J Pharmacol 102:349–354

Christensen AV (1981) Dopamine hyperactivity: effects of neuroleptics alone or in combination with GABA-agonists. In: Perris C, Struwe G, Jansson B (eds) Biological psychiatry. Elsevier, Amsterdam, pp 828–832

Christensen AV, Arnt J, Scheel-Krüger J (1979) Decreased antistereotypic effect of neuroleptics after additional treatment with a benzodiazepine, a GABA agonist and an anticholinergic compound. Life Sci 24:1395–1402

Christensen AV, Arnt J, Scheel-Krüger J (1980) GABA-dopamine/neuroleptic interaction after systemic administration. Brain Res Bull 5 [Suppl 2]:885–890

Christensen AV, Hyttel J (1982) Neuroleptics and the clinical implications of adaptation of dopamine neurons. Pharmacy Int 3:329–332

Creese I, Burt DR, Snyder SH (1976) Dopamine receptor binding predicts clinical and pharmacological potencies of antischizophrenic drugs. Science 192:481–483

Cross AJ, Crow TJ, Owen F (1981) ^{3}H-flupenthixol binding in post-mortem brains of schizophrenics: evidence for a selective increase in D2 receptors. Psychophamacology 74:122–124

Crow TJ, Baker HF Cross AJ, Joseph MH, Lofthouse R, Longden A, Owen F, Riley GJ, Glover V, Killpack WS (1979) Monoamine mechanisms in chronic schizophrenia: post-mortem neurochemical findings. Br J Psychiatry 134:249–256

Crow TJ, Cross AJ, Johnstone EC, Owen F, Owens DGC, Waddington JL (1982) Abnormal involuntary movements in schizophrenia: are they related to the disease process or its

treatment? Are they associated with changes in dopamine receptors? J Clin Psychopharmacol 2:336–340
Fleminger S, Rupniak NMJ, Hall MD, Jennep, Marsden CD (1983) Changes in apomorphine-induced stereotypy as a result of subacute neuroleptic treatment correlate with increased D-2 receptors, but not with increases in D-1 receptors. Biochem Pharmacol 19:2921–2927
Hyttel J (1978) Effects of neuroleptics on ^{3}H-haloperidol and ^{3}H-*cis*(Z)-flupenthixol binding and on adenylate cyclase activity in vitro. Life Sci 23:551–556
Hyttel J (1981) Similarities between the binding of ^{3}H-piflutixol and ^{3}H-flupentixol to rat striatal dopamine receptors in vitro. Life Sci 28:563–569
Hyttel J (1982) Preferential labelling of adenylate cyclase coupled dopamine receptors with thioxanthene neuroleptics. In: Kohsaka M, Shomori T, Tsukada Y, Woodruff GN (eds) Advances in dopamine research. Pergamon, Oxford, pp 147–152 (Advances in the biosciences, vol 37)
Hyttel J (1983) SCH 23390 – The first selective dopamine D-1 antagonist. Eur J Pharmacol 91:153–154
Hyttel J, Christensen AV (1983) Biochemical and pharmacological differentiation of neuroleptic effect on dopamine D-1 and D-2 receptors. J Neural Transm [Suppl] 18:157–164
Hyttel J, Christensen AV, Arnt J (1983) Neuroleptic classification: implications for tardive dyskinesia. In: Bannet J, Belmaker RH (eds) New directions in tardive dyskinesia research. Mod Probl Pharmacopsychiatry 21:49–64
Kebabian JW, Calne DB (1979) Multiple receptors for dopamine. Nature 277:93–96
Lee T, Seeman P (1980a) Elevation of brain neuroleptic/dopamine receptors in schizophrenia. Am J Psychiatry 137:191–197
Lee T, Seeman P (1980b) Abnormal neuroleptic/dopamine receptors in schizophrenia. In: Pepeu G, Kuhar MJ, Enna SJ (eds) Receptors for neurotransmitters and peptide hormones. Raven, New York, pp 435–442
Lee T, Seeman P, Tourtellotte WW, Farley IJ, Hornykeiwicz O (1978) Binding of ^{3}H-neuroleptics and ^{3}H-apomorphine in schizophrenic brains. Nature 274:897–900
Leff S, Lynne A, Hyttel J, Creese I (1981) Kainate lesion dissociates striatal dopamine radioligand binding sites. Eur J Pharmacol 70:71–75
Leysen J (1982) New discoveries in brain receptor research. Receptor binding properties of neuroleptics. In: Lauridsen B, Bech P (eds) Janssenpharmas III psykiatersymposium, Fossum Tryk, Birkerød, pp 21–26
Memo M, Kleiman JE, Hanbauer I (1983) Coupling of dopamine D_1 recognition sites with adenylate cyclase in nuclei accumbens and caudatus of schizophrenics. Science 221:1304–1307
Molloy AG, Waddington JL (1984) Dopaminergic behavior stereospecifically promoted by the D_1 agonist R-SK & F 38393 and selectively blocked by the D_1 antagonist SCH 23390. Psychopharmacology 82:409–410
Nielsen M, Klimek V, Hyttel J (1984) Distinct target size of dopamine D-1 and D-2 receptors in rat striatum. Life Sci 35:325–332
O'Boyle KM, Waddington JL (1984) Loss of rat striatal dopamine receptors with ageing is selective for D-2 but not D-1 sites: association with increased non-specific binding of the D-1 ligand [^{3}H] piflutixol. Eur J Pharmacol 105:171–179
Owen F, Cross AJ, Crow TJ, Longden A, Poulter M, Riley GJ (1978) Increased dopamine-receptors sensitivity in schizophrenia. Lancet II:223–225
Peroutka SJ, Snyder SH (1980) Relationship of neuroleptic drug effects at brain dopamine, serotonin, α-adrenergic, and histamine receptors to clinical potency. Am J Psychiatry 137:1518–1522
Rosengarten H, Schweitzer JW, Friedhoff AJ (1983) Induction of oral dyskinesias in naive rats by D_1 stimulation. Life Sci 33:2479–2482
Stoof JC, Kebabian JW (1982) Independent in vitro regulation by the D-2 dopamine receptor of dopamine-stimulated efflux of cyclic AMP and K^+-stimulated release of acetylcholine from rat neostriatum. Brain Res 250:263–270
Ungerstedt U, Herrera-Marschitz M, Ståhle L, Tossmann U, Zetterström T (1983) Dopamine receptor mechanisms studied by correlating transmitter release and behavior. In: Carlsson A, Nilsson JLG (eds) Dopamine receptor agonists 1. Acta Pharm Suec [Suppl] 1:165–181

Functional Classification of Different Dopamine Receptors

U. Ungerstedt, M. Herrera-Marschitz, L. Ståhle, U. Tossman, and T. Zetterström [1]

Contents

Abstract 19
1 Functional Classification – Sense or Non-Sense 19
2 Experimental Models 20
2.1 Postsynaptic Receptors 21
2.2 Presynaptic Receptors 26
3 An Explanatory Model 28
References 30

Abstract

A series of experiments is described in which behavioral models and intracerebral dialysis were used to study neurotransmitter release and which illustrate the functional properties of different dopamine receptors. Evidence is presented for the existence of postsynaptic D-1 dopamine receptors, which are preferentially stimulated by apomorphine and inhibited by SCH 23390, and postsynaptic D-2 receptors, which are preferentially stimulated by pergolide and inhibited by sulpiride. On the basis of results obtained following systemic and local treatment with picrotoxin it seems probable that D-2 receptors are located on GABA interneurons in the striatum. Furthermore, lesion studies indicate that the D-1 and D-2 receptors are related to different neuronal pathways. In contrast to postsynaptic dopamine receptors, presynaptic autoreceptors, as studied by recording the decrease in exploratory behavior and dopamine release, seem not to differ in their response to apomorphine and pergolide. Sulpiride selectively inhibits dopamine autoreceptors and is equally potent in inhibiting apomorphine and pergolide autoreceptor-dependent responses. In summary, the data strongly support the existence of functionally important D-1 and D-2 receptors.

1 Functional Classification – Sense or Non-Sense

The identity of the dopamine (DA) "receptor" has experienced many changes during the last 10 years. In attempts to achieve a "functional" classification of this receptor, scientists have used a large number of behavioral and biochemical models, which has resulted in a long list of different ways of classifying DA receptors.

In behavioral experiments it is possible to find dopamine receptor agonists and antagonists which induce or inhibit, with considerable specificity, behaviors such as locomotion, exploration, rearing, gnawing, stereotypy, climbing, etc.

---

1 Department of Pharmacology, Karolinska Institutet, P.O. Box 60400, S-10401 Stockholm, Sweden

Dyskinesia – Research and Treatment
(Psychopharmacology Supplementum 2)
Editors: Casey, Chase, Christensen, Gerlach

Additionally, studies of DA-dependent adenylate cyclase stimulation or inhibition have given rise to the concept of a D-1 receptor linked to adenylate cyclase and a D-2 receptor linked not to adenylate cyclase but possibly to an ion channel (Kebabian and Cote 1981). Receptor labeling studies involving binding of radioactive forms of either DA agonists or DA antagonists to membrane preparation (in vitro binding) or to DA-rich areas of the brain (in vivo binding) have also provided evidence for DA receptor multiplicity (Seeman 1981).

In spite of the considerable specificity of the various behavioral and biochemical phenomena related to DA receptor pharmacology, it is possible that some of the DA receptors may represent pharmacological rather than truly physiological phenomena. It is often asked, for example, whether the D-1 receptor has a functional role (e.g., Seeman 1981; Scatton 1982), i.e., whether it has a function in the normal neurophysiology of the animal.

In our own studies we have defined functional as having a response related to an alteration of the activity of a neuron, or a population of neurons, leading to measurable physiological events such as changes in transmitter release or changes in behavior. With this definition in mind we have set out to develop experimental models that may prove suitable for evaluation of the function of pre- and postsynaptic receptors and D-1/D-2 receptors.

2 Experimental Models

The 6-hydroxydopamine (6-OHDA) rotational model (Ungerstedt 1971) allows selective stimulation of forebrain DA receptors that have increased in sensitivity due to the degeneration of the presynaptic DA nerve terminals. The hypersensitivity is achieved by giving a 6-OHDA-injection unilaterally into the bundle of DA axons leaving the mesencephalic DA cell bodies, which produces almost complete degeneration of forebrain DA nerve terminals. With this model, we have performed experiments combining different DA agonists with different antagonists, in an attempt to reveal the existence of different postsynaptic receptors (Herrera-Marschitz and Ungerstedt 1984a).

It may be argued that any pharmacologic manipulations in hypersensitive receptors may not represent conditions in the normal brain. However, it is possible to perform comparative studies measuring rotational behavior elicited in animals by unilateral injection of kainic acid into the striatum. The rotational behavior after DA agonist in such animals is induced by doses similar to those that cause activation and stereotyped behavior in normal animals. This rotational response is in all probability induced by the stimulation of normosensitive DA receptors in the nonlesioned side of the brain (Schwarcz et al. 1979). It is thus possible to directly compare pharmacological experiments using rotating animals with hypersensitive and normosensitive DA receptors.

While the rotational behavior model is useful for studying postsynaptic DA mechanisms, the recording of exploratory behavior can be used to study both pre- and postsynaptic stimulation. It is well known that low doses of various DA agonists inhibit exploratory behavior while higher doses change exploration into stereotyped behavior. The low-dose effect is probably due to specific stimulation of presynaptic DA autoreceptors, while the stereotyped activation after higher doses presumably involves postsynaptic DA receptors. By using a holeboard model (Ljungberg and Ungerstedt 1978) we have recently been able to make a detailed study of the interaction between various doses of DA agonists and exploratory behavior (Ungerstedt et al. 1983). The inhibition of exploration and the induction of stereotyped behavior can be antagonized by various doses of DA-blocking drugs. In combination, the results with rotational behavior and exploratory behavior can be used to compare the effects of various agonists and antagonists on pre- and postsynaptic receptors, respectively.

While the behavioral models reflect an overall functional change, the measurement of transmitter release reflects more specific changes in neuronal activity. We have recently developed a method of intracerebral dialysis for measurement of transmitter release in vivo (Ungerstedt et al. 1983). A thin dialysis tube is implanted into the brain parenchyma and perfused with a physiological solution. The perfusate is then analyzed for DA and DA metabolites by the use of HPLC and electrochemical detection (Zetterström et al. 1983). With this method it is possible to follow the changes in, for example, DA release after stimulation of presynaptic DA receptors. Furthermore, it is possible to directly correlate behavioral events and transmitter release when the experiments are performed on awake animals. The following is an account of experiments performed using the above models aiming at a functional classification of various DA-receptor populations in the rat brain.

2.1 Postsynaptic Receptors

Comparison of the effects of the DA agonists apomorphine and pergolide in the unilaterally 6-OHDA-denervated rat reveals that they differ markedly both in the patterns of rotation and in the dose-response curves that they produce (Figs. 1 and 2). These differences are indicative of differences in the mechanism of action between the two DA agonists. We therefore tested the ability of various DA blockers to inhibit the rotational responses elicited by apomorphine and pergolide (Herrera-Marschitz and Ungerstedt 1984a). We found that the D-1/D-2 antagonist *cis*(Z)-flupentixol blocked both apomorphine and pergolide to similar degrees, while sulpiride, a substituted benzamide devoid of any effect on D-1 receptors, was a poor inhibitor of the apomorphine response. In contrast, sulpiride blocked pergolide rotation at doses 1000 times lower than those needed to block apomorphine rotation (Fig. 3).

These results indicate that apomorphine and pergolide differ in their ability to stimulate D-1 and D-2 receptors. This hypothesis has recently received strong support from our finding that the recently developed D-1 receptor blocker SCH 23390 produces marked inhibition of apomorphine rotation while having no effect on pergolide-induced rotation (Herrera-Marschitz et al. 1984a) (e.g., Fig. 4).

So far, our data indicate a remarkable specificity in the actions of apomorphine and pergolide on D-1 and D-2 receptors. Moreover, our data support the idea that D-1 and D-2 receptors may be associated with different types of behavior. Although both apomorphine and pergolide induce rotational behavior, a

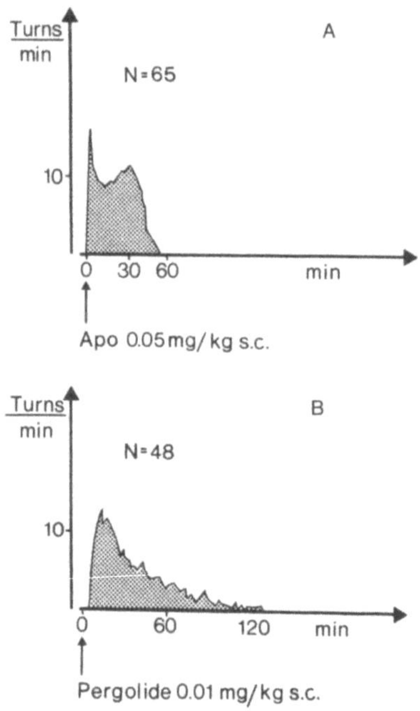

Fig. 1 A, B. Patterns of contralateral rotational behavior induced by apomorphine (**A**) and pergolide (**B**) in 6-OHDA-denervated rats. *Abscissa*, time (min) after SC administration of apomorphine (Apo) or pergolide; *ordinate*, turns/min

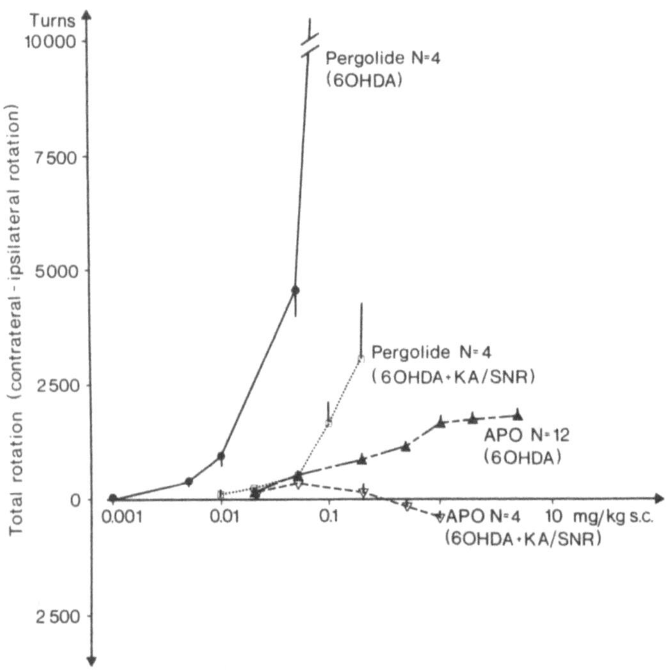

Fig. 2. Dose-dependent rotation induced by apomorphine and pergolide in 6-OHDA-treated rats and in 6-OHDA-treated rats receiving, in addition, kainic acid injected into the ipsilateral substantia nigra reticulata (6-OHDA + KA/SNR). The *curve* induced by pergolide is shifted to the right after the kainic acid treatment through parallel to that with 6-OHDA only, while the apomorphine response (Apo) is reversed towards ipsilateral values. *Abscissa*, doses (mg/kg SC). *Ordinate*, total contralateral-ipsilateral rotation

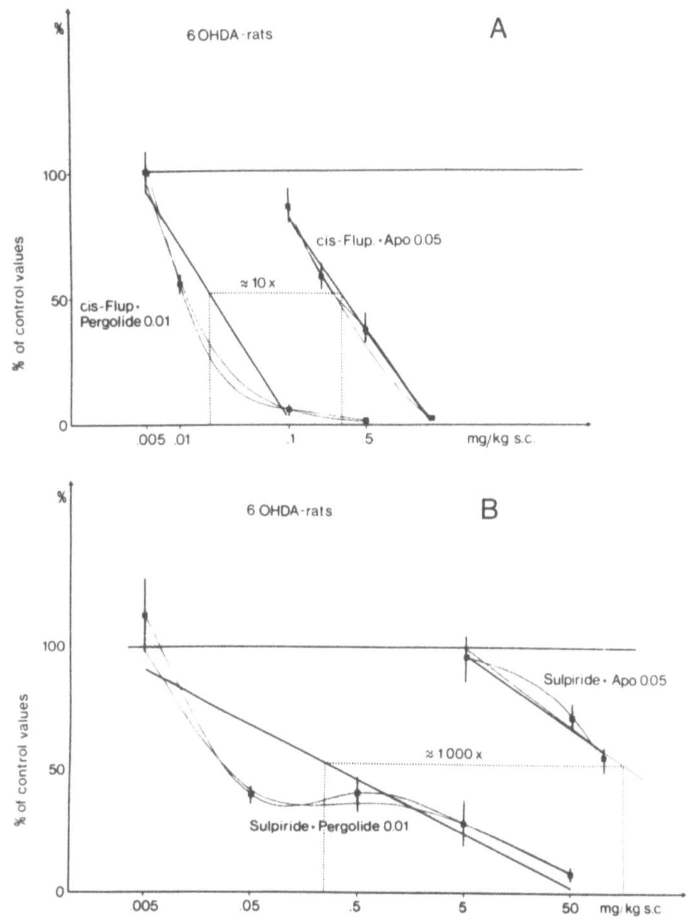

Fig. 3 A, B. Inhibition of apomorphine (Apo) and pergolide rotation in 6-OHDA-treated rats by *cis*(Z)-flupentixol (*cis-Flup*) and sulpiride pretreatments. *Abscissa*, doses (mg/kg, SC); *ordinate*, changes in percentage of the total rotation in relation to control values

detailed analysis reveals important differences in the behavior that accompany the rotational responses. Apomorphine induces a typical two-peak rotational pattern associated with pronounced gnawing, biting, and self-mutilation in higher doses. Pergolide, on the other hand, induces even rotation associated with mild stereotyped sniffing behavior. It seems reasonable to assume that differences in behavior are associated with the involvement of different neuronal pathways in the brain. It therefore seems possible that D-1 and D-2 receptors may be located on different postsynaptic neurons. To test this hypothesis we pretreated animals with the GABA antagonist picrotoxin (Ungerstedt et al. 1983). Picrotoxin increased the response to pergolide, while it decreased the response to apomorphine (Fig. 5). These differences became even more pronounced when picrotoxin was injected directly into one striatum in normal animals before they received an SC injection of pergolide or apomorphine (Herrera-Marschitz and Ungerstedt

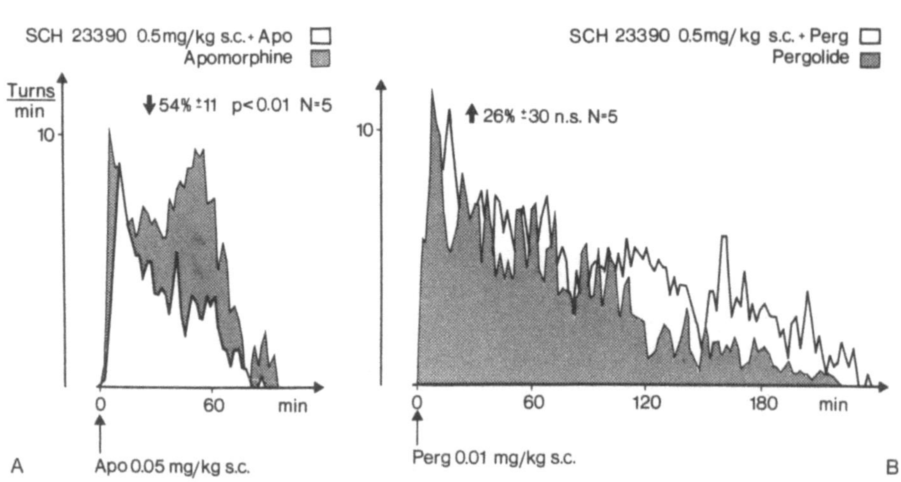

Fig. 4 A, B. Modification of apomorphine (**A**) and pergolide (**B**) patterns of rotation with SCH 23390 0.5 mg/kg SC (*outline figures*). *Bold arrows* indicate percentage inhibition compared with controls (*solid figures*). *Abscissa*, time (min) after the injection of DA agonists; *ordinate*, turns/min

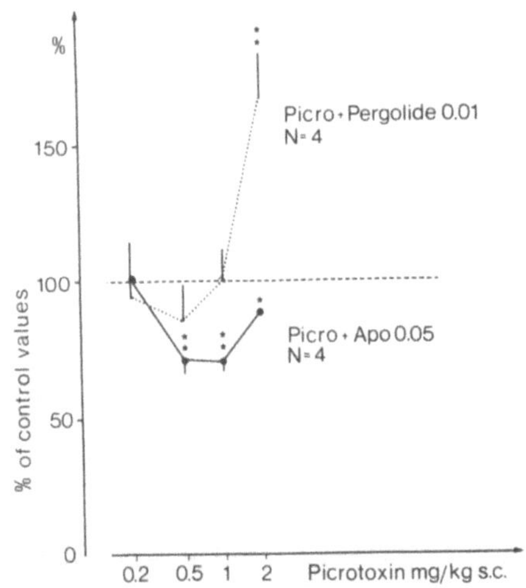

Fig. 5. Change of apomorphine (*Apo*) and pergolide-induced rotation in 6-OHDA-treated rats by picrotoxin (*Picro*) pretreatments. *Abscissa*, doses of picrotoxin in mg/kg SC; *ordinate*, changes in percentage of the total rotation in relation to control values

1984b). In this model pergolide induced contralateral rotation while apomorphine induced ipsilateral rotation (Fig. 6). Similar results were obtained when the GABA antagonist bicuculline was injected intrastriatally instead of picrotoxin. This qualitative difference between the two agonists represents further evidence for their different mechanisms of action.

The picrotoxin experiments indicate differences in the localization of D-1 and D-2 receptors on postsynaptic GABA neurons. If this is the case apomorphine and pergolide ought to affect GABA release differently in the striatum. This was studied by performing intracerebral dialysis with a thin dialysis tube implanted horizontally across the two striata. The tube was perfused with a physiological

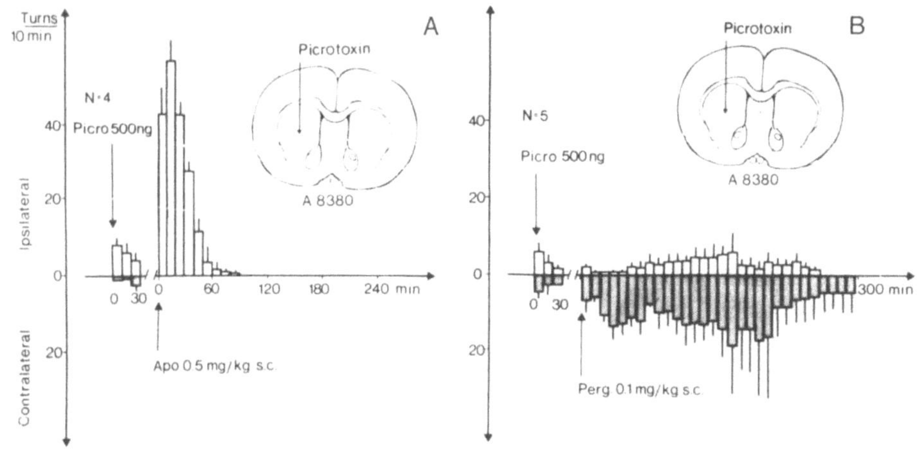

Fig. 6 A, B. Rotational behavior induced by apomorphine (*Apo*) or pergolide (*Perg*) following pictrotoxin (*Picro*) injected into the left striatum in a total volume of 0.5 ul. The position of the tip of the injection needle is indicated by the *arrow* drawn in the corresponding figure from König and Klippel (1963)

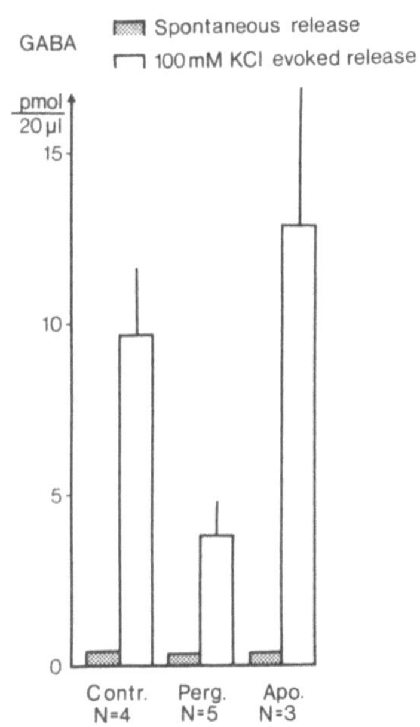

Fig. 7. Effect of saline (*Contr*), apomorphine (*Apo*) and pergolide (*Perg*) perfused into the striata of halothane-anesthetized rats by using a dialysis fiber implanted stereotaxically through the temporal bones on GABA released with 4 m*M* KCl (spontaneous release) and 100 m*M* KCl (evoked release)

Ringer solution containing either apomorphine (10^{-4} *M*) or pergolide (10^{-4} *M*) and in one of two sets of experimental conditions (a) 4 m*M* KCl concentration in the perfusate to measure spontaneous GABA release; and (b) 100 m*M* KCl concentration to evoke GABA release. It was found that pergolide inhibited the evoked GABA release while apomorphine seemed to enhance it, although the difference did not reach statistical significance (Fig. 7). The decreased GABA release following the pergolide perfusion with 100 m*M* KCl was probably due to stimulation of a D-2 receptor exerting inhibition on postsynaptic GABA neurons.

It is thus evident that the results obtained with intracerebral dialysis provide further evidence of a functional dissociation between D-1 and D-2 receptors in the striatum.

2.2 Presynaptic Receptors

The pronounced differences between the effects of apomorphine and pergolide on postsynaptic DA receptors suggested that it would be interesting to test the effects of these drugs on presynaptic dopamine receptor mechanisms. Rats were tested for spontaneous exploratory behavior over 10 min immediately after being placed in an automatic holeboard apparatus (Ljungberg and Ungerstedt 1978). This condition elicited an exploratory behavior which was markedly inhibited when animals were pretreated with various doses of apomorphine and pergolide (Fig. 8).

The dose-response curves are biphasic, since the activity increased after a sharp breakpoint. This increase of acitivity coincides with the development of stereotyped acitivity in the animals. On the basis of previous results (Strömbom 1976; Ljungberg and Ungerstedt 1976) we can assume that the decrease in behavior is due to the stimulation of presynaptic autoreceptors, which inhibits the synthesis and release of dopamine. The qualitative and quantitative change in behavior after the breakpoint in all probability indicates the dose level at which the drug also stimulates postsynaptic receptors.

It seemed conceivable that presynaptic receptors might show a response to apomorphine and pergolide similar to that seen when the effect of these agonists on postsynaptic receptors was measured. The animals were therefore pretreated with various doses of *cis*(Z)-flupentixol and sulpiride. However, the results differed widely from those obtained in the study of postsynaptic mechanisms. Of all the neuroleptics tested, only sulpiride was able to counteract the effects of apo-

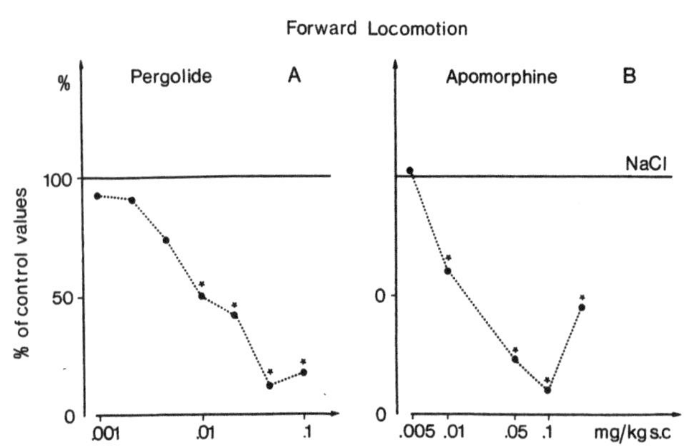

Fig. 8 A, B. Effect of pergolide (**A**) and apomorphine (**B**) on locomotion, recorded in a holeboard. *Abscissa*, doses (mg/kg SC); *ordinate*, percentage in relation to control values

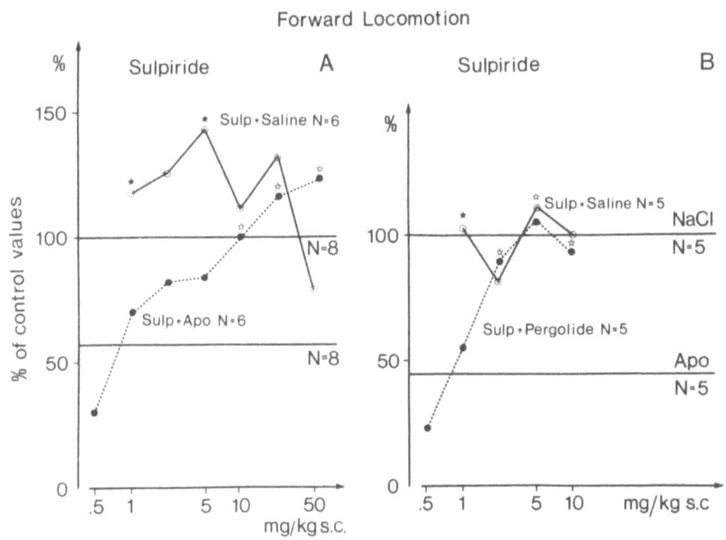

Fig. 9 A, B. Sulpiride (*Sulp*) antagonism of apomorphine (*Apo*) (**A**) and pergolide (**B**) inhibition of locomotion

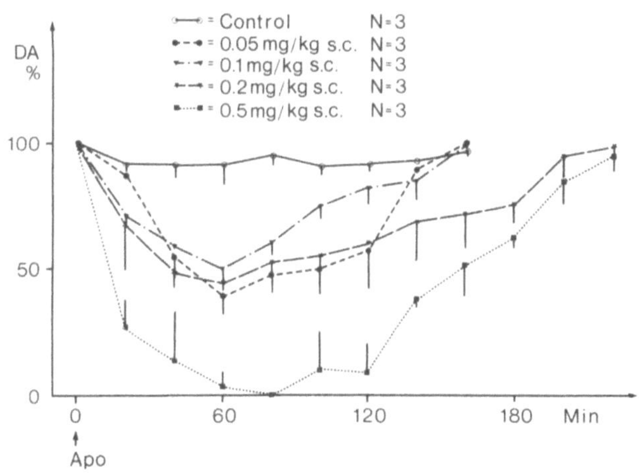

Fig. 10. Time course of the reduction of DA levels in striatal perfusates following apomorphine (*Apo*). Apomorphine 0.05–0.2 mg/kg reduced DA to 50% of the control values, while a dose of 0.5 mg/kg reduced DA levels to undetectable amounts. *Abscissa*, time (min) after the apomorphine injection; *ordinate*, levels of DA, expressed as percentages of the mean of three control samples taken immediately before the injection of apomorphine

morphine and pergolide (Fig. 9). Furthermore sulpiride was equally potent in counteracting apomorphine and pergolide, which is clearly at variance with the postsynaptic findings.

Following the administration of apomorphine, intracerebral dialysis experiments showed a decrease in endogenous DA release, which reached undetectable

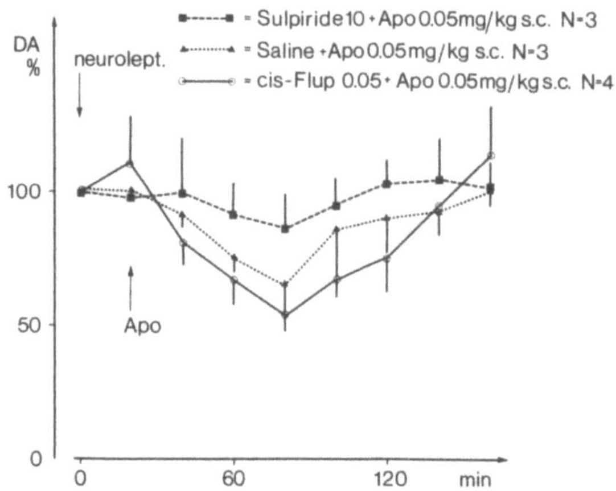

Fig. 11. Ability of sulpiride, but not *cis*(Z)-flupentixol (*cis-Flup*) (injected 20 min before) to counteract the apomorphine (*Apo*)-induced decrease of DA release recovered by intracerebral dialysis. *Abscissa*, time (min) after injection of saline or neuroleptics; *ordinate*, levels of DA expressed as % percentages of the control values

levels at postsynaptic doses (Zetterström and Ungerstedt 1984) (Fig. 10). The effect of a low dose of apomorphine was tested after pretreatment with *cis*(Z)-flupentixol and sulpiride. In agreement with the behavioral studies sulpiride was found to counteract the effect of apomorphine in decreasing the release of dopamine, while *cis*(Z)-flupentixol did not have this effect in the dose tested (Fig. 11).

3 An Explanatory Model

The present paper demonstrates that we are able to record functional changes related to presynaptic dopamine receptors, which seem to be equally affected by apomorphine and pergolide and inhibited specifically by sulpiride. Furthermore, we have presented evidence suggesting the existence of functional postsynaptic D-1 and D-2 receptors. Our data do not directly address the identity of the D-1 and D-2 receptors, but our conclusions are inferred from the use of drugs whose profiles on D-1 and D-2 receptors are known. These two receptors seem to be localized on different postsynaptic neurons. Our behavioral data and the data obtained by measuring GABA release indicate that the D-2 receptors may be located on GABA interneurons while the D-1 receptor may be located on some other type of interneuron, probably an acetylcholine neuron.

Figure 12 shows a hypothetical model of the interconnection between dopamine, GABA, and acetylcholine neurons. It represents the simplest possible neuronal interconnections that could account for our data. *A*, *B*, and *C* represent different neuronal levels, *A* being presynaptic, *B* postsynaptic, and *C* the continuation of neuronal pathways.

At level *C* the diagram (Fig. 12) indicates two efferent outflows from the striatum. This hypothesis is inferred from results of lesioning the substantia nigra reticulata of previously 6-OHDA-denervated rats (Herrera-Marschitz and Ungerstedt 1984 b). In this model, the apomorphine-induced rotation was blocked to the extent that the animal rotated ipsilaterally instead of contralaterally. On the other hand, the effect of pergolide was only decreased, which indicated a contin-

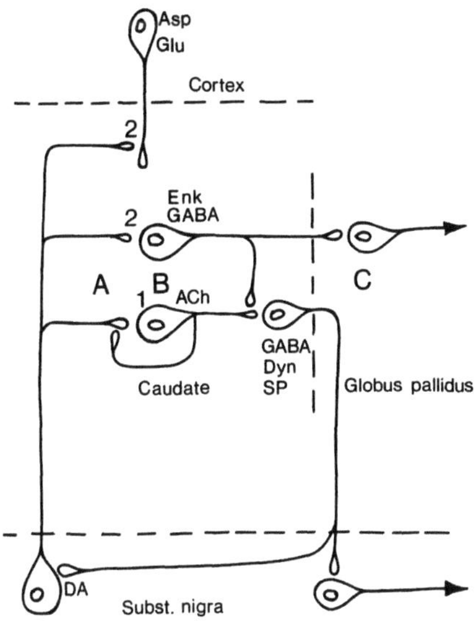

Fig. 12. Hypothetical outline of neuronal connection in the basal ganglia based on the findings reported in the text

ued effect on the ipsilateral denervated striatum (Fig. 2). We interpret these responses as due to different output pathways from the striatal complex, which are differentially affected by apomorphine and pergolide acting on different populations of postsynaptic neurons.

In our model, apomorphine-induced rotation can be elicited by inhibiting a non-GABA neuron, possibly an acetylcholine neuron which, in turn, inhibits a descending striatonigral GABA pathway. The apomorphine inhibition may thus cause a disinhibition of the descending GABA system, which is consistent with the fact that direct GABA receptor stimulation by muscimol injected into the substantia nigra induces contralateral rotational behavior (Herrera-Marschitz et al. 1984b). Pergolide may induce rotation by stimulating a D-2 receptor located on GABA interneurons which, in turn, may have an inhibitory action on a striatopallidal pathway.

Systemic picrotoxin treatment (see above) inhibits the effect of apomorphine by blocking an action on the descending striatonigral GABA pathway. However, it will potentiate pergolide rotation by inhibiting GABA transmission to the globus pallidus, which becomes synergistic to the inhibition induced by stimulating the D-2 DA receptor. Locally injected picrotoxin will have the same effect as systemic picrotoxin on pergolide rotation, inducing an inhibition of GABA transmission and thus in turn an enhancement of pergolide-induced contralateral rotation in both 6-OHDA-denervated rats and normal animals that have received picrotoxin injected into the striatum. The ipsilateral rotation elicited by apomorphine in animals receiving a unilateral injection of picrotoxin into the striatum is more difficult to explain in this model. We have included in our hypothesis a collateral between the GABA interneuron and the acetylcholine neuron. Picrotoxin may inhibit the GABA effect of this collateral on the acetylcholine neuron, thereby counteracting the inhibitory effect of apomorphine on this neuron. This will then diminish the effect of apomorphine in the striatum injected with picrotoxin, whereupon the apomorphine effect on the nondenervated striatum will be more pronounced, leading to ipsilateral rotation.

In conclusion, our results provide support for the existence of functionally important D-1 and D-2 receptors in the rat brain. Furthermore, these two types of receptors appear to elicit behavioral responses by way of different neuronal systems.

References

Herrera-Marschitz M, Ungerstedt U (1984a) Evidence that apomorphine and pergolide induce rotation in rats by different actions on D-1 and D-2 receptor sites. Eur J Pharmacol 98:165–176

Herrera-Marschitz M, Ungerstedt U (1984b) Evidence that striatal efferents relate to different dopamine receptors. Brain Res (to be published)

Herrera-Marschitz M, Hyttel J, Ungerstedt U (1984a) The dopamine D-1 antagonist SCH 23390 inhibits apomorphine but not pergolide-induced rotation. Acta Physiol Scand (to be published)

Herrera-Marschitz M, Hökfelt T, Ungerstedt U, Terenius L, Goldstein M (1984b) Effects of intranigral injections of dynorphin, dynorphin fragments and alfa-neoendorphin on rotational behavior in the rat. Eur J Pharmacol (to be published)

Kebabian JW, Cote TE (1981) Dopamine receptors and cyclic AMP: a decade of progress. TIPS March:69–71

König JFR, Klippel RR (1963) The rat brain: a stereotaxic atlas of the forebrain and lower parts of the brain stem. Krieger, New York

Ljungberg T, Ungerstedt U (1976) Automatic registration of behavior related to dopamine and noradrenalin transmission. Eur J Pharmacol 36:181–188

Ljungberg T, Ungerstedt U (1978) A method for simultaneous recording of eight behavioral parameters related to monoamine neurotransmission. Pharmacol Biochem Behav 8: 483–489

Scatton B (1982) Further evidence for the involvement of D-2, but not D-1 dopamine receptors in dopaminergic control of striatal cholinergic transmission. Life Sci 31:2883–2890

Schwarcz R, Fuxe K, Agnati LF, Hökfelt T, Coyle JT (1979) Rotational behavior in rats with unilateral striatal kainic acid lesions: a behavioral model for studies on intact dopamine (DA)-receptors. Brain Res 170:485–495

Seeman P (1981) Brain dopamine receptors. Pharmacol Rev 32:229–313

Strömbom U (1976) Catecholamine receptor agonists: effects on motor activity and tyrosine hydroxylation in mouse brain. Naunyn Schmiedeberg Arch Pharmacol 292:167–176

Ungerstedt U (1971) Postsynaptic supersensitivity after 6-hydroxy-dopamine induced degeneration of the nigtro-striatal dopamine system. Acta Physiol Scand [Suppl] 367:69–93

Ungerstedt U, Herrera-Marschitz M, Jungnelius U, Ståhle L, Tossman U, Zetterström T (1982) Dopamine synaptic mechanisms reflected in studies combining behavioral recordings and brain dialysis. In: Kohsaka M (eds) Advances in dopamine research. Pergamon, Oxford, pp 219–231

Ungerstedt U, Herrera-Marschitz M, Ståhle L, Tossman U, Zetterström T (1983) Dopamine receptor mechanisms studied by correlating transmitter release and behavior. In: Carlsson A, Nilsson JLG (eds) Dopamine receptor agonists. Swedish Pharmaceutical, Stockholm, pp 165–181

Zetterström T, Ungerstedt U (1984) Effect of apomorphine on the in vivo release of dopamine and its metabolites studied by brain dialysis. Eur J Pharmacol 97:29–36

Zetterström T, Sharp T, Marsden CA, Ungerstedt U (1983) In vivo measurement of dopamine and its metabolites by intracerebral dialysis: changes after d-amphetamine. J Neurochem 41:1769–1773

Pharmacological Properties of Presynaptic Dopamine Receptor Agonists

A. Carlsson[1]

Contents

Abstract 31
1 Introduction 31
2 Summary of Pharmacological Properties of 3-PPP 33
2.1 Agonist Action of 3-PPP on Presynaptic DA Receptors (Autoreceptors) in the Rat Forebrain 33
2.2 Antagonist Action of (−)-3-PPP on Postsynaptic DA Receptors of the Intact Rat Forebrain 33
2.3 Effect of 3-PPP on Prolactin Secretion 34
2.4 Effect of 3-PPP on DA Receptors of the Emetic Trigger Zone 34
2.5 Effect of 3-PPP on Postsynaptic DA Receptors in the Forebrain After Denervation by Intranigral 6-OHDA Injection 34
3 Discussion 35
4 Functional and Clinical Aspects 36
References 37

Abstract

Selective presynaptic dopamine receptor agonists appear to offer promise as putative antipsychotic agents with a low risk of extrapyramidal side-effects, including tardive dyskinesia. However, no such agent with a reasonable degree of selectivity has yet reached the stage of clinical trial.

In the present paper the particular pharmacological profile of presynaptic dopamine receptor (autoreceptor) agonists is described, and underlying mechanisms are discussed. Special attention is paid to the compound 3-(3-hydroxyphenyl-*N*-*n*-propylpiperidine (3-PPP), especially its levotatory enantiomer. This agent shows affinity for both pre- and postsynaptic dopamine receptors. Its intrinsic activity in different locations varies between virtually zero and 100%, leading to a mixture of agonist and antagonist properties. It is suggested that this variability depends on the adaptive properties of the dopamine receptor.

1 Introduction

Presynaptic dopamine (DA) receptor agonists appear to offer some promise as antipsychotic drugs with a low risk of extrapyramidal side-effects, including tardive dyskinesia. However, no such agent, at least none with a reasonable degree of selectivity, has yet reached the stage of clinical trial. Moreover, there are still a number of fundamental questions related to the nature of presynaptic DA

1 Department of Pharmacology, University of Göteborg, P.O. Box 33031, S-40033 Göteborg, Sweden

Dyskinesia – Research and Treatment
(Psychopharmacology Supplementum 2)
Editors: Casey, Chase, Christensen, Gerlach

receptors and for that matter, DA receptors in general, that must be answered before we can understand and interpret the peculiar pharmacological properties of the presynaptic DA receptor agonists known thus far.

The pharmacological profile of a DA agonist acting selectively on presynaptic receptors, or autoreceptors, will largely depend on the degree of selectivity. This, in turn, leads to the question as to whether subtypes of DA receptors are fundamentally different or rather represent alternative conformations of the same molecule.

This presentation will describe some observations that have led us to believe that DA receptors in different locations, despite considerable differences in responsiveness to an agonist, may well be identical in structure and differ only in conformational state or perhaps only in coupling between the receptor and other molecules involved in the response. We feel that the criteria for classification of receptor subtypes, at least insofar as DA receptors are concerned, may need revision in the future.

Needless to say, definite answers to questions related to receptor classification will have to await the isolation and strict chemical characterization of receptor molecules. Nevertheless, it is important for the interpretation of pharmacological data to try to reach a provisional standpoint at an early stage.

The present discussion will be mainly based on observations with 3-(3-hydroxyphenyl)-*N*-*n*-propylpiperidine (3-PPP), especially its levorotatory enantiomer. The reason for focusing on this compound is that no other DA autoreceptor agonist has been studied so extensively. However, in the course of the discussion reference will be made to other selective dopamine autoreceptor agonists.

Our first experiments were made with the racemic mixture of 3-PPP. This compound exhibits the profile of a dopaminergic agonist, acting selectively on the presynaptic dopamine receptors, the so-called autoreceptors, in the rat forebrain, while leaving the postsynaptic dopamine receptors unchanged. Since activation of dopaminergic autoreceptors causes inhibition of presynaptic dopaminergic activity, i.e., firing and transmitter synthesis, release, and metabolism, the most striking physiological change induced by such a compound will be inhibition of motility, especially exploratory behavior (Hjorth et al. 1981).

When the two enantiomers of 3-PPP later became available, they were found to have different profiles. The (+)-form behaved essentially as a classic DA receptor agonist such as apomorphine, i.e., preferential activation of autoreceptors in low dosage and activation also of postsynaptic receptors in higher dosage. The (−)-form was also found to stimulate DA autoreceptors, although to a somewhat lesser extent than the (+)-form, but it behaved as an antagonist on the postsynaptic DA receptors (Hjorth et al. 1983).

We and other workers have subsequently extended the studies to DA receptors at other sites. The pattern thus emerging forms the basis of the present discussion. The most pertinent data will first be summarized.

2 Summary of Pharmacological Properties of 3-PPP

2.1 Agonist Action of 3-PPP on Presynaptic DA Receptors (Autoreceptors) in the Rat Forebrain

Both enantiomers of 3-PPP are agonists on DA autoreceptors, as indicated by reduced dopa formation and DA metabolite levels under conditions where feedback loops have been disconnected [pretreatment with γ-butyrolactone or reserpine (Hjorth et al. 1983) or after axotomy (Magnusson et al. 1983)].

The efficacy of the levorotatory enantiomer is lower than that of the (+)-form or apomorphine, indicating that it is a partial agonist on autoreceptors. The same conclusion has been reached from electrophysiological single-cell recordings of rat nigral neurons (Clark et al. 1984, and unpublished data).

While DA autoreceptors controlling the impulse generation in dendrites/soma and the neurotransmitter synthesis in the nerve terminals are stimulated by 3-PPP, this does not seem to be the case for the autoreceptors controlling the neurotransmitter release by the nerve impulse (Langer et al. 1983; Starke 1984; Markstein and Lahaye 1983). A possible explanation of this anomalous behavior may be that the latter receptors are at least partly located in the synaptic cleft and thus exposed to a high concentration of neurotransmitter (see below).

The two forms of 3-PPP appear to act directly rather than after biotransformation, as indicated by their activity after local application in the rat nucleus accumbens (Svensson and Ahlenius 1983).

2.2 Antagonist Action of (−)-3-PPP on Postsynaptic DA Receptors of the Intact Rat Forebrain

In normal rats (−)-3-PPP inhibits exploratory activity. In contrast to a classic DA receptor agonist, such as apomorphine, this agent exhibits no stimulating properties, e.g., induction of increased motility and stereotyped behavior, even after high doses. It thus seems to be devoid of any stimulating action on postsynaptic DA receptors. This assumption is strengthened by the fact that in reserpine-treated animals (−)-3-PPP causes at most a very slight increase in motility and does not counteract catalepsy. Thus, if this agent has any intrinsic activity on postsynaptic DA receptors in the rat forebrain, it amounts to only a few percent of the maximum response elicited, for example, by apomorphine (Hjorth et al. 1983).

That (−)-3-PPP has affinity for postsynaptic DA receptors is supported both by pharmacological and biochemical data. This agent antagonizes the behavioral actions of DA agonists, such as apomorphine, (+)-3-PPP, and amphetamine (Hjorth et al. 1983). Moreover, it is capable of displacing the DA agonist dipropyl-5,6-ADTN from striatal DA receptor sites in vivo (Table 1). Feenstra et al. (1983) have demonstrated that the receptor sites showing up under these experimental conditions are entirely or predominantly postsynaptic. In vitro binding of 3-PPP to DA receptor sites has also been demonstrated and will be discussed below.

Table 1. Displacement of dipropyl-5,6-ADTN[a] from rat striatal binding sites in vivo

Drug (mg/kg SC)		Displacement (%)
Haloperidol	(1)	61[b]
(−)-3-PPP	(14)	67[b]
(+)-3-PPP	(14)	9
BHT 920	(3)	12

[a] Dipropyl-5,6-ADTN 0.25 μmol/kg was given SC 1 h before test drug and rats were killed 40 min after test drug. Mean differences from controls are shown (striatum minus cerebellum, $n = 6$)
[b] Differs from control at $p < 0.001$

Table 1 shows data on the ability of several other dopaminergic drugs to displace dipropyl-5,6-ADTN in vivo. Haloperidol and (−)-3-PPP, both given in apparently maximally active doses, caused approximately the same degree of displacement, although the former agent was more potent. (+)-3-PPP was considerably less active. In fact, several in vitro studies indicate a lower affinity of the (+)-form than of the (−)-form for dopaminergic binding sites (e.g., Koch et al. 1983). BHT 920 also proved to have very low displacing activity in a dose exceeding those shown to cause strong activation of DA autoreceptors, in agreement with pharmacological data indicating a high degree of selectivity for presynaptic receptors (Andén et al. 1984). Unfortunately, this agent also shows a fairly high affinity for α-adrenergic receptors.

2.3 Effect of 3-PPP on Prolactin Secretion

Both enantiomers of 3-PPP act as equipotent, strong agonists on the DA lactotroph receptors in the anterior pituitary (Eriksson et al. 1983). Again the (−)-form tends to have a lower efficacy than the (+)-form (Mikuni et al. 1984).

2.4 Effect of 3-PPP on DA Receptors of the Emetic Trigger Zone

Both enantiomers of 3-PPP elicit emesis after IV injection to dogs (Martin et al. 1981; Arnt et al. 1982; G. Paalzow et al., personal communication). However, the response appears to be less pronounced than after apomorphine treatment. Certain observations suggest that the (−)-form is less active than the (+)-form (G. Paalzow, personal communication).

Both enantiomers of 3-PPP can antagonize the emetic action of apomorphine, suggesting that they are partial agonists on the emetic DA receptors (Arnt et al. 1983).

2.5 Effect of 3-PPP on Postsynaptic DA Receptors in the Forebrain after Denervation by Intranigral 6-OHDA Injection

After unilateral destruction of the nigrostriatal DA pathway by intranigral injection of 6-OHDA, both enantiomers of 3-PPP elicited contralateral turning of an intensity comparable to apomorphine. The two enantiomers were approximately equipotent. The effects are blocked by DA receptor antagonists (Arnt et al. 1983; Oberlander and Boissier 1983). Subsequent studies showed that both enantiomers of 3-PPP behaved as DA receptor agonists on bilaterally denervated receptors (Arnt and Hyttel 1984).

Observations somewhat similar to those summarized above have been reported in an investigation on transdihydrolisuride (Wachtel and Dorow 1983).

3 Discussion

The data briefly summarized above suggest that there is a relationship between the intrinsic activity of (−)-3-PPP and the degree of agonist occupancy on the receptor during a period preceding the experiments. On the normal postsynaptic DA receptor in the rat forebrain, where the agonist occupancy can be assumed to be high, (−)-3-PPP acts as an antagonist with at most a slight intrinsic activity. Even after reserpine pretreatment 18 hours beforehand, which can be assumed to induce a certain, albeit slight degree of receptor supersensitivity, (−)-3-PPP did not show more than a trace of intrinsic activity.

On the other hand, on receptors where the agonist occupancy can be assumed to be low, since these receptors are largely or entirely located outside the synaptic cleft, (−)-3-PPP showed up as an agonist with an intrinsic activity approaching or comparable to that of its dextrorotatory enantiomer and to that of apomorphine. This is true of dopaminergic autoreceptors, lactotroph receptors, and denervated postsynaptic receptors. In the emetic trigger zone, which may or may not receive a small dopaminergic input, (−)-3-PPP appears to behave like a partial agonist (see Fig. 1).

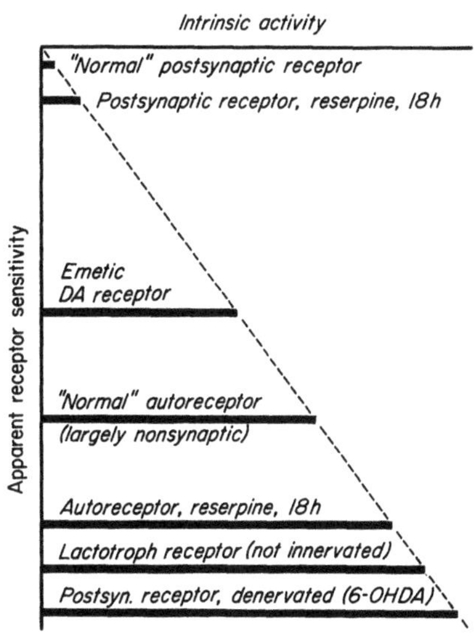

Fig. 1. Intrinsic activity of (−)-3-PPP in different localities: a possible function of the adaptive state of the dopamine receptor

These data invite the speculation that the DA receptor molecules are basically the same in all the locations mentioned; their different responsiveness to an agonist such as (−)-3-PPP is a result of the adaptability of the receptor molecule, or of a component in the receptor complex. A change in agonist occupancy on the receptor may induce a slow conformational change in the receptor molecule or in a nearby molecule, influencing the overall responsiveness of the receptor complex. In this way the same receptor agonist will show a varying intrinsic activity, depending on the state of the receptor.

Establishment of the time taken to reach a new equilibrium after a change in receptor occupancy needs further investigation. The intrinsic activity of (−)-3-PPP on autoreceptors is significantly elevated as soon as 18 hours after administration of reserpine (unpublished data recorded in this laboratory). However, agonistic properties of this compound on postsynaptic receptors became obvious only about a week after denervation by 6-hydroxydopamine or initiation of chronic reserpine treatment (Arnt and Hyttel 1984).

It was previously proposed that receptor hypersensitivity following denervation was due to an increase in the number of receptors without any concomitant change in receptor properties. For example, the affinity of the receptor for the agonist is generally thought to be unchanged. The increase in the number of receptor molecules hardly exceeds 50% after denervation (see review by Seeman 1980). It is difficult to envisage such a small increase to account for a drastic change in intrinsic acitivity, from virtually zero to 100%, as described above for (−)-3-PPP. A qualitative change somewhere in the receptor complex seems more likely.

A preliminary report by George et al. (1983) is of interest in this context. In vitro binding experiments with ^{3}H-spiperone in the presence or absence of Na^{+} indicated that in the pituitary both enantiomers of 3-PPP behave as agonists, while in the caudate nucleus the (+)-form seemed to be an agonist and the (−)-form an antagonist. These observations are thus in agreement with the in vivo data described above.

The intrinsic activity of partial adrenergic agonists has been reported to differ considerably in different tissues. Local tissue factors influencing the coupling between receptor molecules and response have been assumed to account for these differences, which obviously do not form a sufficient basis for a subclassification of receptors (Kenakin 1982). Future work will decide to what extent such differences are determined by a varying receptor occupancy, according to the hypothesis proposed above.

4 Functional and Clinical Aspects

The possible usefulness of DA autoreceptor agonists must await future clinical studies. The pharmacological profile of (−)-3-PPP suggests that this compound is an efficient antipsychotic agent; especially its ability to counteract amphetamine-induced stimulation supports this view. Moreover, the absence of catalepsy suggests the absence of extrapyramidal side-effects. The ability of 3-PPP, and especially its levorotatory enantiomer, to alleviate experimental tardive dyskinesia in monkeys is a further pointer in the same direction (Häggström et al. 1983). Further interest in this context attaches to the neuroleptic-like, stereospecific effect of (−)-3-PPP on brain glucose metabolism, as revealed by autoradiography with ^{14}C-2-deoxyglucose (Palacios and Wiederhold 1984).

Certain aspects of the pharmacological profile of 3-PPP and its enantiomers are difficult to explain at this time. As shown in Table 1, (−)-3-PPP appears to be as effective as haloperidol in displacing dipropyl-5,6-ADTN from striatal binding sites in vivo. Why does not the former agent, like the latter, cause catalepsy? It should be noted that the intrinsic activity of (−)-3-PPP on normal postsynaptic receptors appears to be virtually zero and that this agent is unable to counteract catalepsy in reserpine-treated animals. No explanation can yet be offered for this apparent discrepancy. Maybe there is a difference of some kind, in the binding to or interaction with the striatal postsynaptic DA receptors, between a classic neuroleptic such as haloperidol and a compound derived from a family of DA receptor agonists, like (−)-3-PPP. Future work is needed to clarify whether such a difference does indeed exist and, if so, its nature. Finally, the question must be addressed as to whether such a difference in drug-receptor interaction is also relevant for the antipsychotic activity. Further aspects, e.g., regional aspects of the problem, have been discussed by Hjorth et al. (1983).

Since the intrinsic activity of a partial DA receptor agonist appears to depend on the state of the receptor, the question arises as to whether this state can be influenced by pathological processes or by therapeutic interventions. For example, hypersensitive receptors probably occur in Parkinson patients, and such receptors may recognize a postsynaptic DA receptor antagonist such as (−)-3-PPP as an agonist. In fact, this might have therapeutic applications (cf. also Carlsson 1983). On the other hand, if hypersensitive DA receptors exist in schizophrenia or other psychotic states – a controversial issue at present – an agent like (−)-3-PPP might worsen the condition.

References

Andén NE, Ålander T, Grabowska-Andén M, Liljenberg B, Lindgren S, Thornström U (1984) The pharmacology of pre- and postsynaptic dopamine receptors; differential effects of dopamine receptor agonists and antagonists. In: Usdin E, Carlsson A, Dahlström A, Engel JA (eds) Catecholamines, vol. B. Liss, New York, p 19

Arnt J, Hyttel J (1984) Postsynaptic dopamine agonistic effects of 3-PPP enantiomers revealed by bilateral 6-hydroxydopamine lesions and by chronic reserpine treatment in rats. Neural Transm 60

Arnt J, Christensen AV, Hyttel J, Larsen JJ, Svendsen O (1982) Effects of putative dopamine autoreceptor agonists in pharmacological models related to dopaminergic and neuroleptic activity. Eur J Pharmacol 86:185–198

Arnt J, Bögesö KP, Christensen AV, Hyttel J, Larsen JJ, Svendsen O (1983) Dopamine receptor agonistic effects of 3-PPP enantiomers. Psychopharmacology 81:199–207

Carlsson A (1983) Are "on-off" effects during chronic L-dopa treatment due to faulty feedback control of the nigrostriatal dopamine pathway? J Neural Transm [Suppl] 19:153–161

Clark D, Engberg G, Pileblad E, Svensson TH, Carlsson A, Freeman AS, Bunney BS (1984) The effect of novel dopaminergic agonists on the nigrostriatal dopamine system. Proceedings of the 14th CINP congress. Clin Neuropharmacol (to be published)

Eriksson E, Modigh K, Carlsson A (1983) Dopamine receptors involved in prolactin secretion pharmacologically characterized by use of 3-PPP enantiomers. Eur J Pharmacol 96:29–36

Feenstra MGP, Rollema H, Mulder TBA, Westerink BHG, Horn AS (1983) In vivo dopamine receptor binding studies with a non-radioactively labeled agonist, dipropyl-5,6-ADTN. Life Sci 32:1313–1323

George SR, Watanabe M, Seeman P (1983) The brain D_2 receptor differs from the pituitary D_2 receptor. Abstracts of the 13th annual meeting. Society for Neuroscience, Boston

Häggström JE, Gunne LM, Carlsson A, Wikström H (1983) Antidyskinetic action of 3-PPP, a selective dopaminergic autoreceptor agonist, in Cebus monkeys with persistent neuroleptic-induced dyskinesias. J Neurol Transm 58:135–142

Hjorth S, Carlsson A, Wikström H, Lindberg P, Sanchez D, Hacksell U, Arvidsson LE, Svensson U, Nilsson JLG (1981) 3-PPP, a new centrally acting DA receptor agonist with selectivity for autoreceptors. Life Sci 28:1225–1238

Hjorth S, Carlsson A, Clark D, Svensson K, Wikström H, Sanchez D, Lindberg P, Hacksell U, Arvidsson LE, Johansson A, Nilsson JLG (1983) Central dopamine receptor agonist and antagonist actions of the enantiomers of 3-PPP. Psychopharmacology 81:89–99

Kenakin TP (1982) Organ selectivity of drugs. Alternatives to receptor selectivity. TIPS April 1982:153–156

Koch SW, Koe BK, Bacopoulos NG (1983) Differential effects of the enantiomers of 3-(3-hydroxyphenyl)-*N-n*-propylpiperidine (3-PPP) at dopamine receptor sites. Eur J Phar macol 92:279–283

Langer SZ, Arbilla S, Kamal L, Cantrill R (1983) Peripheral and central dopamine receptors modulating the release of neurotransmitters. Acta Pharm Suec [Suppl] 1:108–117

Magnusson T, Carlsson A, Lindberg P, Sanchez D (1983) Evidence for activation of dopaminergic autoreceptors by (−)-3-PPP. Acta Pharm Suec [Suppl] 1:16–18

Markstein R, Lahaye D (1983) In vitro effect of the racemic mixture and the (−)enantiomer of *N-n*-propyl-3-(3-hydroxyphenyl) piperidine (3-PPP) on postsynaptic dopamine receptors and on a presynaptic autoreceptor. J Neural Transm 58:43–53

Martin GE, Haubrich DR, Williams M (1981) Pharmacological profiles of the putative dopamine autoreceptor agonists 3-PPP and TL-99. Eur J Pharmacol 76:15–23

Mikuni M, Gudelsky GA, Simonovic M, Meltzer HY (1984) Interaction of (+)- and (−)-3-PPP with the dopamine receptor in the anterior pituitary gland. Life Sci 34:239–246

Oberlander C, Boissier JR (1983) Postsynaptic striatal dopamine agonist or antagonist actions of (+) or (−) 3-PPP and modification after receptor deafferentation. J Pharmacol (Paris) 14:401–404

Palacios JM, Wiederhold KH (1984) Presynaptic dopaminergic agonists modify brain glucose metabolism in a way similar to the neuroleptics. (to be published)

Seeman P (1980) Brain dopamine receptors. Pharmacol Rev 32:229–313

Starke K (1984) Functional in vitro comparison of striatal pre- and postsynaptic dopamine receptors. In: Usdin E, Carlsson A, Dahlström A, Engel JA (eds) Catecholamines, vol. B. Liss, New York, p 5

Svensson L, Ahlenius S (1983) Suppression of exploratory locomotor activity in the rat by the local application of 3-PPP enantiomers into the nucleus accumbens. Eur J Pharmacol 88:393–397

Wachtel H, Dorow R (1983) Dual action on central dopamine function of transdihydrolisuride, a 9,10-dihydrogenated analogue of the ergot dopamine agonist lisuride. Life Sci 32:421–432

Influence of GABA Mimetics and Lithium on Biochemical Manifestations of Striatal Dopamine Target Cell Hypersensitivity

B. Scatton, D. Fage, A. Oblin, B. Zivkovic, S. Arbilla, S. Z. Langer, and G. Bartholini [1]

Contents

Abstract 39
1 Introduction 39
2 Potential Mechanisms Involved in the GABA-Mimetic-Induced Modulation of Striatal Dopaminergic Transmission 40
3 Similarity of the Effects of GABA Mimetics and Lithium on Striatal DA Target Cell Hypersensitivity 43
4 Concluding Remarks 44
References 44

Abstract

The potential mechanisms whereby GABA mimetics and the antimanic agent lithium stabilize dopaminergic transmission are discussed. Evidence is presented that GABA mimetics, and in particular progabide, affect dopamine-mediated events in the basal ganglia on at least three levels. First, they reduce dopamine neuron activity in both the basal and the activated states. Secondly, on a long-term basis, they antagonize the proliferation of striatal dopamine receptors subsequent to chronic neuroleptic treatment. Thirdly, they modulate the expression of dopamine receptor activation by acting distally to the dopaminergic synapse. Lithium and GABA mimetics have the last two properties in common. These effects may represent the biochemical basis for the therapeutic action of GABA mimetics in iatrogenic dyskinesias. Moreover, the similarity between the biochemical effects of GABA mimetics and lithium suggest that the former drugs may have a therapeutic potential in mania.

1 Introduction

Tardive dyskinesias are known to develop gradually during the course of prolonged treatment with neuroleptic agents in schizophrenic patients. A connection between this iatrogenic disorder and the development of the hypersensitivity of dopamine (DA) target cells induced by protracted blockade of striatal dopaminergic transmission by neuroleptics has been suggested (Tarsy and Baldessarini 1977). During the past few years, extensive effort has been devoted to the search for drugs that might alleviate these abnormal involuntary motor movements. Recent clinical evidence has been provided that GABA-mimetic drugs (e.g., progabide, muscimol, sodium valproate, γ-acetylenic GABA) exert a beneficial action in this iatrogenic condition (Linnoila et al. 1976; Bartholini et al. 1979;

1 Synthélabo-L.E.R.S., Biology Department, 31 Avenue Paul Vaillant Couturier, F-92220 Bagneux, France

Dyskinesia – Research and Treatment
(Psychopharmacology Supplementum 2)
Editors: Casey, Chase, Christensen, Gerlach

Tamminga et al. 1979; Morselli et al. 1980; Casey et al. 1980). This action also occurs in animal models of dyskinesia induced either by dopaminomimetics or by neuroleptics (see Lloyd et al., this volume; Lloyd and Worms 1980). For instance, the simultaneous repeated administration of a GABA agonist and haloperidol greatly antagonizes the hypersensitivity of the stereotyped response to apomorphine and the tolerance to neuroleptic catalepsy which occur upon repeated administration of the neuroleptic. In the present paper, we briefly discuss the potential mechanisms whereby GABA mimetics stabilize dopaminergic transmission and the neuroanatomical sites of their action. The action of progabide will be compared with that of the antimanic agent lithium, which has also been reported to abolish hypersensitivity to dopaminomimetics induced by chronic neuroleptic treatment (Pert et al. 1978; Le Douarin et al. 1983).

2 Potential Mechanisms Involved in the GABA-Mimetic-Induced Modulation of Striatal Dopaminergic Transmission

It is now well established that GABA-agonist agents have an inhibitory action on DA neuron activity (Bartholini et al. 1979; Scatton et al. 1980, 1982). Thus, at anticonvulsant doses, progabide and other GABA mimetics depress (a) the rate of synthesis and utilization of striatal DA in the rat (tyrosine hydroxylase activity, DOPA accumulation and α-methyltyrosine induced DA disappearance); (b) the release of DA from the cat caudate nucleus perfused by means of the push-pull cannula; and (c) the levels of 3-methoxytyramine, an index of DA release, in the rat striatum (unpublished data). GABA mimetics reduce DA neuron activity not only in the basal state but also, and more efficiently, in the activated state occurring after DA receptor blockade by neuroleptics. Thus, they antagonize the elevation of DA turnover (tyrosine hydroxylase activity and DA release in the striatum) induced by neuroleptics (Bartholini et al. 1979; Scatton et al. 1980, 1982). The observations made in behavioral studies are also consistent with an inhibitory action of GABA mimetics on DA neuron function. Thus, haloperidol-induced catalepsy is potentiated by these drugs (Worms et al. 1982): this effect is probably related to a reduction of the feedback activation of DA neurons, leading to a decrease of DA release from nerve terminals and thus to further impairment of dopaminergic transmission.

In addition to the antagonism of the activation of dopaminergic neurons induced by a single administration of neuroleptics, GABA mimetics also attenuate the development of dopaminergic supersensitivity due to the prolonged administration of these drugs. As shown in Table 1, repeated treatment with haloperidol for 14 days and subsequent withdrawal increased the high-affinity binding of ^{3}H-spiroperidol to DA receptors in the rat striatum by 57% while the dissociation constant (Kd) remained unchanged. When progabide was administered concomitantly with the neuroleptic the increase in the density of ^{3}H-spiroperidol binding sites was almost totally prevented (Table 1). This suggests that progabide prevents the proliferation of striatal DA receptors induced by chronic neuroleptic treatment. These biochemical changes may explain pharmacological findings

Table 1. Effect of repeated administration of Progabide[a] on the haloperidol-induced alterations in high affinity ^{3}H-spiroperidol binding in the striatum and substance *P* levels in the substantia nigra in rat

Treatment	^{3}H-Spiroperidol binding (striatum)		Substance *P* (substantia nigra)
	B_{max} (fmol/mg protein)	Kd (n*M*)	ng/g
Controls	51 ± 9	0.05 ± 0.01	1986 ± 76
Haloperidol	80 ± 8 [b]	0.05 ± 0.01	1606 ± 51 [b]
Progabide	49 ± 9	0.05 ± 0.01	1981 ± 109
Haloperidol plus progabide	56 ± 7 [c]	0.14 ± 0.08	1789 ± 53 [c]

[a] Progabide (400 mg/kg IP, b.i.d.) was co-administered with vehicle (0.1% Tween 80) or with haloperidol (2 mg/kg IP) for 14 consecutive days. Rats were sacrificed 48 h after the last injection of haloperidol. Apparent dissociation constants (Kd) and the maximal binding (B_{max}) were determined by Scatchard analysis. Results are means ± SEM of data obtained in 9–11 animals per group.
[b] $p < 0.05$ compared with to controls
[c] $p < 0.05$ compared with haloperidol alone

showing that progabide antagonizes the haloperidol-induced supersensitivity to apomorphine and the development of tolerance to the cataleptogenic action of neuroleptic (Lloyd and Worms 1980).

GABA mimetics have also been reported to diminish dopaminomimetic-induced behavior (Lloyd et al. 1984, this volume). In the rat, progabide and muscimol block the stereotypies induced by apomorphine in normal animals as well as the rotation caused by this dopaminomimetic in animals bearing a unilateral 6-hydroxydopamine-induced lesion of the nigrostriatal dopaminergic pathway. In cat and monkey, progabide also prevents dopaminomimetic-induced dyskinetic movements. These results suggest another site of action for progabide distally to the DA receptor in the chain of neurons responsible for the expression of DA receptor activation.

In an attempt to identify the mechanisms involved in GABA-mimetic-induced prevention of the homeostatic changes occurring after chronic neuroleptic administration, the effect of concurrent treatment with progabide and haloperidol on neurochemical indices of striatal DA target cell supersensitivity have been studied. Another consequence of the striatal dopaminergic supersensitivity induced by repeated treatment with neuroleptics is the development of tolerance to the increase in DA synthesis and tyrosine hydroxylase activation (Scatton et al. 1975; Table 2). Progabide co-administered for 11–14 days with haloperidol fails to affect the tolerance to the elevation of these biochemical parameters (Table 2). Therefore, the mechanism(s) whereby progabide prevents dopaminergic supersensitivity may not be related to an action on the neuronal feedback processes involved in the regulation of the activity of the nigrostriatal dopaminergic neurons, but may rather involve a site of action postsynaptic to the DA neurons.

A large body of evidence indicates that striatal cholinergic neurons, among others, are target cells for the nigrostriatal dopaminergic system (for review see Lloyd 1978). Striatal cholinergic neurons also appear to play a key role in deter-

Table 2. Effect of repeated treatment with progabide on haloperidol-induced development of tolerance of dopamine synthesis and tyrosine hydroxylase activation and ACh level diminution in the rat striatum

Repeated treatment	Challenge treament	Accumulation of dopa [a] (ng/g/30 min)	Tyrosine hydroxylase [b] (nmol/h/mg protein)	ACh [a] (nmol/g)
Vehicle	Vehicle	1312 ± 56	1.44 ± 0.03	30.0 ± 0.7
Vehicle	Haloperidol	5501 ± 319 [c]	4.21 ± 0.15 [c]	16.1 ± 0.8 [c]
Haloperidol	Haloperidol	4535 ± 166 [d]	3.31 ± 0.17 [d]	23.6 ± 0.9 [d]
Haloperidol plus progabide	Haloperidol	5063 ± 68	3.22 ± 0.13 [d]	22.9 ± 1.0 [d]

[a] Progabide (400 mg/kg IP, b.i.d.) was co-administered with vehicle (0.1% Tween 80) or with haloperidol (2 mg/kg IP once daily) for 14 consecutive days. At 48 h after the last injection rats were challenged with haloperidol (0.5 mg/kg IP), with sacrifice 1 h later. NSD-1015 (100 mg/kg IP) was injected 30 min before sacrifice

[b] Progabide (400 mg/kg IP, b.i.d.) was co-administered with vehicle (0.1% Tween 80) or with haloperidol (2 mg/kg IP once daily) for 11 consecutive days. On the day of the experiment rats received only a haloperidol injection and were sacrificed 2 h thereafter.
Results are mean ± SEM of data obtained in eight rats per group

[c] $p < 0.001$ vs vehicle-treated group

[d] $p < 0.01$ vs acute haloperidol

mining the motor patterns of striatal origin, and as such represent a site where progabide may act to prevent dopaminergic hypersensitivity. Prolonged treatment with haloperidol leads to an attenuation of the decrease of striatal acetylcholine (ACh) levels (which reflects increased cholinergic transmission) caused by a single injection of the neuroleptic (Table 2), a phenomenon thought to be connected with DA receptor hypersensitivity (see Le Douarin et al. 1983). When co-administered with haloperidol (2 mg/kg IP), progabide (400 mg/kg IP, b.i.d.) failed to prevent the neuroleptic-induced changes in ACh concentrations. Thus, the striatal cholinergic system develops the tolerance that is usually seen during repeated treatment with the neuroleptic alone. These findings suggest that striatal cholinergic neurons are not implicated in the mechanism of progabide-induced stabilization of dopaminergic hypersensitivitiy and that the site of action of progabide is beyond the dopaminergic and cholinergic synapses.

One of the major outputs from the striatum, the striatonigral pathway, includes well – defined neurons which use substance P (SP) as the neurotransmitter. There is evidence that these neurons are also target cells for the nigrostriatal dopaminergic neurons. Thus, destruction of the nigrostriatal dopaminergic pathway leads to reduction of the nigral content of SP (Hanson et al. 1981), probably as a result of an enhanced release of the peptide from striatonigral nerve terminals. Repeated treatment with neuroleptics similarly diminishes SP levels in substantia nigra (Hanson et al. 1981; Le Douarin et al. 1983; Table 1). As several days of neuroleptic treatment are needed before this effect is observed, it is probable that changes in the sensitivity of DA receptors located on SP-ergic neurons may play a role in determining the response patterns on the SP-ergic system after subacute neuroleptic treatment. As shown in Table 1, the decrease of nigral SP induced by prolonged haloperidol treatment is markedly attenuated by progabide co-administration. This suggests a restoration of normal nigral SP-ergic transmission by the GABA mimetic. Since the striatonigral SP-ergic neurons appear to represent output pathways for the expression of DA-receptor-mediated events (Le Douarin et al. 1983), it is conceivable that progabide attenuates the dopaminergic behavioral hypersensitivity elicited by chronic exposure to neuroleptics by normalizing an enhanced nigral SP-ergic transmission. This hypothesis would be consistent with the inhibitory influence of GABA on nigral SP release (Jessell 1978). However, striatonigral SP-ergic neurons may not be the only ones involved. In fact, there is evidence that both striatonigral and nigrothalamic GABA neurons also play a role in the behavioral expression of striatal DA receptor activation. Moreover, afferents to the striatum, e.g., the corticostriatal (glutamatergic) and the raphé-striatal (serotonergic) neurons are involved in extrapyramidal motor function, and their activities are reduced by progabide and other GABA mimetics (Scatton and Bartholini 1980; Scatton et al. 1982). Thus, both striatal afferent and efferent neurons may be implicated in the action of progabide on the dopaminergic supersensitivty induced by prolonged neuroleptic administration.

3 Similarity of the Effects of GABA Mimetics and Lithium on Striatal DA Target Cell Hypersensitivity

Lithium (Li) is known to prevent manic episodes, in which increased dopaminergic transmission and enhanced response to DA have been proposed as possible pathogenetic factors (Murphy et al. 1971). Recent evidence has been provided that Li may affect DA receptor hypersensitivity. Thus, prolonged exposure of an animal to Li prevents behavioral manifestations of the striatal hypersensitivity to dopaminomimetics (viz. exaggerated stereotyped response to DA agonists) induced by chronic treatment with neuroleptics (Pert et al. 1978). Moreover, chronic Li treatment prevents the increase in striatal DA receptor density induced by prolonged administration of neuroleptics (Pert et al. 1978). Electrophysiological studies have suggested that Li also blocks the development of DA autoreceptor hypersensitivity (Gallager et al. 1978).

We have recently investigated the effect of Li on different neurochemical indices of striatal DA target cell supersensitivity (Le Douarin et al. 1983). Chronic administration of dietary Li (2.5 g LiCl/kg food) together with haloperidol (delivered at a rate of 2.5 μg/h by means of osmotic minipumps) did not influence tolerance to the increase in DA turnover or to the diminution of ACh levels in the striatum of the rat, which normally occur during prolonged neuroleptic treatment. However, in similar experimental conditions, Li prevented the fall of nigral SP levels induced by the neuroleptic (ng/g: controls 2457 ± 72, chronic haloperidol 2102 ± 63; difference from controls significant at $P < 0.01$; chronic Li + haloperidol 2484 ± 77; difference from result with chronic haloperidol alone significant at $P < 0.01$). These data taken together indicate a striking similarity between Li and GABA mimetics with respect to their effects on behavioral and neurochemical indices of striatal DA target cell hypersensitivity.

4 Concluding Remarks

A hypothesis for the pathogenesis of neuroleptic-induced dyskinesia postulates two mechanisms for the increase in dopaminergic transmission: (a) the increase in DA release induced by the neuroleptic; and (b) the hypersensitivity of the striatal DA target cell developing during prolonged neuroleptic treatment. L-Dopa-induced involuntary movements have also been linked with an exaggerated striatal dopaminergic transmission. The present experimental results suggest that there are at least three possible mechanisms for the reported therapeutic action of GABA mimetics in L-dopa- and neuroleptic-induced dyskinesias. First, GABA mimetics may tune down an exaggerated activity of nigrostriatal dopaminergic neurons. Secondly, on a long-term basis, these drugs may antagonize the proliferation of striatal postsynaptic DA receptor density. Thirdly, GABA mimetics may prevent the expression of DA receptor activation at sites distal to the dopaminergic synapses, possibly by modulating striatonigral SP-ergic output pathways.

Clinical evidence suggests that hyperactivity of central dopaminergic pathways may be an important factor in the etiology of manic states (Murphy et al. 1971), and it has been proposed that the antimanic action of Li may be related, at least in part, to its ability to reduce DA receptor responses (Pert et al. 1978). The striking similarities between the reducing effects of GABA mimetics and Li on both behavioral and neurochemical indices of dopaminergic hypersensitivity suggest that the former drugs may also have a therapeutic potential in mania. Clinical evaluation of progabide in mania is not yet available. However, sodium valproate has been shown to exert a beneficial effect in manic patients that is comparable in magnitude to that observed with Li treatment (Emrich et al. 1983). Conversely, the ability of Li to reduce DA target cell hypersensitivity suggest a therapeutic potential of this drug in iatrogenic dyskinesias. The report by Reda et al. (1975) that Li carbonate may be of value in the treatment of tardive dyskinesias is consistent with this proposal.

References

Bartholini G, Scatton B, Zivkovic B, Lloyd KG (1979) On the mode of action of SL 76002, a new GABA receptor agonist. In: Krogsgaard-Larsen P, Scheel-Krüger J, Kofod H (eds) GABA-Neurotransmitters. Munksgaard, Copenhagen, pp 326–339

Casey DE, Gerlach J, Magelund G, Christensen TR (1980) γ-Acetylenic-GABA in tardive dyskinesia. Arch Gen Psychiatry 37:1376–1379

Emrich HM, Altmann H, Dose M, von Zerssen D (1983) Therapeutic effects of GABAergic drugs in affective disorders. A preliminary report. Pharmacol Biochem Behav 19:369–372

Gallager DW, Pert A, Bunney WE Jr (1978) Haloperidol-induced presynaptic dopamine supersensitivity is blocked by chronic lithium. Nature 273:309–311

Hanson GR, Alphs L, Wolf W, Levine R, Lovenberg W (1981) Haloperidol-induced reduction of nigral substance-P like immunoreactivity: a probe for the interactions between dopamine and substance P neuronal systems. J Pharmacol Exp Ther 218:568–578

Jessell TM (1978) Substance P release from the rat substantia nigra. Brain Res 151:469–473

Le Douarin C, Oblin A, Fage D, Scatton B (1983) Influence of lithium on biochemical manifestations of striatal dopamine target cell supersensitivity induced by prolonged haloperidol treatment. Eur J Pharmacol 93:55–62

Linnoila M, Viukari M, Hietala O (1976) Effect of sodium valproate on tardive dyskinesia. Br J Psychiatry 129:114–129
Lloyd KG (1978) Neurotransmitter interactions related to central dopamine neurons. In: Youdim MBH, Lovenberg W, Sharman DF, Lagnado JR (eds) Essays in neurochemistry and neuropharmacology, vol 3. Wiley, New York, pp 131–207
Lloyd KG, Worms P (1980) Sustained γ-aminobutyric acid receptor stimulation and chronic neuroleptic effects. In: Cattabeni F, Racagni G, Spano PF, Costa E (eds) Long term effects of neuroleptics. Raven, New York, pp 252–258
Lloyd KG, Zivkovic B, Scatton B, Bartholini G (1984) Evidence for functional roles of GABA pathways in the mammalian brain. In: Bowery NG (ed) Actions and interactions of GABA and benzodiazepines. Raven, New York, pp 59–79
Morselli PL, Bossi L, Henry JF, Zarifian E, Bartholini G (1980) On the therapeutic action of SL 76002, a new GABAmimetic agent: preliminary observations in neuropsychiatric disorders. Brain Res Bull 5 [Suppl 2]:411–414
Murphy DL, Brodie HKH, Goodwin F, Bunney WE Jr (1971) Regular induction of hypomania by L-DOPA in bipolar manic-depressive patients. Nature 299:135–137
Pert A, Rosenblatt JE, Sivit C, Pert CB, Bunney WE Jr (1978) Long term treatment with lithium prevents the development of dopamine receptor supersensitivity. Science 201:171–174
Reda FA, Escobar JI, Scanlan JM (1975) Lithium carbonate in the treatment of tardive dyskinesia. Am J Psychiatry 132:560–562
Scatton B, Bartholini G (1980) Modulation by GABA of cholinergic transmission in the striatum. Brain Res 183:211–216
Scatton B, Garret C, Julou L (1975) Acute and subacute effects of neuroleptics on dopamine synthesis and release in the rat striatum. Naunyn Schmiedebergs Arch Pharmacol 289:419–434
Scatton B, Zivkovic B, Bartholini G (1980) Differential influence of GABAergic agents on dopamine metabolism in extrapyramidal and limbic systems of the rat. Brain Res Bull 5 [Suppl 2]:421–425
Scatton B, Zivkovic B, Dedek J, Lloyd KG, Constantinidis J, Tissot R, Bartholini G (1982) γ-Aminobutyric acid (GABA) receptor stimulation. III. Effect of progabide (SL 76002) on norepinephrine, dopamine and 5-hydroxytryptamine turnover in rat brain areas. J Pharmacol Exp Ther 220:678–688
Tamminga CA, Crayton JW, Chase TN (1979) Improvement in tardive dyskinesia after muscimol therapy. Arch Gen Psychiatry 36:595–598
Tarsy D, Baldessarini RJ (1977) The pathophysiologic basis of tardive dyskinesia. Biol Psychiatry 12:431–441
Worms P, Depoortere H, Durand A, Morselli P, Lloyd KG, Bartholini G (1982) γ-Aminobutyric acid (GABA) receptor stimulation. I. Neuropharmacological profiles of progabide (SL 76002) and SL 75102, with emphasis on their anticonvulsant spectra. J Pharmacol Exp Ther 220:660–671

New Aspects on the Role of Dopamine, Acetylcholine, and GABA in the Development of Tardive Dyskinesia

J. Scheel-Krüger[1] and J. Arnt[2]

Contents

Abstract 46
1 The Differential Role of DA in the Dorsal Versus the Ventral Regions of Striatum for Oral Stereotyped Activities 46
2 Role of the Mesolimbic and Mesocortical DA Systems in Tardive Dyskinesia 49
3 New Aspects on DA-Acetylcholine Interaction 51
4 Dopamine and the GABA Systems 55
References 56

Abstract

In this paper various new findings on the possible anatomical substrates of tardive dyskinesia will be presented. The results show that the striatum is heterogeneously organized, and the syndromes of biting, gnawing, and licking activities in the rat model involve a complex balance between various dopamine (DA), cholinergic, and GABAergic systems within the striatum and the mesolimbic and mesocortical systems.

1 The Differential Role of DA in the Dorsal Versus the Ventral Regions of Striatum for Oral Stereotyped Activities

Anatomical studies on the afferent and efferent connections of the striatum (nucleus caudatus, putamen) and biochemical studies on the differential distribution of striatal transmitters strongly suggest that the striatum is organized as a heterogeneous structure. Several functional and behavioral studies provide further support for this conclusion (Cools and Van Rossum 1980; Costall et al. 1980; Scheel-Krüger et al. 1981; Scheel-Krüger 1983, 1985). The different brain regions innervated by the DA systems (i.e., the striatum, the nucleus accumbens, the olfactory tubercle, and the mesocortical systems) participate to various extents in the behavioral elements seen after the systemic injection of DA stimulants. It has been found that the ventromedial region of the striatum is involved in the development of oral licking and gnawing activities. Iversen and Koob (1977) reported that a 6-hydroxydopamine (6-OHDA) lesion of the ventral striatum (but not a dorsal 6-OHDA lesion) abolished the stereotyped licking/gnawing response after

1 Psychopharmacological Research Laboratory, Department E, Saint Hans Mental Hospital, DK-4000 Roskilde, Denmark
2 Department of Pharmacology and Toxicology, H. Lundbeck A/S, Ottiliavej 7–9, DK-2500 Copenhagen-Valby, Denmark

Dyskinesia – Research and Treatment
(Psychopharmacology Supplementum 2)
Editors: Casey, Chase, Christensen, Gerlach

amphetamine, and Costall et al. (1980) found that DA and the DA agonist 2-(*N*,*N*-dipropyl)-amino-5,6-dihydroxytetralin produced biting activity within the posterior ventromedial region of the striatum.

We found that a DA receptor blockade in the ventromedial region of striatum produced a complete blockade of apomorphine-induced oral stereotypy, whereas DA receptor blockade within the anterodorsal region of striatum *increased* apomorphine induced licking/gnawing activities. A series of neuroleptic drugs have been tested following intracerebral injection into the ventromedial region of the striatum (Arnt 1984, unpublished) and all the potent DA antagonists (including *cis*(Z)-flupentixol, fluphenazine, haloperidol, spiroperidol, (−)sulpiride, and SCH 23390) antagonized the stereotyped licking/gnawing induced by systemic injection of apomorphine. Among the neuroleptic drugs (−)sulpiride was found to be the most potent. This drug produced blockade of apomorphine (0.5–2.5 mg/kg SC) following intracerebral injection of doses within the range of 1–125 ng (Arnt 1984, unpublished). We have tested the effect of (−)sulpiride (31 ng) following intracerebral injection into various regions of the striatum (Table 1). The results showed clearly that (−)sulpiride injected into the ventromedian region of striatum localized 0.5–1 mm rostral to the globus pallidus blocked the licking/gnawing stereotypy. The injection of (−)sulpiride into the most anterior and ventromedian region of striatum, i.e., the nucleus accumbens, produced a blockade of the locomotor activity, but not of the licking/gnawing activities induced by apomorphine (data not shown). (−)Sulpiride injected into the dorsal

Table 1. Effects of dorsal and ventral intrastriatal injections of dopamine antagonists on apomorphine stereotypy

Treatments	*n*	Striatal region	Percentage of rats demonstrating various behavorial effects							
			Locomotion	Rearing	Rating groups of stereotypy [a]					
					A	B	C	D	E	[b]
31 ng (−)Sulpiride	7	Dorsal	0	57	0	0	0	0	100	$P<0.01$
2 µg SCH 23390	6	Dorsal	0	0	0	0	17	33	50	$P<0.05$
1 µg SCH 23390	6	Dorsal	67	33	0	17	0	17	50	
Saline	14	Dorsal	78	65	14	14	36	29	7	
31 ng (−)Sulpiride	9	Ventral	67	67	78	0	0	0	0	$P<0.01$
1 µg SCH 23390	6	Ventral	0	100	100	0	0	0	0	$P<0.01$
Saline	11	Ventral	100	91	27	9	27	18	18	

n, number of rats. All rats received apomorphine 0.50 mg/kg SC in the neck immediately after the bilateral intrastriatal injection of the dopamine antagonists (−)sulpiride or SCH 23390 (dissolved in 0.9% saline) into the ventral [coordinates Ant. 7.1–7.8, Lat. 2.4–3, DV −(0.8–1.2)] or dorsal [Ant. 7.8–9.4, Lat. 2.3–2.8, DV +(1–1.5)] regions of the striatum. The placebo groups received 0.5 µl saline into the dorsal or ventral striatum

[a] Rats were observed continuously after the injection of apomorphine, and the behavior and stereotypy classified according to the following rating groups: (A) continuous sniffing; (B) continuous sniffing plus episodes of licking; (C) continuous sniffing plus episodes of licking and gnawing; (D) continuous licking; (E) continuous stereotyped gnawing plus licking

[b] The Kruskal-Wallis one-way analysis of variance by ranks

regions of the striatum at various anterior-posterior coordinates produced *no* blockade of apomorphine stereotypy. Rather, within the most anterior dorsal region (Table 1) (−)sulpiride in fact produced *an intensification* of the apomorphine licking/gnawing syndrome! This last finding is new and has not previously been reported by other investigators.

Rosengarten et al. (1983) reported that "vacuum chewing" and perioral movements in the rat can be mediated by the D-1 DA receptor and by an imbalance between D-1/D-2 DA receptor activity. Christensen et al. (this volume) have also shown the involvement of the D-1 DA receptor in the induction of the stereotyped gnawing syndrome in rat and mouse during acute and chronic treatments with neuroleptic drugs. Since (−)sulpiride is a highly specific antagonist of the D-2 DA receptor, it may be speculated that our findings within the dorsal striatum may be due to a change in the balance between the D-1 and the D-2 DA receptors, because apomorphine stimulates both D-1 and D-2 receptors. This possibility was directly tested with the specific D-1 DA antagonist SCH 23390. However, SCH 23390 injected into the dorsal or ventral regions of the striatum produced the same results as were obtained with (−)sulpiride: antagonism of apomorphine stereotypy within the ventromedian striatum and an increase of apomorphine-induced stereotyped gnawing/licking activities within the anterodorsal striatal region (Table 1).

The results demonstrate that the striatum is functionally heterogeneously organized, and that DA has a dual functional role within the striatum with regard to the influence on the oral stereotyped gnawing/licking activities: these oral activities may depend on the balance between the anterodorsal striatal region and the ventromedian striatal region, since the former suppresses and the latter facilitates the syndrome induced by apomorphine. This hypothesis is supported by the fact that various lesions (mechanical, electrolytic, or induced by kainic acid) restricted to the dorsal region of the striatum have been found to enhance amphetamine- or apomorphine-induced locomotor or stereotyped oral activities (Mason et al. 1978; Neill and Herndon 1978; Wolfarth 1974), whereas lesions restricted to the caudoventral part of the striatum abolish the apomorphine-induced gnawing syndrome (Wolfarth 1974). Although direct comparisons would be premature, it is striking that our findings show certain similarities to the hypothesis put forward by Cools (Cools and Van Rossum 1980; Cools 1983) on the heterogeneous distribution of two distinct types of DA receptors (or maybe systems?) each characterized by their functional properties: the excitation-mediating (DAe) and the inhibition-mediating (DAi) DA receptors. In the cat, Cools et al. have found the DAi receptors present within the anterodorsal part of the caudate nucleus and the DAe receptors within the rostromedial part of the caudate nucleus. A detailed topographical analysis on the possible distribution of the DAe, DAi systems has not yet been performed in the rat (AR Cools, personal communication), although it is considered that the DAe system seems to be related to the striatum and the DAi system to the mesolimbic DA system.

2 Role of the Mesolimbic and Mesocortical DA Systems in Tardive Dyskinesia

The majority of investigators consider that the development of tardive dyskinesia is related to an increased and abnormal DA receptor function within the striatum, produced by the long-term treatment with neuroleptic drugs. However, various clinical observations cannot readily be explained with reference to this model, since hypersensitivity in the animal models disappears within a relatively short time after withdrawal of the neuroleptic drugs. In some patients the symptoms seem to be permanent and irreversible in nature, especially in elderly subjects, and some may have dyskinesia without prior exposure to neuroleptics. Patients may even have concomitant symptoms of parkinsonism and tardive dyskinesia (Gerlach 1979; Cools 1983). Animal experiments suggest that dysfunction or brain damage in the structures innervated by the mesolimbic and mesocortical DA systems can modify the development of oral dyskinetic symptoms triggered from striatal DA receptors. There is anatomical support for this idea, since the major efferent pathways from the median prefrontal cortex, the nucleus accumbens, and the central nucleus of the amygdala all include major projections that directly innervate the substantia nigra, zona compacta (SNC), and zona reticulata (SNR) (Fig. 1). The prefrontal cortex, the nucleus accumbens, and the amygdala thus have the potential ability to regulate the activity of the nigrostriatal DA system

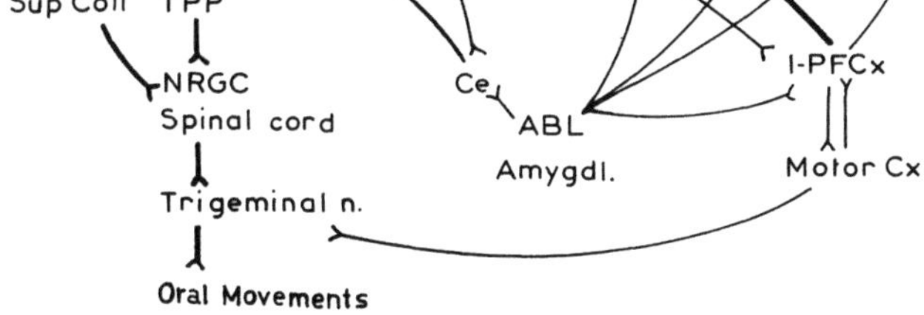

Fig. 1. Anatomical connections between the mesolimbic, mesocortical, and striatal systems, which may be relevant for the syndrome of tardive dyskinesia. The limbic part of the dopamine system originating in the ventral tegmental area (*VTA*) includes projections to the ventral striatum (*Vent. Str.*); nucleus accumbens (*N. Acc.*), central nucleus of amygdala (*Ce*) and the medial prefrontal cortex (*mPFCx*) and lateral prefrontal cortex (*lPFCx*). The lPFCx is interconnected with the region of motor cortex involved in oral activities and also projects directly to the ventral striatal region related to DA-induced oral activities. All major efferents from the limbic DA system are directed towards the DA neurons of SNC, which innervate the dorsal striatum and thus influence the nondopaminergic SNR neurons of substantia nigra, which projects to the superior colliculus (*Sup. Coll.*), the tegmental pedunculopontine nucleus (*TPP*), and finally reach the nucleus reticularis gigantocellularis (*NRGC*), the spinal cord and the trigeminal motor nucleus

and in addition to control directly the output system from striatum localized to the SNR efferent neurons (see later discussion). Several new findings support this concept.

Prefrontal Cortex. There is substantial evidence that the prefrontal DA systems influence behavior related to the subcortical DA systems. In fact, lesions of the prefrontal cortex enhance striatal DA transmission, increase amphetamine oral stereotypies and locomotor activity, and antagonize the immobility and catalepsy induced by the systemic injection of neuroleptics. (For further discussion and reviews, see Bannon and Roth 1983; Carter and Pycock 1980b; Pycock et al. 1980; Scatton et al. 1982.) Rats with prefrontal cortex lesions develop chewing movements, which increase markedly following the chronic administration of neuroleptics (Gunne et al. 1982). In the rat the motor cortex for facial movements is interconnected with the DA-innervated lateral prefrontal cortex, i.e., the sulcal cortex which projects directly to the ventromedian region of the striatum, where DA agonists/antagonists given by intracerebral injection respectively induce/suppress licking and gnawing activities (results discussed in this paper).

Amygdala. The amygdaloid complex also participates in the expression of the gnawing syndrome, since lesions of this structure attenuate the syndrome produced by both amphetamine and apomorphine (Carter and Pycock 1980a; Costall and Naylor 1972). There are also differential actions of classic and atypical neuroleptic drugs on neuronal activity in the amygdala (Rebec et al. 1983). It is known that electrical stimulation of the amygdala or the sulcal cortex initiates a jaw-closing or a jaw-opening reflex, respectively (Nakamura and Kubo 1978). Since the amygdala is involved in stress (Scheel-Krüger and Petersen 1983) it seems likely that the amygdala-prefrontal cortex systems may participate in the stress-provoked accentuation of tardive dyskinesia.

Nucleus Accumbens. It is well known that lesions of the nucleus accumbens do not abolish the licking/gnawing syndrome induced by DA agonists. However, such findings do not exclude a role of nucleus accumbens. Costall et al. (1977) found that several new putative DA agonists induced an oral dyskinetic biting syndrome following injection into the nucleus accumbens. The local injection of GABA agonists (muscimol, THIP) into the "ventral pallidum" (a major output station from the nucleus accumbens) also induced chewing movements (Scheel-Krüger, unpublished). In fact, Cools suggests (Cools and Van Rossum 1980; Cools 1983) that the syndrome of orofacial dyskinesia provoked after chronic neuroleptic treatment mainly involves a disturbance in the balance between the DA systems, i.e., hypoactivity in the nigrostriatal DAe system and hyperactivity in the mesolimbic DAi system. Injection of various drugs affecting noradrenaline, GABA, the DAi, DAe systems, etc. into the nucleus accumbens also influences the development of oral stereotypies induced by the systemic injection of DA agonists (Cools 1983; Scheel-Krüger et al. 1977).

DA Systems and Tardive Dyskinesia: Concluding Comments

The data summarized briefly in this paper suggest that the development of oral stereotyped activities in animal models depends on a balance between several distinct anatomical substrates innervated by various DA systems. Consequently it is suggested that the syndrome of tardive dyskinesia in clinical practice may also depend on a disturbed balance between these systems due to the long-term neuroleptic treatment. Biochemical studies support this hypothesis, since regional studies have shown that tolerance develops more easily in the striatum than in certain limbic areas including the nucleus accumbens. The prefrontal cortical regions are minimally affected and may even show lack of tolerance to the effect of chronically administered DA antagonists. There are also differential regional effects of classic versus atypical antipsychotic drugs (Bannon and Roth 1983; Matsumoto et al. 1983; Rupniak et al. 1983; White and Wang 1983). The present findings suggest the significance of maintained DA receptor blockade within the anterior dorsal striatum and the prefrontal cortex, development of tolerance within the ventromedian striatum, and a modulatory influence of nucleus accumbens and amygdala.

3 New Aspects on DA-Acetylcholine Interaction

Clinical pharmacology indicates opposite effects of DA and acetylcholine in various diseases related to the basal ganglia system, tardive dyskinesia, parkinsonism, Huntington's disease, and possibly also schizophrenia, and various animal models support this concept. The striatum has traditionally been considered the major anatomical target for the DA-acetylcholine interaction, but within the last few years several major and "new" cholinergic pathways have been well documented, which now represent an obvious challenge for future functional and experimental studies. The major cholinergic system in the brain is localized as a continuum of cholinergic neurons throughout the entire extent of the basal forebrain from the median septum, nucleus of diagonal band, nucleus basalis magnocellularis (NBM), and substantia innominata (Saper 1984; Satoh et al. 1983 reviews). The cholinergic neurons of NBM, which innervate the entire cortex, represent the origin of the most massive cholinergic system of the brain and form a crucial link in the circuitry for direct and indirect DA-acetylcholine interactions. A direct interaction may be localized to the frontal and prefrontal cortex between DA and cholinergic nerve terminals, and the outcome of this cortical intervention is directed towards the striatum and nucleus accumbens. The efferents from nucleus accumbens, ventral striatum (Scheel-Krüger 1983, 1985), and prefrontal cortex (Saper 1984) are directed towards ventral pallidum, NBM, and substantia innominata, and the DA terminal regions may consequently indirectly control the activity of the cholinergic cells. The cholinergic fibers originating in the dorsal tegmental reticular formation including the pedunculopontine nucleus (TPP) represent another interesting system, because the efferents are directed towards all the output stations of the basal ganglia, the substantia nigra, subthalamic nucleus, globus pallidus, thalamus, and prefrontal cortex (Jackson and Crossman 1983; Satoh et al. 1983). The cholinergic systems may obviously represent crucial elements in the mesolimbic, mesocortical, and nigrostriatal circuits, which directly and/or indirectly influence behavior related to DA functions following the systemic administration of cholinergic/anticholinergic agents (Fig. 2).

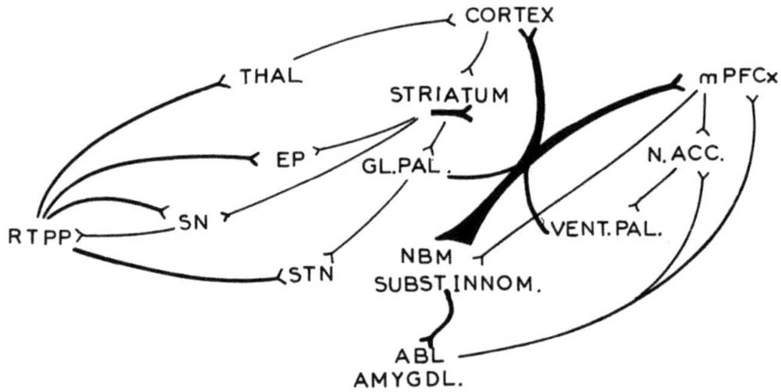

Fig. 2. Anatomical substrates for DA-acetylcholine interconnections. The major cholinergic system is localized in nucleus basalis magnocellularis (*NBM*) and includes minor regions of globus pallidus (*GL. PALL.*) and ventral pallidum (*Vent. Pall.*). The NBM has projections to the entire cortex, including the DA-innervated medial prefrontal cortex (*mPFCx*) and the basolateral nucleus of amygdala (*ABL*). The *mPFCx* has direct projections towards the *NBM*, *ABL* and nucleus accumbens (*N. Acc.*). The *NBM*-cholinergic system is thus directly and indirectly interconnected with the mesolimbic/mesocortical DA systems and the striatal DA system, which receives afferents from the cortex. The reticular tegmental pedunculopontine nucleus (*Ret. TPP*) provides a cholinergic projection towards the thalamus and probably also substantia nigra (*SN*), the entopeduncular nucleus (*EP*), and the subthalamic nucleus (*STN*). The DA interaction with the striatal cholinergic interneurons may only represent a minor system

Striatal Cholinergic Neurons. In recent years it has been established that the cholinergic neurons of the striatum are interneurons and represent only 1%–5% of the total cell population of the striatum (see Lehmann and Langer 1983; Satoh et al. 1983; Scheel-Krüger 1985, for reviews). In contrast, the noncholinergic medium-sized spiny neurons constitute the vast majority of the cells (i.e., 90%–95%) within the striatum and represent in addition the efferent neurons of the striatum, projecting to the pallidal nuclei and substantia nigra, using GABA, enkephalin and substance P as transmitters. It is thus obvious from a quantitative point of view that the role of the cholinergic interneurons in the traditional DA-acetylcholine-GABA nigrostriatal loop becomes much uncertain (Scheel-Krüger 1985). It even seems to be doubtful whether the DA terminals directly innervate the cholinergic interneurons (Lehmann and Langer 1983).

Functional Role of Striatal Acetylcholine. The net role of acetylcholine for striatal functions still remains uncertain and complex. Numerous biochemical studies have shown that DA agonists produce inhibition and neuroleptics, facilitation of striatal acetylcholine release. In contrast, almost no biochemical knowledge seems available on the effect of acetylcholine on the striatal efferent neurons, which actually mediate the DA-related function. Furthermore, various functional effects considered to be related to stimulation or blockade of striatal DA receptors cannot be reproduced by local injection of cholinergic antagonists/agonists into the striatum; injection of the cholinergic agonist carbachol (1–5 μg) did not produce a cataleptic syndrome, as did the systemic injection of neuroleptics, and the antimuscarinic drug methylscopolamine (10–20 μg) injected into various regions of the striatum produced no antagonism of the cataleptic effect induced by haloperidol (0.50 mg/kg SC). Nor did intrastriatal injection of methylscopolamine produce the symptoms of licking/gnawing activities characteristic for the DA agonists (DeMontis et al. 1979; Scheel-Krüger 1985).

Dorsal and Ventral Regions of the Striatum. The experiments showed differential functional roles of acetylcholine within the dorsal and the ventral parts of striatum (Table 2). Carbachol (1–2.5 μg) injected locally into the dorsomedian region of the striatum strongly *increased* apomorphine-induced stereotyped licking/gnawing activity, whereas methylscopolamine (10–20 μg) injected into this region produced antagonism. In contrast, injection of carbachol (2.5–5 μg) into the ventromedian region of the striatum produced complete *blockade* of apomorphine stimulation and stereotypy, whereas methylscopolamine (10–20 μg) injected into this site produced an increase of apomorphine-induced oral stereotypies. In fact, the distinct effects on apomorphine oral stereotypies induced by carbachol injected into the dorsal or ventral regions of the striatum closely resemble the differential effects found following administration of the DA antagonists (–)sulpiride and SCH 23390. Other investigators have also reported differential regional effects of cholinergic agents on DA-related function following local injection into the striatum. Wolfarth and Kolasiewicz (1977) found that cholinergic agonists injected into the dorsal striatum increased apomorphine-induced stereotyped gnawing in rabbit, and Neill and Grossman (1970) and Neill and Herndon (1978) also found facilitatory cholinergic systems in the dorsal part and inhibitory cholinergic systems in the ventral part of the rat striatum. Cools and

Table 2. Effect of intrastriatal injections of cholinergic drugs on apomorphine stereotypy

Treatment	*n*	Striatal region	Percentage of rats demonstrating various behavioral effects							
			Loco-motion	Rearing	Rating groups of stereotypy [a]					
					A	B	C	D	E	[b]
2.5 μg Carbachol	7	Dorsal	28	28	0	0	0	0	100	$P<0.001$
5 μg Carbachol	7	Dorsal	28	14	0	0	0	0	100	$P<0.001$
20 μg Methyl-scopolamine	5	Dorsal	80	40	60	20	0	20	0	
Aqua dest.	12	Dorsal	83	42	25	33	33	8	0	
2.5 μg Carbachol	10	Ventral	10	10	0	0	0	0	0	$P<0.001$
20 μg Methyl-scopolamine	5	Ventral	20	20	0	0	60	0	40	$P<0.05$
Aqua dest.	10	Ventral	90	40	30	40	30	0	0	

n, number of rats. All rats received apomorphine 0.50 mg/kg SC in the flank immediately after bilateral injection of cholinergic drugs into the central part of the striatum [coordinates Ant. 7–7.4 Lat. 2.3–2.6 within the dorsal region DV (1.5–2) or ventral region DV– (0.6–1.2)]

[a] Rats were observed continuously after the injection of apomorphine and the behavior and stereotypy classified according to the following rating groups: (A) continuous sniffing; (B) continuous sniffing plus episodes of licking; (C) continuous sniffing plus episodes of licking and gnawing; (D) continuous licking; (E) continuous gnawing plus licking

[b] Kruskal-Wallis one-way analysis of variance by ranks

van Rossum (1980) and Cools (1983) consider the distinct cholinergic systems related to the DAe and DAi systems in his studies in cat and monkey.

Substantia Nigra. A minor but interesting cholinergic system is present within the substantia nigra. Electrophysiological data have shown that the non-DA zona reticulata neurons (SNR) are excited by and very sensitive to muscarinic agonists, whereas the zona compacta DA neurons are relatively insensitive to acetylcholine. (For references see Scheel-Krüger 1985.) The dorsal tegmental area, including the tegmental pedunculopontine nucleus (TPP) may contain the cholinergic neurons which innervate the substantia nigra (Jackson and Crossman 1983; Satoh et al. 1983). Our findings suggest that the functional and pharmacological interaction between DA and acetylcholine may also include an interaction between acetylcholine and the efferent GABA neurons localized at the level of the output station of SNR (Arnt and Scheel-Krüger 1980; DeMontis et al. 1979; Scheel-Krüger et al. 1981; Scheel-Krüger 1983, 1985). DA-related functional effects are thus mediated via the striatonigral GABA-ergic neurons by a GABA-ergic inhibition of the nondopaminergic SNR efferent neurons (see later discussion). In support of the hypothesis we found that stimulation of muscarinic receptors in the SNR induced neuroleptic-like behavioral effects, such as immobility, catalepsy, and antagonism of apomorphine-induced stereotyped behavior (DeMontis et al. 1979; Scheel-Krüger 1985). The syndrome of a strong and rigid catalepsy was seen immediately after injection of carbachol (2.5–5 μg, duration 45–60 min) or oxotremorine (5–10 μg, duration 5–15 min) into the caudal region of SNR. A few of the rats that received carbachol and most of the rats that received oxotremorine also showed (during the immobile cataleptic period) dyskinetic oral movements and teeth chattering. The injection of carbachol (2.5–5 μg) into the SNC induced only a short-lived catalepsy (due to diffusion to the SNR?), followed by a long period of locomotor stimulation. Oxotremorine (5–10 μg) induced no catalepsy, but mainly locomotor stimulation following the injection into the SNC, an effect probably due to stimulation of the nigrostriatal DA neurons. Methylscopolamine (10–20 μg) injected into the caudal part of SNR induced an apomorphine/amphetamine-like behavioral stimulation, including the characteristic stereotyped side-to-side movements of the head, sniffing, and licking and gnawing activities. The stereotyped licking/gnawing syndrome induced by methylscopolamine was found completely independent of DA activity, since pretreatment with haloperidol (1 mg/kg SC) or reserpine (5 mg/kg SC) plus α-methyltyrosine (250 mg/kg IP) induced no blockade, but rather a further enhancement of these oral stereotypies. The catalepsy and immobility induced by the pretreatment with haloperidol or reserpine plus α-MT was found to be antagonized immediately after the injection of methylscopolamine (10–20 μg) into the SNR (Scheel-Krüger 1985). Injection of carbachol into the caudal SNR induced a partial (2.5 μg) or complete (5 μg) inhibition of the stimulation and stereotypy induced by the systemic injection of apomorphine (0.50 mg/kg). We also observed that the apomorphine-like stereotyped licking/gnawing activities induced by the GABA agonist muscimol injected into the SNR was completely antagonized by the systemic injection of oxotremorine (0.25 mg/kg SC) (Scheel-Krüger and Arnt, unpublished).

DA-Acetylcholine: Concluding Comments

The present findings suggest the participation of the non-dopaminergic SNR neurons as an anatomical target for the functional antagonism between DA and acetylcholine seen after the systemic injections of drugs which are known to be relevant for the clinical pharmacological treatment of tardive dyskinesia, Parkinson's disease etc. The effects produced by the cholinergic drugs were mainly found related to the nondopaminergic efferent SNR GABA neurons, and cannot be interpreted as a direct influence on the activity of the nigrostriatal DA neurons. The effects induced by the DA agonist apomorphine are independent of DA neuronal activity. Cholinergic agonists may thus produce a blockade of the DA-mediated licking/gnawing syndrome by effects directly related to the output systems localized within the ventromedian striatum and also the efferent SNR neurons.

4 Dopamine and the GABA Systems

Recent studies have shown that the efferent GABA neurons from striatum and nucleus accumbens mediate DA-related functions. DA receptor stimulation thus produces an activation of the principal GABA-containing output pathways, the striatopallidoentopeduncular (EP), the striatonigral (SN) and the nucleus accumbens-ventral pallidum GABA-ergic pathways. DA-related functions are thus further transmitted via a GABA-ergic inhibition of the efferent nondopaminergic neurons localized in the major output stations: EP, SNR, and ventral pallidum. In contrast, the GABA-ergic projection from striatum to globus pallidus acts distinctly, since dopamine controls this system inhibitorily. It remains for future experiments to test whether this differential organization of the striatopallidal system versus the striato-SNR, EP, and GABA-ergic systems can explain the different functions of DA and acetylcholine in dorsal versus ventral striatal regions. The balance between these systems may also be relevant for tardive dyskinesia. The efferent GABA-ergic neurons from striatum and nucleus accumbens also include projections towards the DA cells in SNC and this ("feedback") effect of GABA participates in the regulatory control of the DA neurons projecting towards the striatum. In summary, it can be concluded that GABA, due to its effects on nondopaminergic and dopaminergic neurons, is an important mediator and moderator of DA-related functions in the striatal and limbic systems (Scheel-Krüger et al. 1981; Scheel-Krüger 1983).

GABA Systems and Tardive Dyskinesia. Experiments in the rat model have established the SNR as an important relay center for the expression of oral activities elicited by DA via the efferent GABA neurons localized within the ventromedial striatum. Dyskinesia related to the limbs, in contrast, seems mainly to involve the pallidoentopeduncular nucleus (EP) (Scheel-Krüger 1983). The efferent neurons from SNR and EP are also GABA-ergic neurons. Recent studies have shown that DA-induced oral activities depend on a striatonigral GABA-ergic inhibition of the SNR efferent GABA-ergic neurons projecting towards the superior colliculus (deeper layer) and the tegmental pedunculopontine nucleus (TPP). The multisynaptic pathways finally involve projections to the nucleus reticularis gigantocellularis, which sends efferents to the spinal cord and the trigeminal motor nucleus to activate the oral movements directly (Fig. 1). The conclusions, briefly summarized, indicate that in addition to the "dopamine hypothesis" for various diseases of the basal ganglia system, a "dopamine-GABA" hypothesis should be considered, including dysfunctions within the efferent GABA-ergic pathways. However, the presence of distinct and multiple GABA systems connected in series, which exert mutually opposing actions, still causes obvious problems for predictions of a therapeutic strategy using GABA-ergic agents in clinical practice (Christensen et al. 1980; Scheel-Krüger and Christensen 1980; Scheel-Krüger 1983).

References

Arnt J, Scheel-Krüger J (1980) Intranigral GABA antagonists produce dopamine-independent biting in rats. Eur J Pharmacol 62:51–61

Bannon MJ, Roth RH (1983) Pharmacology of mesocortical dopamine neurons. Pharmacol Rev 35:53–68

Carter CJ, Pycock CJ (1980a) 5,7-Dihydroxytryptamine lesions of the amygdala reduce amphetamine- and apomorphine-induced stereotyped behavior in the rat. Naunyn Schmiedebergs Arch Pharmacol 312:235–238

Carter CJ, Pycock CJ (1980b) Behavioral and biochemical effects of dopamine and noradrenaline depletion within the medial prefrontal cortex of the rat. Brain Res 192:163–176

Christensen AV, Arnt J, Scheel-Krüger J (1980) GABA-dopamine/neuroleptic interaction after systemic administration. Brain Res Bull 5:885–890

Cools AR (1983) Mesolimbic system and tardive dyskinesia: new perspectives for therapy. In: Bannet J, Belmaker RH (eds) Modern problems of pharmacopsychiatry, vol 21. Karger, Basel, pp 111–123

Cools AR, van Rossum JM (1980) Multiple receptors for brain dopamine in behavior regulation: concept of dopamine-E and dopamine-I receptors. Life Sci 27:1237–1253

Costall B, Naylor RJ (1972) Possible involvement of a noradrenergic area of the amygdala with stereotyped behavior. Life Sci 11:1135–1146

Costall B, Naylor RJ, Cannon JG, Lee T (1977) Differentiation of the dopamine mechanisms mediating stereotyped behavior and hyperactivity in the nucleus accumbens and caudate-putamen. J Pharm Pharmacol 29:337–342

Costall B, De Souza CX, Naylor RJ (1980) Topographical analysis of the actions of 2-(N,N-dipropyl)amino-5,6-dihydroxytetralin to cause biting behavior and locomotor hyperactivity from the striatum of the guinea-pig. Neuropharmacology 19:623–631

DeMontis GM, Olianas MC, Serra G, Tagliamonte A, Scheel-Krüger J (1979) Evidence that a nigral GABA-ergic-cholinergic balance controls posture. Eur J Pharmacol 53:181–190

Gerlach J (1979) Tardive dyskinesia. Thesis. Dan Med Bull 26:209–245

Gunne LM, Growdon J, Glaeser B (1982) Oral dyskinesia in rats following brain lesions and neuroleptic drug administration. Psychopharmacology 77:134–139

Jackson A, Crossman AR (1983) Nucleus tegmenti pedunculopontinus: Efferent connections with special reference to the basal ganglia, studied in the rat by anterograde and retrograde transport of horseradish peroxidase. Neuroscience 10:725–765

Iversen SD, Koob GF (1977) Behavioral implications of dopaminergic neurons in the mesolimbic system. In: Costa E, Gessa GL (eds) Advances in biochemical psychopharmacology, vol 16. Raven, New York, pp 209–214

Lehmann J, Langer SZ (1983) The striatal cholinergic interneuron: synaptic target of dopaminergic terminals? Neuroscience 10:1105–1120

Mason ST, Sanberg PR, Fibiger HC (1978) Kainic acid lesions of the striatum dissociate amphetamine and apomorphine stereotypy: similarities to Huntington's chorea. Science 201:352–355
Matsumoto T, Uchimura H, Hirano M, Kim JS, Yokoo H, Shimomura M, Nakahara T, Inoue K, Oomagari K (1983) Differential effects of acute and chronic administration of haloperidol on homovanillic acid levels in discrete dopaminergic areas of rat brain. Eur J Pharmacol 89:27–33
Nakamura Y, Kubo Y (1978) Masticatory rhythm in intracellular potential of trigeminal motoneurons induced by stimulation of orbital cortex and amygdala in cats. Brain Res 148:504–509
Neill DB, Grossman SP (1970) Behavioral effects of lesions or cholinergic blockade of the dorsal and ventral caudate of rats. J Comp Physiol Psychol 71:311–317
Neill DB, Herndon JG Jr (1978) Anatomical specificity within rat striatum for the dopaminergic modulation of DRL responding and activity. Brain Res 153:529–538
Pycock CJ, Carter CJ, Kerwin RW (1980) Effects of 6-hydroxydopamine lesions of the medial prefrontal cortex on neurotransmitter systems in subcortical sites in the rat. J Neurochem 34:91–99
Rebec GV, Gelman J, Alloway KD, Bashore TR (1983) Cataleptogenic potency of the antipsychotic drugs is inversely correlated with neuronal activity in the amygdaloid complex of the rat. Pharmacol Biochem Behav 19:759–763
Rosengarten H, Schweitzer JW, Friedhoff AJ (1983) Induction of oral dyskinesias in naive rats by D-1 stimulation. Life Sci 33:2479–2482
Rupniak NMJ, Jenner P, Marsden CD (1983) The effect of chronic neuroleptic administration on cerebral dopamine receptor function. Life Sci 32:2289–2311
Saper CB (1984) Organization of cerebral cortical afferent systems in the rat. II. Magnocellular basal nucleus. J Comp Neurol 222:313–342
Satoh K, Armstrong DM, Fibiger HC (1983) A comparison of the distribution of central cholinergic neurons as demonstrated by acetylcholinesterase pharmacohistochemistry and choline acetyltransferase immunohistochemistry. Brain Res Bull 11:693–720
Scatton B, Worms P, Lloyd KG, Bartholini G (1982) Cortical modulation of striatal function. Brain Res 232:331–343
Scheel-Krüger J (1983) The GABA receptor and animal behavior. In: Enna SJ (ed) GABA receptors. Humana, Clifton, pp 114–137
Scheel-Krüger J (1984) New aspects on the functional role of acetylcholine in the basal ganglia system. Interactions with other neurotransmitters. In: Singh MM,Warburton DM, Lal H, (eds) Central cholinergic mechanisms and adaptive dysfunctions. Plenum, New York, pp 105–139
Scheel-Krüger J, Christensen AV (1980) The role of gamma-aminobutyric acid in acute and chronic neuroleptic action. In: Cattabeni F, Racagni G, Spano PF, Costa E (eds) Long-term effects of neuroleptics. Adv Biochem Psychopharmacol 24:233–243
Scheel-Krüger J, Petersen EN (1983) Anticonflict effect of the benzodiazepines mediated by a GABA-ergic mechanism in the amygdala. Eur J Pharmacol 82:115–116
Scheel-Krüger J, Cools AR, van Wel PM (1977) Muscimol, a GABA-agonist injected into the nucleus accumbens, increases apomorphine stereotypy and decreases the motility. Life Sci 21:1697–1702
Scheel-Krüger J, Magelund G, Olianas MC (1981) Role of GABA in the striatal output system: globus pallidus, nucleus entopeduncularis, substantia nigra and nucleus subthalamicus. In: DiChiara G, Gessa GL (eds) GABA and the basal ganglia. Adv Biochem Psychopharmacol 30:165–186
White FJ, Wang RY (1983) Differential effects of classical and atypical antipsychotic drugs on A9 and A10 dopamine neurons. Science 221:1054–1057
Wolfarth S (1974) Reactions to apomorphine and spiroperidol of rats with striatal lesions: the relevance of kind and size of the lesion. Pharmacol Biochem Behav 2:181–186
Wolfarth S, Kolasiewicz A (1977) The effects of intrastriatal injections of atropine and methacholine on the apomorphine induced gnawing in the rabbit. Pharmacol Biochem Behav 6:5–10

Discussion Section

Differential Effects of Dopamine D-1 and D-2 Agonists and Antagonists in 6-Hydroxydopamine-Lesioned Rats

J. Arnt [1]

With regard to the dopamine (DA) D-1 and D-2 receptor classification by Ungerstedt and his colleagues, using the unilaterally 6-OHDA lesioned rat as a model, I would like to show recent results from our laboratories. In our experiments we have measured the contralateral circling behavior induced by the specific DA D-1 agonist SK & F 38393 (4.3 μmol/kg SC) and the DA D-2 agonist pergolide (0.05 μmol/kg SC), and the ipsilateral circling behavior induced by amphetamine (14 μmol/kg SC). While the amphetamine-induced circling is induced by release of DA, with subsequent stimulation of normosensitive DA receptors in the intact side of the brain, the circling induced by direct DA agonists is mediated by hypersensitive DA receptors (Ungerstedt et al., this volume). In agreement with the data of Ungerstedt et al., we found that the effect of D-1- and D-2-selective compounds could be differentiated.

Table 1. Inhibition of circling behavior in rats with unilateral 6-OHDA lesions (Arnt and Hyttel 1984)

Test compound	ED_{50} (μmol/kg SC)		
	SK & F 38393	Pergolide	Amphetamine
SCH 23390	0.006	3.5	0.03
cis(Z)-Flupentixol	0.18	0.03	0.04
cis(Z)-Clopenthixol	1.2	0.047	0.10
Spiroperidol	14	0.04	0.04
Clebopride	19	0.03	0.51

As shown in Table 1 the selective D-1 antagonist SCH 23390 potently blocks the circling induced by SK & F 38393, whereas the D-2 antagonists, spiroperidol and clebopride, had weak activity. In contrast, the D-2 antagonists were potent blockers of pergolide, whereas SCH 23390 had a weak effect. The ratios between the ED50 values in the two models were at least 350 for the selective antagonists. The mixed D-1 and D-2 antagonists, *cis*(Z)-flupentixol and *cis*(Z)-clopenthixol, were effective in both models, as expected. These results indicate that the circling behavior induced by D-1 and D-2 agonists are mediated through different sites. However, these may anyhow be closely connected, as *both* D-1 and D-2 antagonists equally well block the circling induced by amphetamine. This result is diffi-

1 Department of Pharmacology and Toxicology, H. Lundbeck A/S, Ottiliavej 7–9, DK-2500 Copenhagen-Valby, Denmark

Dyskinesia – Research and Treatment
(Psychopharmacology Supplementum 2)
Editors: Casey, Chase, Christensen, Gerlach

cult to explain if circling induced by stimulation of D-1 and D-2 receptors is conveyed through different output pathways in the striatum. Selective antagonists would then be expected to only partially inhibit circling induced by the mixed D-1 and D-2 receptor activation, as is probably the case after amphetamine administration. We suggest, alternatively, that the denervation process is responsible for the functional dissociation of closely related DA D-1 and D-2 receptors, which in the innervated DA synapse cannot be differentiated by antagonists. Our view is also supported by data obtained in stereotypy experiments (Arnt, unpublished): While SCH 23390 and spiroperidol potently block the stereotyped behavior induced by apomorphine or pergolide in normal rats, SCH 23390 has no effect against pergolide-induced hyperactivity in rats with bilateral 6-OHDA lesions, while spiroperidol retains its inhibitory potency. In contrast, while SK & F 38393 does not induce stereotyped licking/biting in normal rats, strong hyperactivity is induced in rats with bilateral 6-OHDA lesions. This effect is blocked by SCH 23390, but not affected by spiroperidol, and again indicates a differentiation between D-1 and D-2 receptor functions only in denervated rats.

Reference

Arnt J, Hyttel J (1984) Differential inhibition by dopamine D-1 and D-2 antagonists of circling behavior induced by dopamine agonists in rats with unilateral 6-hydroxydopamine lesions. Eur J Pharmacol 102:349–354

Clinical Aspects

Is Tardive Dyskinesia a Unique Disorder?

C. D. Marsden [1]

Contents

Abstract . . . 64
1 Introduction . . . 64
2 Clinical Features of Tardive Dyskinesia . . . 65
3 Movement Disorders in Schizophrenia . . . 65
4 Prevalence of Tardive Dyskinesias Relative to That of Spontaneous Dyskinesias . . . 67
5 Chronic Neuroleptic Treatment as the Cause for the Precipitant of Tardive Dyskinesia 69
6 The Problem of Persistent Tardive Dyskinesias . . . 70
7 Conclusion . . . 71
References . . . 71

Abstract

The role of neuroleptics in causing the tardive dyskinesia syndrome is controversial. To properly assess the contribution of drugs as the etiology of dyskinesias, the effects of aging, the natural history of psychosis, and characteristics of spontaneous dyskinesias must be considered. Though the buccolinguo-masticatory triad is seen more often in tardive than in spontaneous dyskinesias, these two disorders have many symptoms in common. Other dyskinesias, such as idiopathic and tardive dystonia or tardive Tourette's syndrome and dyskinesias in untreated schizophrenia, are poorly understood. Chronic neuroleptic treatment may only precipitate TD in those already predisposed to develop such movement disorders. Tardive dyskinesia is not a unique movement disorder, but rather spans several clinical and epidemiological phenomena which must be considered in a balanced evaluation of how much of the permanent dyskinesias should be attributed to neuroleptic drugs.

1 Introduction

Tardive dyskinesias are those involuntary abnormal movements that appear in a proportion of patients during chronic antipsychotic drug treatment. They are seen most commonly among patients with schizophrenia, but are not specific to that psychiatric diagnosis. From their first recognition, soon after chlorpromazine was introduced into psychiatric practice in the 1950s, there have been questions as to whether tardive dyskinesias are a separate nosological entity amongst movement disorders and, by implication, whether neuroleptic drugs really are their cause. Two issues have raised argument. First, disorders of move-

1 University Department of Neurology, Institute of Psychiatry and King's College Hospital Medical School, de Crespigny Park, London SE5 8AF, England

Dyskinesia – Research and Treatment
(Psychopharmacology Supplementum 2)
Editors: Casey, Chase, Christensen, Gerlach

ment are known to occur in the untreated schizophrenic patient. So, are the abnormal movements that occur during chronic neuroleptic therapy no more than those of schizophrenia, or are they really associated with chronic drug intake? Second, the abnormal movements of tardive dyskinesia resemble many spontaneously occurring movement disorders. So, are tardive dyskinesias merely incidental?

To prove that the entity of tardive dyskinesia is distinct requires demonstration that its characteristics differ from those of the movement disorders of untreated schizophrenia, and that it occurs with a greater frequency amongst chronic neuroleptic-treated patients than in the general population. Both problems require definition of the clinical characteristics of tardive dyskinesias.

2 Clinical Features of Tardive Dyskinesia

The clinical features of tardive dyskinesia have been described elsewhere (Marsden et al. 1975). The commonest form is the bucco-linguo-masticatory syndrome of mouth, tongue and jaw movement, characterised by chewing, lip sucking and tongue movements. The prevalence of the bucco-linguo-masticatory syndrome in those receiving chronic neuroleptic treatment increases with age (Smith and Baldessarini 1980). Amongst younger patients a different clinical picture may appear, with spasms of muscle contraction affecting axial and limb muscles to produce a picture of torsion dystonia (tardive dystonia). A few patients have developed isolated or even generalised tics, sometimes with vocalisation (tardive Tourette). Thus, a range of movement disorders has been described under the rubric of tardive dyskinesias. To what extent do they resemble the disorders of movement seen in untreated schizophrenia?

3 Movement Disorders in Schizophrenia

Disorders of movement were mentioned in the first descriptions of schizophrenia. Kraepelin (1907, 1919) commented on abnormal movements in his original monograph on *Dementia Praecox*: 'Some of them resemble movements of expression, wrinkling of the forehead, distortion of the corners of the mouth, irregular movements of the tongue and lips, twisting of the eyes, opening them wide, and shutting them tight, in short, those movements which we bring together under the name of "making faces" or grimacing; they remind one of the corresponding disorders of choreic patients... Several patients continually carried out peculiar sprawling irregular, choreiform, out-spreading movements, which I think I can best characterise by the expression "athetoid ataxia".'

A casual reading of this and of the many other psychiatric texts containing similar statements might suggest that those dyskinesias familiar to neurologists as chorea and athetosis occur in patients with schizophrenia. However, this is not so. Psychiatrists have used the words chorea and athetosis to describe what they see in schizophrenic patients, but what they have seen has not been the same as occurs in Huntington's disease or dystonia musculorum deformans. The majority of abnormal movements seen in schizophrenia are best described as 'stereotypies' or 'mannerisms'. Kraepelin (1919) defined a stereotypy as persistence of the same movement or action, either as a continued position or as a repetition of the same movement. He defined a mannerism as an adornment of volitional action, causing unnatural and affected expression. Stereotypies thus are purposeless, repetitive motor acts, while mannerisms are goal-directed actions carried out in unusual and unnecessarily bizarre ways. Stereotypies and mannerisms frequently co-exist and often merge one with the other. They were formerly seen most commonly in patients with catatonic schizophrenia (Kahlbaum 1973; originally published in 1874) as many as a quarter of whom might exhibit such motor phenomena. However, catatonic schizophrenia is now relatively infrequent, so the florid stereotypies and mannerisms that illustrated earlier texts on schizophrenia are rarely seen today.

Confused terminology is a plague in this area. Many stereotypies and mannerisms, because of their repetitive character, might be called tics by some observers, particularly if they can be temporarily suppressed by the patient. Other, more persistent stereotypies may resemble dystonias. Thus, a head tilt might be called a stereotypy by one group, torticollis by another, and a tic by still others.

There have been other difficulties in interpreting reports of disorders of movement in schizophrenia before the advent of neuroleptic drugs. Many organic neurological diseases, which may themselves produce movement disorders, can on occasion also cause a schizophreniform psychosis. Most important was the epidemic of encephalitis lethargica that beset the world in the 1920s and 1930s, leaving in its wake many individuals with a combination of a movement disorder and a psychotic illness. Such patients, and others with neurosyphilis and undiagnosed Huntington's disease, were probably often included in descriptions of schizophrenia in an earlier age.

All these factors have contributed to make it difficult to assess the significance of reports of disorders of movement in schizophrenia prior to the neuroleptic era. Since the advent of neuroleptics, it has proved extremely difficult to study large groups of schizophrenic patients who are guaranteed never to have received these drugs in the course of their illness. This has made it particularly difficult to judge, by modern criteria, the prevalence and type of movement disorders in the untreated patient. Yet, despite all these difficulties, it remains generally true that no neurologist with experience in movement disorders is convinced that neurological dyskinesias are consistently present in patients with schizophrenia. Indeed, the presence of a typical neurological movement disorder would, today, lead the neurologist to doubt a diagnosis of primary schizophrenia and to seek secondary neurological causes.

Finally, it has already been noted that identical tardive dyskinesias can occur in patients who are receiving chronic neuroleptic treatment and do not have schizophrenia (Klawans et al. 1978). The neurologist meets this problem in two common situations. First, the patient who suffers an episode of acute vestibular failure whose vertigo is so intense as to require some form of vestibular sedative commonly has a phenothiazine, or a related drug, prescribed, and although the vertigo settles spontaneously, the patient continues to take the drug for long periods until a tardive dyskinesia appears. Second, neuroleptic drugs are now commonly used to treat a variety of chronic gastrointestinal disorders, and such patients again may present after years of therapy with tardive dyskinesia.

From this evidence it must be concluded that tardive dyskinesias are not unique to schizophrenia, do not represent the disorders of movements that may occur in the untreated schizophrenic, and are "associated" with chronic neuroleptic drug treatment.

4 Prevalence of Tardive Dyskinesias Relative to That of Spontaneous Dyskinesias

The problem still remains, that the clinical syndromes of tardive dyskinesia resemble similar disorders that may occur spontaneously in patients who have never been exposed to neuroleptic drugs. Thus, the bucco-linguo-masticatory syndrome occurs spontaneously in many elderly subjects; tardive dystonia is indistinguishable from idiopathic (primary) torsion dystonia; and tardive tics, whether simple or multiple, are identical with their spontaneous counterparts, including those of the syndrome of Gilles de la Tourette. Proof that tardive dyskinesias are precipitated by chronic neuroleptic treatment thus depends on epidemiology. In other words, the point prevalence of a given type of tardive dyskinesia must be in excess of that of the similar spontaneous dyskinesia in drug-free populations if neuroleptics are to be incriminated.

Such evidence is only available for the bucco-linguo-masticatory form of tardive dyskinesia. The prevalence of tardive dystonia and tardive Tourette's disease is relatively low amongst patients receiving chronic neuroleptic treatment, and that of spontaneous torsion dystonia and Gilles de la Tourette syndrome is not well established.

The point prevalence of the bucco-linguo-masticatory dyskinesia amongst patients receiving chronic neuroleptic treatment has been reported to vary from 0.5% to 65% (Task Force Report). Such wide variations reflect differences in diagnostic criteria as well as differences in patient populations. Many surveys have been based on standardised rating scales to document the presence of a dyskinesia, but ordinal scoring systems cannot reliably distinguish between mild normal lip-smacking, particularly in those with a dry mouth and no teeth, and obvious and unequivocal abnormal mouth movements (Tab. 1). Other unresolved problems include the relation of the prevalence of tardive dyskinesias to the duration of treatment and the total dose of neuroleptic ingested. However, one factor that consistently emerges from most studies is that the prevalence of bucco-linguo-masticatory dyskinesia increases with age, both for tardive dyskinesias in chronically neuroleptic-treated populations, and for spontaneous forms of the syndrome (Smith and Baldessarini 1980; Klawans and Barr 1982).

The point prevalence figure for bucco-linguo-masticatory tardive dyskinesias averages out at about 20% of patients receiving chronic neuroleptic treatment (Task Force Report; Kane and Smith 1982; Tab. 2). The point prevalence of spontaneous similar dyskinesias is about 5% and is unlikely to exceed 8% (Kane and Smith 1982; Tab. 3). Comparison of age-matched groups of patients currently receiving and not receiving drug treatment suggests that at all ages tardive

Table 1. Influence of criterion of diagnosis on prevalence of tardive dyskinesia. (Smith et al. 1979)

AIMS Score	Prevalence of TD (%)	
	In-patients (n = 293)	Out-patients (n = 213)
2.0 (mild)	62.2	72.3
2.5	45.9	40.9
3.0 (moderate)	30.2	33.7
3.5	13.8	8.6
4.0 (severe)	6.9	2.4

AIMS, abnormal involuntary movement scale

Table 2. Prevalence [a] of tardive dyskinesia. (Jenner and Marsden 1983)[b]

Reference [c]	Number of patients	% TD
Uhrbrand and Faurbye (1960)	500	6.6
Dincmen (1966)	1700	3.4
Degkwitz (1967)	1209	22
Heinrich et al. (1968)	554	17
Paulson (1968)	500	10
Eckmann (1968)	804	3
Villeneuve et al. (1969)	3280	2
Dynes (1970)	1200	8
Hippius and Lange (1970)	531	32
Brandon et al. (1971)	625	24
Crane (1970)	926	17
Bell and Smith (1978)	1329	26
Simpson et al. (1978)	3319	10.8
Smith et al. (1979)	506	42

[a] Mean prevalence 20% (± 14%)
[b] Full references cited in original paper
[c] Only studies of 500 or more drug-treated patients have been included. Kane and Smith (1982) reviewed 56 studies involving a total of 34555 patients

Table 3. Prevalence [a] of spontaneous BLM dyskinesias. (Jenner and Marsden 1983)[b]

Reference [c]	Number of patients	% BLM
Degkwitz (1967)	912	1.5
Heinrich et al. (1968)	201	3
Hippius and Lange (1970)	137	14
Brandon et al. (1970)	285	19
Crane (1973)	196	0.5
Delwaide and Desseilles (1977)	240	36.7
Klawans and Barr (1982)	423	6.8

[a] Mean prevalence 5% (± 9%)
[b] Full references cited in original paper
[c] Kane and Smith (1982) reviewed 19 studies involving a total of 11000 patients

Table 4. Prevalence of tardive and spontaneous dyskinesias

Age (years)	Tardive dyskinesias [a] (%)	Spontaneous dyskinesias [b] (%)
< 40	16	—
40–49	33	—
50–59	44	0.8
60–69	57	6
70+	53	7.8

[a] American Psychiatric Association (1980) Task Force 18 ($n = 506$)
[b] Klawans and Barr (1982) ($n = 423$)

dyskinesias are substantially commoner than their spontaneous counterpart (Klawans and Barr 1982; Table 4).

So, the bucco-linguo-masticatory tardive dyskinesia really does seem to be more common amongst those receiving chronic neuroleptic treatment than would be expected from its frequency in the drug-free population (although not all would agree; see Owens et al. 1982). However, this does not necessarily mean that the neuroleptic therapy was the *cause* of the tardive dyskinesia.

5 Chronic Neuroleptic Treatment as the Cause for the Precipitant of Tardive Dyskinesia

Use of the word "cause" implies that chronic drug treatment has produced these movement disorders in patients who otherwise would not have developed them. The alternative, and equally valid contention, is that tardive dyskinesias are precipitated by chronic drug treatment in patients who already possess the substrate for their development. It is difficult to resolve this debate on the basis of current evidence. A similar dilemma faces the interpretation of neuroleptic-induced parkinsonism. There are good reasons to suppose that those who develop drug-induced parkinsonism do so because their dopaminergic reserve is less than those who do not. Given a large enough dose of a neuroleptic, probably any one of us would develop pseudo-parkinsonism. However, only about a third of those treated with conventional doses exhibit signs of parkinsonism, and it can be argued that these are at risk of doing so because of lower dopaminergic reserve. Indeed, the age-related prevalence of pseudo-parkinsonism parallels that of idiopathic Parkinson's disease.

Whether similar considerations apply to the problem of tardive dyskinesias is not known. However, there are suspicions that they may do so. For example, the age-related prevalence of the bucco-linguo-masticatory syndrome parallels that of spontaneous bucco-linguo-masticatory dyskinesias, while the age-related prevalence of tardive dystonia also parallels that of the idiopathic disease. Some resolution of this dilemma might come from an analysis of the chances of chronic neuroleptic treatment causing permanent dyskinesias.

6 The Problem of Persistent Tardive Dyskinesias

Many patients who develop a tardive dyskinesia during chronic neuroleptic treatment recover when the offending drug is withdrawn. However, it is accepted that, in some cases, the tardive dyskinesia may persist for years, or even permanently, despite drug withdrawal. However, this does not prove that the drug treatment caused the tardive dyskinesia. Again, the argument is epidemiological. The crucial issue is whether the point prevalence of persistent dyskinesias exceeds that of the spontaneously occurring forms in the drug-free population. Such an analysis, of course, demands a definition of persistence. At what point after drug withdrawal is there little or no hope of recovery?

Information on this crucial point is incomplete. However, there is much suggestive evidence to indicate that the longer one waits after withdrawal of drugs, the greater the proportion of patients who remit (Tab. 5). Indeed, from

Table 5. Remission of tardive dyskinesias on withdrawal of neuroleptic drugs. (Jenner and Marsden 1983) [a]

Reference	Number of patients	% Recovering	Period of follow-up (months)
Paulson (1968)	33	0	3
Hershon et al. (1972)	23	0	4
Edwards (1970)	19	5	12
Crane (1970)	39	8	6–24
Itoh and Yagi (1979)	19	10	3
Degkwitz (1969)	273	19	7–10
Uhrbrand and Faurbye (1960)	17	35	4–22
Yagi et al. (1976)	19	53	12–24
Jeste et al. (1979)	21	57	13
Itoh and Yagi (1979)	14	64	60
Quitkin et al. (1977)	12	92	1–24

[a] Full references cited in original paper

personal experience, one can say that it may take 3–5 years for a tardive dyskinesia to disappear after the withdrawal of neuroleptic treatment. On present evidence, albeit scanty, one may say that approximately 60% of tardive dyskinesias will disappear when drugs are withdrawn.

A mathematical exercise can be undertaken. If the prevalence of tardive dyskinesias amongst drug-treated patients averages 20%, and 60% of these will recover when drugs are withdrawn, then the point prevalence of persistent tardive dyskinesia is about 8%. This may turn out to be not significantly higher than the estimates of the point prevalence of spontaneous dyskinesias at around 5%. So, on present evidence it can be suggested that the concept of permanent tardive dyskinesias caused by neuroleptic drugs is not proven.

7 Conclusion

A review of the present evidence suggests the following conclusions:

1. Tardive dyskinesias are not the movement disorders of untreated schizophrenia.
2. The bucco-linguo-masticatory form of tardive dyskinesia occurs more commonly than its spontaneous counterpart, which it otherwise resembles.
3. Whether other forms of tardive dyskinesia, such as tardive dystonia or tardive Tourette, are chance associations with neuroleptic treatment is unknown.
4. Chronic neuroleptic treatment may precipitate tardive dyskinesias in those already predisposed to development of such movement disorders.
5. Tardive dyskinesias may be permanent, but the case that they are caused by chronic neuroleptic treatment is unproven.
6. Tardive dyskinesias cannot be considered to be unique movement disorders.

References

Jenner P, Marsden CD (1983) Neuroleptic and tardive dyskinesia. In: Coyle JT, Enna SJ (eds) Neuroleptics: neurochemical, behavioral and clinical perspectives. Raven, New York, pp 223–253

Kahlbaum KL (1973) Catatonia. Johns Hopkins University Press, Baltimore

Kane JM, Smith JM (1982) Tardive dyskinesia. Prevalence and risk factors, 1959–1979. Arch Gen Psychiatry 39:473–481

Klawans HL, Barr A (1982) Prevalence of spontaneous lingual-facial-buccal dyskinesia in the elderly. Neurology 32:558–559

Klawans HL, Bergen D, Bruyn GW, Paulson GW (1978) Neuroleptic-induced tardive dyskinesias in nonpsychotic patients. Arch Neurol 30:338–339

Kraepelin EL (1907) Die Psychiatrie. 7th ed. English edition: McMillan, London

Kraepelin EL (1919) Textbook of psychiatry, vol 3, dementia praecox, Livingstone, Edinburgh, part 2

Marsden CD, Tarsy D, Baldessarini RJ (1975) Spontaneous and drug-induced movement disorders in psychotic patients. In: Benson DF, Blumer D (eds) Psychiatric aspects of neurologic disease. Grune and Stratton, New York, pp 219–266

Owens DGC, Johnstone EC, Frith CD (1982) Spontaneous involuntary disorders of movement in neuroleptic treated and untreated chronic schizophrenics – prevalence, severity and distributions. Arch Gen Psychiatry 39:452–461

Smith JM, Baldessarini RJ (1980) Change in prevalence, severity and recovery of tardive dyskinesia with age. Arch Gen Psychiatry 37:1368–1373

Smith JM, Kucharski KT, Eblen C, Knutsen E, Linn C (1979) An assessment of tardive dyskinesia in schizophrenic outpatients. Psychopharmacology 64:99–104

Tardive Dyskinesia (1980) Task force report 18 of the American Psychiatric Association, Washington

Tardive Dyskinesia: Prevalence, Incidence, and Risk Factors [1]

J. M. Kane, M. Woerner, and J. Lieberman [2]

Contents

Abstract 72
1 Epidemiology 72
1.1 Prevalence 72
1.2 Incidence 74
1.3 Risk Factors 75
2 Conclusion 77
References 77

Abstract

Tardive dyskinesia remains a major concern in psychiatry. Epidemiologic data suggest that the prevalence of the disorder has increased over the past two decades. The average prevalence of TD across various populations is 15%–20%. Abnormal involuntary movements appear to be at least three times more prevalent in neuroleptic-treated patients than in patients not exposed to such drugs.

The incidence of TD in a young adult (mean age 27) population is 14% after 4 years of cumulative neuroleptic exposure. The majority of these cases are mild and the condition does not appear to progress in most individuals despite continued neuroleptic exposure.

Age remains the single most important risk factor for the development of TD. Recent investigations suggest that patients with affective illness may also be more vulnerable.

1 Epidemiology

1.1 Prevalence

It is hoped that epidemiological studies will provide important clues to risk factors and ultimately to etiology and pathophysiology; however, in the area of tardive dyskinesia methodological differences and problems make successful integration of the information available somewhat difficult. Prevalence estimates may be influenced by the diagnostic criteria and assessment technique used, patient characteristics (e.g., age and sex), presence or absence of other neuromedical conditions, and treatment history characteristics (e.g., age at first treatment, length of neuroleptic exposure). In addition, the fact that administration of neuroleptics can mask the presence of the condition also complicates prevalence estimates. It is not surprising, therefore, that the prevalence estimates have ranged

1 This work was supported by NIMH contract NO 278-81-0032 and NIMH grant 32369
2 Department of Psychiatry, Long Island Jewish-Hillside Medical Center, Glen Oaks, NY 11004, USA

Dyskinesia – Research and Treatment
(Psychopharmacology Supplementum 2)
Editors: Casey, Chase, Christensen, Gerlach

from 0.5% to 57%. Kane and Smith (1982), in reviewing 56 studies, reported a mean (unweighted) prevalence of 20% among neuroleptic-treated samples. Jeste and Wyatt (1982), reviewing 37 studies (selected for minimum methodological requirements), found a weighted mean prevalence of 17.6%. It is likely that some proportion of these cases had movements which were not neuroleptic induced; however, it appears that abnormal involuntary movements are at least three times more prevalent in neuroleptic-treated patients than in patients not exposed to such drugs. It must be emphasized, however, that the drug-treated and non-drug-treated populations referred to when such comparisons are made are frequently not matched for important variables. The ideal study for assessment of the extent of the neuroleptic drug effect would involve random assignment to drug or placebo for a prolonged period of time – clearly not a practical design. The epidemiologic data, despite their limitations, provide compelling evidence that neuroleptic treatment is the single most important etiologic factor for involuntary movements in these patient populations.

Both the reviews cited above (Kane and Smith 1982; Jeste and Wyatt 1982) found a substantial increase in reported prevalence over the past 20 years, and the authors concluded that despite numerous methodological problems a true increase in prevalence probably has occurred.

The reported prevalence of "spontaneous dyskinesias" in untreated populations has also varied widely (Kane and Smith 1982), with an unweighted mean of 5%. The highest rates have been reported in elderly, institutionalized patients, suggesting that age is an important factor. However, many individuals included in such surveys have suffered from a variety of neuromedical conditions, including various types of senile dementia, complicating any comparisons with neuroleptic-treated patients.

We have had the opportunity of examining two groups of healthy elderly volunteers in the community. The first series involved 127 individuals with an average age of 72, among whom 4% had abnormal involuntary movements (Kane et al. 1982a). In a second series 400 individuals (average age 73) were examined, yielding a prevalence of 1.2% (Lieberman et al. 1984).

Klawans and Barr (1982) reported on 661 patients between the ages of 50 and 79 who had no history of neuroleptic exposure or known CNS disease and who were referred for neurologic evaluation not involving movement disorders (e.g., migraine, back pain, etc.). The prevalence of abnormal involuntary movement was 0.8% between 50 and 59 years of age, 6% between 60 and 69 years of age, and 7.8% between 70 and 79 years of age. It is difficult to tell, however, whether comparable "thresholds" for identifying a "case" of spontaneous dyskinesias were used in these different investigations.

Varga et al. (1982) reported a somewhat higher prevalence (10%) in a sample of 365 elderly individuals. A large proportion of these subjects (236) were patients in nursing homes. Medication histories were not available on those individuals with no dyskinetic symptomatology and therefore, the denominator for the prevalence of spontaneous dyskinesias in untreated individuals was only estimated. In addition, the large proportion of nursing home residents raises the possibility that neuromedical conditions which might play a role in the development of movement disorders were present in this population.

To explore this possibility further we examined 370 elderly individuals residing in a geriatric chronic care facility, 79 of whom had been or were being treated with neuroleptic drugs. The mean age of the entire sample was 84 (SD 8) and 82% were female. Among the neuroleptic-treated patients the prevalence of abnormal involuntary movements was 16.5%, as against 4.8% among those who had never been exposed to neuroleptics. This prevalence for the neuroleptic-treated patients is significantly higher than the 1.2% found among the healthy elderly volunteers, though the mean age in the neuroleptic-treated group was significantly lower (73, SD 7). This finding could support the suggestion that a variety of neuromedical illnesses in the elderly might contribute to the higher prevalence rate of abnormal movements seen in institutionalized elderly individuals. Among the 79 patients with neuroleptic exposure the mean age of first treatment with neuroleptics was 83 and the mean duration of exposure 18 months. Given the 16.5% prevalence rate with relatively brief exposure this suggests that the incidence of TD is much higher in this age group than among younger psychiatric samples.

Toenniessen et al. (1984), in a retrospective review of 57 elderly subjects, came to a similar conclusion and also suggested that the incidence of TD may begin to decline among elderly subjects after the first 2 years of neuroleptic exposure.

In general, data from these studies suggest that spontaneous dyskinesias do occur in the elderly but not to a degree that could fully account for the high prevalence of presumptive TD observed in neuroleptic-treated elderly patients. Whether or not there is a higher proportion of false-positive TD diagnoses in elderly than in nonelderly drug-treated populations remains to be determined. These findings certainly underscore the importance of attempting a careful differential diagnosis and assessing as far as possible the direct causal relationship between drug exposure and onset of movements. In addition, one cannot emphasize enough the importance of careful examination prior to initiation of neuroleptic treatment to determine the presence or absence of pre-existing movement disorders.

The question as to whether the schizophrenic illness itself may be responsible for abnormal movements is difficult to address now that the overwhelming majority of well-diagnosed schizophrenics have had some exposure to neuroleptics. Owens et al. (1982) reported on a group of chronically institutionalized schizophrenics who had apparently not received neuroleptics. A substantial proportion (53%) of these 47 individuals received positive ratings on assessment scales for abnormal involuntary movements. It should be noted that the average age of these patients was 67 and the average length of institutionalization 27 years.

1.2 Incidence

Few reports have focused on the prospective assessment of TD among psychiatric patients. Prevalence surveys provide useful information, but the limitations of retrospective data collection make the identification of possible risk factors difficult. In addition, point prevalence does not provide information on the duration or course of the movement disorder. For example, the prevalence of TD may be higher in the elderly because the condition is more persistent in that population

(Smith and Baldessarini 1980), whereas the incidence may not be increased to the same extent.

We have reported preliminary results (Kane et al. 1982b, 1983, 1984) from an ongoing prospective study of TD development involving over 800 psychiatric patients (mean age 27, median length of drug exposure at study entry 10 months). Patients were selected without consideration of diagnosis or drug treatment history. Therefore, approximately 10% of the entire sample have never received neuroleptics. These patients serve as a control group and allow us to keep the raters blind to treatment history. Patients are systematically re-examined every 3 months on rating scales to assess TD and drug-induced parkinsonism. A presumptive diagnosis of TD is made when three independent raters agree, after separate examinations, that the patient has at least mild TD based on a global judgement item included in a modified version of the Simpson Dyskinesia Scale. At that point the patient undergoes a battery of clinical laboratory tests and a neurological evaluation to rule out other possible causes of movement disorder. An attempt is made to reduce or preferably discontinue neuroleptic drug treatment, and patients are followed biweekly whenever possible, in the hope that a longitudinal perspective will be useful in validating the diagnosis as well as relating risk factors not only to incidence but also to outcome.

The results of a life-table analysis involving the first 554 at-risk (i.e., neuroleptic-treated) subjects indicates that after 4 years of cumulative neuroleptic exposure the incidence of TD is 14% (95% confidence interval 10%–18%). According to the categories included in the research diagnoses for TD (Schooler and Kane 1982), 47% of the cases that have developed are considered persistent in that their symptoms continued for at least 3 months (either receiving or not receiving neuroleptics). Three months is a brief and somewhat arbitrary period, and longer follow-up is necessary to characterize the ultimate course of the disorder. In addition, the outcome will vary depending upon the criteria used to define remission and duration of follow-up; for example, a remission following drug discontinuation could be followed by a recurrence and subsequent persistence with renewed neuroleptic medication.

It is also very important to note that among the patients developing TD in our sample, after an average length of follow-up of 30 months, in 49% it was never rated as more than mild; 24% had more than one rating of moderate, and only 8% ever had a rating of moderately severe. This suggests that in this population, despite the continued presence of symptoms in many cases, there is little evidence of substantial progression or worsening of symptoms. Recent reports from other investigators (Casey 1983, Gardos et al. 1983) also support this conclusion. There is a subgroup of patients, however, who do develop a very severe form of the disorder, and it has been our impression that many of these cases evolve very rapidly and may represent a distinct subtype. An intensive study of these patients may prove to be particularly revealing in terms of risk factors (Kane et al. 1980).

1.3 Risk Factors

It is apparent from epidemiologic reviews that the majority of neuroleptic-treated patients do not develop TD. To allow the disorder to be prevented from developing, the identification of the factors contributing to individual vulnerability would be very helpful. Numerous studies have suggested a variety of risk factors, but in general the data available in the literature are limited by important methodological problems, such as use of different criteria for the diagnosis of TD, varying efforts to rule out false positives, and retrospective collection of data on treatment history variables. In addition, it is difficult to find ideal controls since patient groups which are similar in any one characteristic may differ significantly in other important variables.

Despite this, some important leads have been suggested. The single most frequently implicated risk factor is patient age. The onset of TD is difficult to date, however, making overestimation of age at TD onset somewhat likely. Despite this, the evidence seems quite strong that increasing age among neuroleptic-treated patients increases both the risk of developing TD and the severity and persistence of the condition.

Female sex is the second most frequently suggested risk factor. It does appear that women have somewhat higher overall prevalence than men; however, samples of men and women were not always matched on other relevant variables (e.g., age). In addition, the ratio of women to men increases with increasing strictness of the criteria used to define TD, so that it appears that more severe forms of the disorder are likely to develop in women. Whether sex differences in TD vulnerability reflect differences in other factors, such as treatment history or underlying biological differences, remains to be determined.

Drug type is an important issue, both on clinical and on heuristic grounds. At present there are very few data to implicate specific drugs or drug classes as clearly increasing the risk of TD. Enormous methodological problems are involved in studying this issue. To establish relative risk, it would essentially be necessary to assume some randomness in drug assignment as well as controlling for dosage and other relevant variables. In addition, given enormous interindividual differences in drug absorption and metabolism, blood levels would be ideal for making comparisons, particularly in view of the possibility that blood levels following similar oral doses may be higher in patients with TD than in controls (Jeste et al. 1979). (The role of blood levels remains controversial, however, and further work is needed to clarify this issue.)

Cumulative drug exposure will be determined by both dosage and duration of administration. Given the epidemiologic evidence implicating neuroleptic drugs in the etiology of TD, it has generally been assumed that the risk of TD would increase with increasing cumulative exposure. As Kane and Smith (1982) have suggested, attempts at identifying dose-response curves for TD are made difficult by the relative infrequency of the condition (i.e., 15% corrected prevalence), the retrospective nature of most available data, and the methodological problems inherent in assessing pharmacologic variables. It is not surprising, therefore, that relatively few studies have been able to demonstrate a statistically significant relationship between increasing drug exposure and risk of TD.

Other risk factors that have been discussed in the literature include the presence of organic brain dysfunction, the vulnerability to early clinically significant extrapyramidal side-effects, the prolonged use of anticholinergic medications, neuroleptic-free intervals, and diagnosis.

Data from our prospective study suggest that susceptibility to the development of early clinically significant extrapyramidal side-effects may indicate susceptibility to the subsequent development of TD, particularly for those patients who develop TD with relatively brief (less than 2 years) neuroleptic exposure.

We have also found that diagnosis does appear to be a risk factor. A life-table analysis based on length of drug exposure and comparing the cumulative incidence of TD in patients with affective or schizoaffective disorder with that in patients diagnosed as schizophrenic suggests that the former have a significantly greater incidence of TD after 6 years of total neuroleptic exposure (26% $\pm$ 13% for affective and schizoaffective compared with 18% $\pm$ 7% for schizophrenics).

Evidence supporting these factors remains limited and, again, is complicated by major methodological difficulties. [Risk factors have been reviewed by Jeste and Wyatt (1982) and Kane and Smith (1982).]

2 Conclusion

A good deal has been learned in recent years regarding the prevalence, incidence, and course of tardive dyskinesia. In terms of risk factors, however, there is relatively little new information. Recent studies have added to earlier evidence suggesting age as an important factor, but much remains to be learned about individual susceptibility and ultimate prevention.

References

Casey DE (1983) Tardive dyskinesia: what is the natural history? Int Drug Therapy Newsletter 18:13–16

Gardos G, Perenyi A, Cole JO (1983) Tardive dyskinesia: changes after three years. J Clin Psychopharmacol 3:315–318

Jeste DV, Wyatt RJ (1982) Understanding and treating tardive dyskinesia. Guilford, New York

Jeste DV, Rosenblatt JE, Wagner RL, et al (1979) High serum neuroleptic levels in tardive dyskinesia? N Engl Med 301:1184

Kane JM, Smith JM (1982) Tardive dyskinesia: prevalence and risk factors, 1959–1979. Arch Gen Psychiatry 39:473–481

Kane JM, Struve FA, Weinhold B, Woerner M (1980) Strategy for the study of patients at high risk for tardive dyskinesia. Am J Psychiatry 137:1265–1267

Kane JM, Weinhold P, Kinon B, Wegner J, Leader M (1982a) Prevalence of abnormal involuntary movements ("spontaneous dyskinesias") in the normal elderly. Psychopharmacology 77:105–108

Kane JM, Woerner M, Weinhold P (1982b) A prospective study of tardive dyskinesia development: preliminary results. J Clin Psychopharmacol 2:345–349

Kane JM, Rifkin A, Woerner M, Reardow G, Sarantakos S, Schiebel D, Ramos-Lorenzi J (1983) Low-dose neuroleptic treatment of outpatient schizophrenics. Arch Gen Psychiatry 40:893–896

Kane JM, Woerner M, Weinhold P (1984) Incidence of tardive dyskinesia: five year data from a prospective study. Psychopharmacol Bull (to be published)

Klawans HL, Barr A (1982) Prevalence of spontaneous lingual-facial-buccal dyskinesias in the elderly. Neurology 32:558–559

Lieberman J, Kane JM, Woerner M (1984) Prevalence of tardive dyskinesia in elderly samples. Psychopharmacol Bull (to be published)

Owens DGC, Johnstone FC, Frith CD (1982) Spontaneous involuntary disorders of movement. Arch Gen Psychiatry 39:452–461
Schooler NR, Kane JM (1982) Research diagnoses for tardive dyskinesia. Arch Gen Psychiatry 39:486–487
Smith JM, Baldessarini RJ (1980) Changes in prevalence, severity and recovery in tardive dyskinesia with age. Arch Gen Psychiatry 37:1368–1373
Toenniessen LM, Casey DE, McFarland BH (1984) Tardive dyskinesia in the aged: Duration of treatment relationships. Arch Gen Psychiatry (to be published)
Varga E, Sugerman AA, Varga V, Zomorodi A, Zomorodi W, Menken M (1982) Prevalence of spontaneous oral dyskinesia in the elderly. Am J Psychiatry 139:329–331

Involuntary Disorders of Movement in Chronic Schizophrenia – The Role of the Illness and Its Treatment

D. G. Cunningham Owens [1]

Contents

Abstract . . . 79
1 Introduction . . . 79
2 Methods . . . 80
3 Results . . . 81
4 Discussion . . . 84
References . . . 86

Abstract

The prevalence and distribution of involuntary movements in age-matched chronic schizophrenics treated and not treated with neuroleptics were compared. While exposure to neuroleptic drugs in the past was important, high rates of movement disorder were associated with the severe, untreated illness. Ventricular enlargement correlated with severe movement disorder but not with past neuroleptic exposure. It is suggested that in the context of schizophrenia neuroleptic drugs may act to promote what are features of the illness for some, and that in the search for predisposing factors illness, as well as treatment variables, is worthy of consideration.

1 Introduction

Spontaneous involuntary movement disorder has become a major source of interest to psychiatrists practising in the era of the neuroleptic drugs. Tardive dyskinesia has been the subject of intense study, though facts concerning predisposition, correlates, and course remain few. The concept of tardive dyskinesia clearly implies that the risk is highest in those exposed to neuroleptics for long periods. In practice, this essentially means chronic schizophrenics receiving these preparations for long-term maintenance. Research to date has almost exclusively focused on the drug component of the equation. Little or no attention has been paid to the possibility that movement disorder occurring in the context of schizophrenia may relate to aspects of the illness itself.

We are not the first generation of practitioners to express interest in the problem of involuntary movements. The line can be traced back to Griesinger, who wrote of "the persistent, automatic grimacing" and "chorea-like movements" which augured a bad prognosis "in adult lunatics" (Griesinger 1857). Since the delineation of dementia praecox a number of authors have commented

1 Northwick Park Hospital and Clinical Research Centre, Watford Road, Harrow, Middlesex HA1 30J, UK

Dyskinesia – Research and Treatment
(Psychopharmacology Supplementum 2)
Editors: Casey, Chase, Christensen, Gerlach

on involuntary motor activity in schizophrenics (Reiter 1926; Jones and Hunter 1969; Brandon et al. 1971; Yarden and DiScipio 1971). Kraepelin, who paid great attention to neurological status, described features which "in no way bear the stamp of voluntary movements" (Kraepelin 1919), and even the analytical Bleuler could write of patients performing "grimaces of all kinds, (and) extraordinary movements of the tongue and lips" (Bleuler 1911). Kraepelin too noted the facial distribution of such abnormalities – the "grimacing movements" of facial expression and the "smacking" and "clicking" lip and tongue activity – but in addition noted a peripheral component he referred to as "athetoid ataxia" (Kraepelin 1919).

With the passing of the great age of descriptive psychiatry the above references were largely forgotten, and the whole question has been overtaken by the problem of tardive dyskinesia. The widespread use of neuroleptics in schizophrenia now makes it difficult to separate the long-term effects of the illness from those of its treatment.

This report addresses three main questions:

1. Can schizophrenia, unmodified by neuroleptic drugs, be associated with the development of involuntary movements? *If so,*
2. What is the relationship between these and movements in schizophrenics whose illness has been modified by neuroleptics? *and*
3. Can involuntary movements tell us anything about the cerebral basis of the illness itself?

2 Methods

The basic study population comprised all the chronic schizophrenic patients receiving long-term care in one mental hospital who conformed to both the St. Louis (Feighner et al. 1972) and PSE (Wing et al. 1974) criteria for schizophrenia and who had been hospitalized continuously for at least 1 year at the time of identification. Because of differing treatment policies within the hospital, a number of patients had no history of exposure to neuroleptic drugs. Details of this population, including the reasons for accepting their drug histories as valid, have been presented elsewhere (Owens and Johnstone 1980; Owens et al. 1982). Standardized rating scales were used to record the findings of examinations focusing

Table 1. Conventions for rating neuroleptic exposure

None	Never given	
Some: For 1 year or less	Chlorpromazine	100 mg t.i.d.
	Thioridazine	100 mg t.i.d.
	Trifluoperazine	5 mg t.i.d.
	Perphenazine	4 mg b.d.
	Depot fluphenazine	25 mg 2-weekly
	Depot fluphenthixol	40 mg 2-weekly
Much	More than the above	

specifically on involuntary movement disorders. This presentation concerns results from Abnormal Involuntary Movement Scale (AIMS) data.

Past neuroleptic exposure was graded according to the arbitrarily defined criteria shown in Table 1. These encompass both a dosage element and a component reflecting the duration of treatment.

Age was significantly related to both the prevalence and the severity of movement disorder in this sample, and subjects falling in the categories of past neuroleptic exposure differed considerably in mean age, those heavily treated ('Much') being the youngest while those never exposed ('None') were the oldest. Subsequent analyses were conducted on age-restricted subgroups of the total sample to account for the interposing effects of age.

3 Results

Figure 1 shows the prevalence of abnormality (i.e., at least one rating of 2 or more on any AIMS item) in each of the three categories for past neuroleptic exposure. A high prevalence (45.2%) can be seen to be associated with the unmodified illness. Despite this, a clear effect of past neuroleptic exposure can be demonstrated. A trend analysis reveals a significant linear relationship between the prevalence of abnormal movements and categories of past neuroleptic exposure ($z = 2.54$; $P = 0.005$[2]). Likewise, more severe abnormality is found in patients with a history of neuroleptic treatment than in those with no such history ($z = 2.2$; $P = 0.013$).

The distribution of abnormality (2 or more) on each of the seven AIMS items in each category of past neuroleptic treatment is shown in Fig. 2. The distribution in the neuroleptic-free subjects can be seen to be very similar to that of the rest,

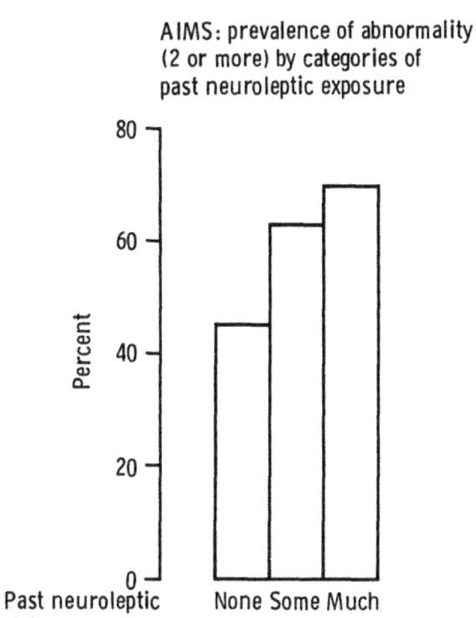

Fig. 1. Abnormal Involuntary Movement Scale: prevalence of abnormality (score of 2 or more) by category of past neuroleptic exposure

2 All P values 1-tailed

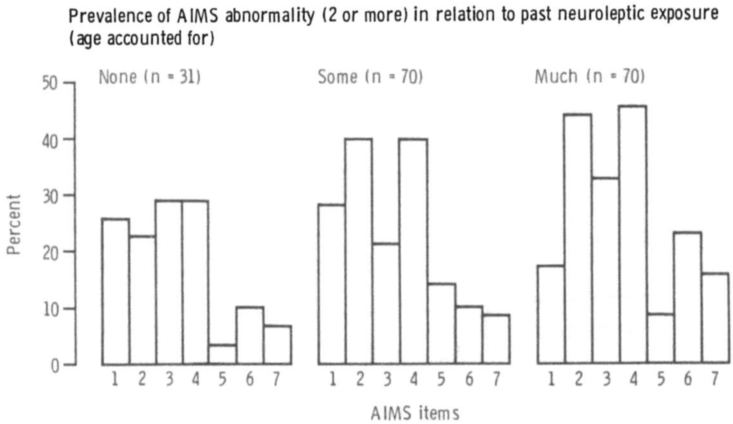

Fig. 2. Abnormal Involuntary Movement Scale: prevalence of abnormality (score of 2 or more) in relation to category of past neuroleptic exposure (age accounted for)

being predominantly orofacial. Trend analysis, however, showed significant linear relationships with increasing degrees of past exposure for item 2 (lips: $z = 1.9$; $P = 0.027$) and item 6 (lower limbs: $z = 2.04$; $P = 0.019$), with the relationships for items 4 (tongue: $z = 1.54$; $P = 0.06$) and 7 (axial/girdle muscles: $z = 1.51$; $P = 0.06$) narrowly missing conventional significance.

Figure 3 shows the prevalence of abnormality (2 or more) on each item, comparing those never exposed to neuroleptics with those exposed regardless of degree (above) and those heavily treated compared with the other two categories combined. It is only with heavy degrees of past exposure that the drug effects begin to become generalized.

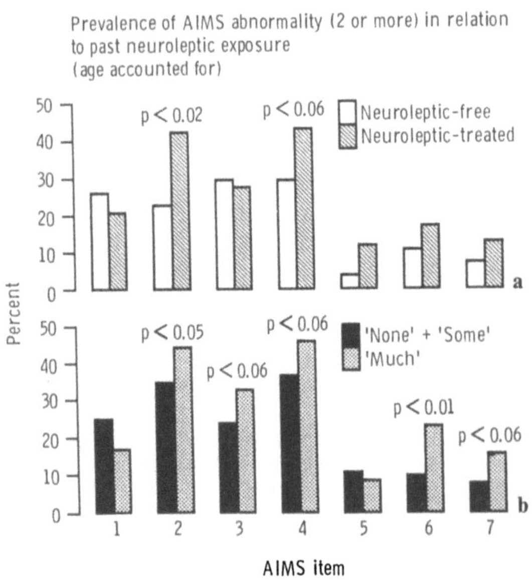

Fig. 3a, b. Abnormal Involuntary Movement Scale: age-corrected prevalence (age accounted for) of abnormality (score of 2 or more) in relation to past neuroleptic exposure. **a** No history of neuroleptic treatment vs exposure regardless of degree. **b** Heavy past treatment vs mild and no exposure

When the severity of the disorder was considered with reference to neuroleptic exposure, more of those treated with these drugs in the past scored 3 or more and 4 on lips/perioral and lower limb items ($P < 0.02$ both items) with a similar trend emerging on tongue and axial/girdle muscles ($P < 0.1 > 0.05$).

Figure 4 illustrates the prevalence of at least a single 2 in combinations of items in terms of the neuroleptic history. Trend analysis showed a significant linear relationship between prevalence (face, $z = 1.68$; $P = 0.04$: BML triad,

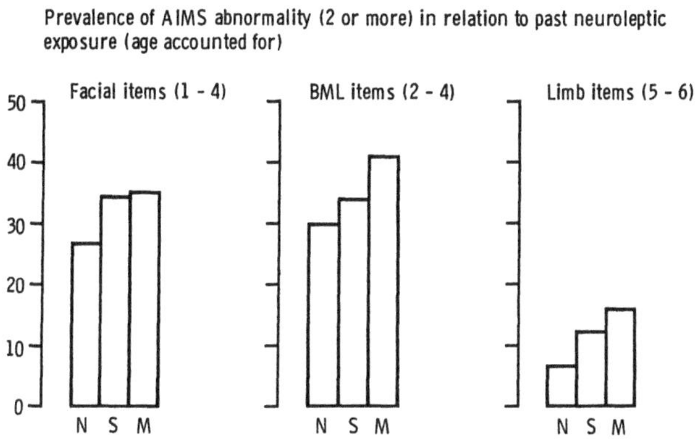

Fig. 4. Abnormal Involuntary Movement Scale: relationship between abnormality (score of 2 or more) and past neuroleptic exposure in different regional subscores (age accounted for)

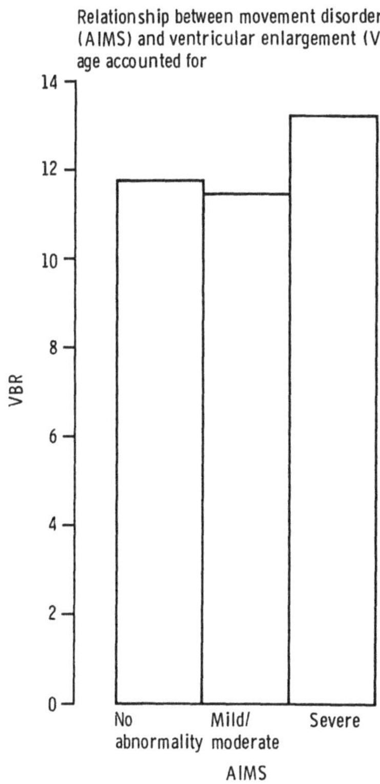

Fig. 5. Relationship between movement disorder (AIMS) and ventricular enlargement (VBR) (age accounted for)

$z = 2.45$; $P = 0.007$: limbs, $z = 1.8$; $P = 0.03$) and severity (face, $z = 1.96$; $P = 0.023$: BML triad, $z = 2.73$; $P = 0.003$: limbs, $z = 1.87$; $P = 0.029$) of movement disorder and categories of past neuroleptic exposure.

Of the 411 patients constituting the total sample, 110 had CT scans performed. Relationships were sought between movement disorder and ventricular enlargement assessed by calculation of the ventricular/brain ratio (VBR).

No significant relationships could be established between VBR and categories of past neuroleptic exposure. The patients in the scanned sample were divided on the basis of AIMS total scores into three groups: no abnormality, mild/moderate disorder, and severe disorder. Analysis of covariance was conducted to assess the relationship between abnormal movements and ventricular size, independent of age. The significant group differences that emerged ($F = 3.85$; $df = 2.106$; $P < 0.025$) arose because those with severe movement disorder had significantly larger ventricles than the rest (Newman-Keuls test: $P < 0.05$, all comparisons). The corrected VBRs in each range of AIMS total scores are shown in Fig. 5.

4 Discussion

The results presented here suggest that spontaneous involuntary disorders of movement with a predominantly orofacial distribution can be associated with severe, long-standing schizophrenia. The prevalence in the unmodified illness was high. Approximately half had at least "mild" disorder, and one third scored at least a single rating of "moderate" (3) severity.

The literature unfortunately gives little guidance as to how the rates found here compare with those of other specific diagnostic and normal groups of similar age. Estimates from pooled data suggest a spontaneous dyskinesia rate of approximately 5% (Jeste and Wyatt 1981; Kane and Smith 1982), though the pooled data technique is unsuitable for application in the above point owing to the widely differing characteristics of the study samples. Kane et al. (1982) reported a 4% prevalence of abnormal movements in a "normal" elderly population, most of which were orofacial and all of which were mild in degree. The present population had a prevalence of *severe* disorder alone that was twice[3] that found by Kane et al.

Some recent reports have found higher prevalences ranging from 10%–29% in retirement home residents (Delwaide and Desseilles 1977; Bourgeois et al. 1980; Varga et al. 1982). For technical and methodological reasons comparisons are difficult, though even these figures are lower than those reported here. The 38% found by Delwaide and Desseilles in a group of inpatients "with varying degrees of senile dementia" is comparable to the prevalences in the present population (Delwaide and Desseilles 1977), and it is of interest that this very high frequency was found in a homogeneous group with a specific psychiatric diagnosis whose implication is one of etiology rooted in organic brain dysfunction.

3 Results from Simpson Scale data not used in this presentation but mentioned here for comparability with the study of Kane et al. (1982)

As has been discussed (Owens et al. 1982), it is unlikely that the high prevalence of abnormal involuntary movements in this population is the result of nonspecific factors such as rater bias, and it is suggested that it is genuine and related to some aspect of the schizophrenic illness per se.

Nonetheless, even accepting this, the effects of neuroleptic drugs could be clearly demonstrated. Previous exposure to neuroleptics produced a striking increase in both the prevalence and the severity of abnormal movements. The division of past neuroleptics into "some" and "much" was totally arbitrary and must not be overemphasized, but the usefulness of such a distinction was shown in the differences that emerged.

Neuroleptic effects were detectable in most body parts. Only the upper limbs showed no demonstrable drug effects. Lip/perioral and leg activity seemed particularly susceptible, with tongue and postural antigravity musculature being affected to a lesser extent. It is of interest that no neuroleptic effects could be found in the muscles of facial expression. Many of the early reports going back to Griesinger emphasized that a prominent part of what they were seeing was "making faces" or "grimacing."

The conclusion possible from the literature to date is that no specific neuroleptic variable in terms of dosage, duration of treatment, etc., can be consistently shown to be of relevance with regard to tardive dyskinesia (Kane and Smith 1982). In the present work a stepwise increase in abnormality could be shown with increasing past exposure. Indeed, as far as the individual AIMS items are concerned, it is only with heavy past exposure that the neuroleptic effects start to become generalized. Whether these relationships reflect the dosage or the duration component of the criteria – or both – is unclear.

While examination of the individual components of rating scales can be of interest, it is hardly physiological. Compilation of items into something approaching clinically recognizable syndromes showed that in statistical terms the buccomasticatory/lingual or BML triad is particularly susceptible to past neuroleptic exposure. While this therefore does appear to have some validity in the context of neuroleptic usage, it must be recalled that BML disorder was also found in 30% of those never treated with these drugs.

CT scanning has been used surprisingly infrequently to study TD. Studies to date have been small and reported either no abnormalities (Gelenberg 1976; Jeste et al. 1980) or only minor abnormalities (Famuyiwa et al. 1979) in dyskinetic subjects. The present results indicate that within this population there is a group of schizophrenics with severe movement disorders who have lateral ventricular enlargement. This association is not an artifact of age or past exposure to neuroleptics.

These results suggest that the writings of the early descriptive psychiatrists should not be overlooked. Schizophrenia in its severe, long-standing untreated state can be associated with involuntary movements which appear similar in type and distribution to those found in patients treated with neuroleptics. There is no part of the body where movements develop solely as a consequence of neuroleptics. It appears that the drugs act to promote or exacerbate a tendency to develop spontaneous motor disorder inherent in at least some forms of the illness. In this regard, Jeste and Wyatt's comments are apposite:

"There are probably few clinical entities that only the man-made drugs can produce. Usually the drugs produce syndromes similar to the naturally occurring ones, although the frequency may be different" (Jeste and Wyatt 1981).

In the present work, heavy past neuroleptic exposure and ventricular enlargement both correlated with severe movement disorder, but not with each other, while there is now good evidence that schizophrenia itself (or at least certain types) is associated with enlargement of the lateral ventricles. Furthermore, it has been suggested elsewhere (Owens et al. 1982) that schizophrenia may also be associated with a tendency to develop involuntary movements. In patients such as those studied here, it is possible that aspects of the illness per se may be associated with an increased likelihood of developing both ventricular enlargement and involuntary movements, the drugs in this situation acting as a sort of catalyst (Fig. 6). In the search for predisposing factors to the development of involuntary movement disorders in schizophrenia, it may be profitable to explore aspects of the illness as well as its treatment.

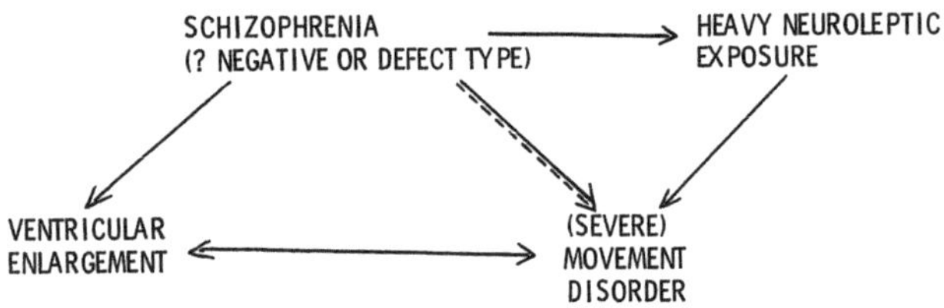

Fig. 6. Possible connections between schizophrenia, neuroleptic exposure, ventricular enlargement, and movement disorder

References

Bleuler E (1911) Dementia praecox or the group of schizophrenias. International Universities Press, New York

Bourgeois M, Bouilh P, Tignol J, Yesavage J (1980) Spontaneous dyskinesias vs. neuroleptic-induced dyskinesias in 270 elderly subjects. J Nerv Ment Dis 168:177–178

Brandon S, McClelland HA, Protheroe C (1971) A study of facial dyskinesia in a mental hospital population. Br J Psychiatry 118:171–184

Delwaide PJ, Desseilles M (1977) Spontaneous buccolinguofacial dyskinesia in the elderly. Acta Neurol Scand 56:256–262

Famuyiwa OO, Eccleston D, Donaldson AA, Garside RF (1979) Tardive dyskinesia and dementia. Br J Psychiatry 135:500–504

Feighner JP, Robins E, Guze SB, Woodruff RA, Winokur G, Munoz R (1972) Diagnostic criteria for use in psychiatric research. Arch Gen Psychiatry 26:57–63

Gelenberg AJ (1976) Computerised tomography in patients with tardive dyskinesia. Am J Psychiatry 133:578–579

Griesinger W (1857) Mental pathology and therapeutics. New Sydenham, London

Jeste DV, Wyatt RJ (1981) Changing epidemiology of tardive dyskinesia: an overview. Am J Psychiatry 138:297–309

Jeste DV, Wagner RL, Weinberger DR, Rieth KG, Wyatt RJ (1980) Evaluation of CT scans in tardive dyskinesia. Am J Psychiatry 137:247–248

Jones M, Hunter R (1969) Abnormal movements in patients with chronic psychiatric illness. In: Crane GE, Gardner J (eds) Psychotropic drugs and dysfunctions of the basal ganglia. NIMH, Bethesda, Public Health Service publication no 1938

Kane JM, Smith JM (1982) Tardive dyskinesia: prevalence and risk factors, 1959–1979. Arch Gen Psychiatry 39:473–481

Kane JM, Weinhold P, Kinon B, Wegner J, Leader M (1982) Prevalence of abnormal involuntary movements ("spontaneous dyskinesias") in the normal elderly. Psychopharmacology 77:105–108

Kraepelin E (1919) Dementia praecox and paraphrenia. Krieger, Huntington

Owens DGC, Johnstone EC (1980) The disabilities of chronic schizophrenia – their nature and factors contributing to their development. Br J Psychiatry 136:384–395

Owens DGC, Johnstone EC, Frith CD (1982) Spontaneous involuntary disorders of movement: their prevalence, severity and distribution in chronic schizophrenics with and without treatment with neuroleptics. Arch Gen Psychiatry 39:452–461

Reiter PJ (1926) Extrapyramidal motor disturbances in dementia praecox. Acta Psychiatry Neurol Scand 1:287–310

Varga E, Sugerman AA, Varga A, Zomorodi A, Zomorodi W, Menken M (1982) Prevalence of spontaneous oral dyskinesia in the elderly. Am J Psychiatry 139:329–331

Wing JK, Cooper JE, Sartorius N (1974) The measurement and classification of psychiatric symptoms: an instruction manual for the P.S.E. and catego program. Cambridge University Press, London

Yarden PE, DiScipio WJ (1971) Abnormal movements and prognosis in schizophrenia. Am J Psychiatry 128:317–323

Tardive Dyskinesia: Reversible and Irreversible [1]

D. E. Casey [2]

Contents

Abstract 88
1 Introduction 88
2 Methods 91
3 Results 92
4 Discussion 94
References 96

Abstract

The long-term prognosis of tardive dyskinesia (TD) has been insufficiently studied. Symptoms are reversible in many patients, but an irreversible course is widely believed to be the expected outcome. This pessimistic view has led to the assumption that neuroleptics should not be used in patients with TD because these drugs will produce an inevitable aggravation of TD. To clarify this issue, 27 patients were serially evaluated over 5 years for changes in neuroleptic treatment, TD, and mental status. Ten patients were able to discontinue medications; 15 required continued low-dose neuroleptic therapy [average 223 mg/day chlorpromazine (CPZ) equivalents], and two needed high doses (1000–2000 mg/day CPZ equivalents) to control psychosis. The majority of patients improved by more than 50% in both treated and untreated groups. In 8 of 27 patients (29.6%) TD resolved; in 1 patient TD increased by 25%. Younger patients improved the most. Prognosis was most favorable if neuroleptics were discontinued, but improvement was still possible with low to moderate doses (less than 600 mg/day CPZ equivalents). The large majority of patients with schizophrenia or schizoaffective illness relapsed, and required continued drug treatment. TD must be evaluated over several years to monitor the resolving/persisting course. Control of psychosis and improvement of TD during low-dose neuroleptic treatment suggest the antipsychotic and neurological effects of neuroleptics may involve different thresholds or mechanisms of action.

1 Introduction

The disturbing trend of increasing TD prevalence rates, which are now perhaps as high as 20%, poses a critical problem for maintenance drug treatment of chronic psychosis. With no uniformly safe and effective treatment for TD, the indications for and appropriate uses of neuroleptic medications have been reconsidered (Baldessarini et al. 1980; Casey and Gerlach 1984).

---

1 This research was supported in part by funds from the Veterans Administration Career Development Award and Merit Review Program, and NIMH Grant no 36657
2 Psychiatric Service, VA Medical Center, Portland, OR 97207, USA

Dyskinesia – Research and Treatment
(Psychopharmacology Supplementum 2)
Editors: Casey, Chase, Christensen, Gerlach

Since neuroleptic drugs are considered to be the cause of TD, difficult clinical choices must be made when treating patients who benefit from these drugs. With continued therapy, TD may develop or existing TD may be aggravated, while the psychosis is controlled. Without drug treatment, TD may stabilize or gradually improve, but the psychosis may exacerbate. Just as there are risks of TD with continued neuroleptic treatment, so too are there risks of psychotic exacerbation with no treatment.

The potential irreversibility of TD has led to admonitions against using neuroleptic drugs in patients with this syndrome. Though the reversible course of TD has been regularly noted since the initial publications identifying the syndrome (Schönecker 1957; Sigwald et al. 1959; Uhrbrand and Faurbye 1960), this optimistic outcome is less well known.

Two readily accepted assumptions about TD have led to a restrictive and overly pessimistic view of treating psychosis when TD is present. The first assumption is that TD will constantly increase in severity if neuroleptics are continued, since these agents are thought to be the cause of the disorder. Second, the irreversibility of TD has led to a fear of using neuroleptic drugs in patients who benefit from them and has fostered an unduly negative view of the prognosis of TD. These beliefs, however, are based on very few clinical data, and may be incorrect.

The initial report about TD by Schönecker (1957) noted, "We have observed oral automatisms with licking and smacking of the lips, frequently in older (occasionally also younger) patients on chlorpromazine-reserpine medication... These phenomena are mostly reversible after discontinuation of medication... (but) with three of our patients the syndrome continued for weeks and months..." Shortly thereafter Uhrbrand and Faurbye (1960) provided the first English-language report about TD. They noted that 6 of 17 patients who discontinued neuroleptics had TD resolve in 10 days to 4 months. In 2 of 12 patients who continued neuroleptics, the TD resolved when the drug dosage was reduced.

Existing data about the natural history of TD are not adequate to guide clinical practice. When neuroleptics are discontinued, the trend has been for symptoms to stabilize or slowly improve, though a few reports note aggravation of symptoms (Schönecker 1957; Sigwald et al. 1959; Uhrbrand and Faurbye 1960; Paulson 1968; Yagi et al. 1976; Quitkin et al. 1977; Itoh and Yagi 1979; Jeste et al. 1979; Jus et al. 1979; Carpenter et al. 1980; Gardos and Cole 1980; Levine et al. 1980; Smith and Baldessarini 1980; Pyke and Seeman 1981; Seeman 1981; Smith et al. 1981; Wegner and Kane 1982). There is considerably less information about the effect on TD when neuroleptic drugs are continued, but at lower doses. These findings also suggest that TD decreased or remained unchanged, but again some patients had more severe symptoms (Uhrbrand and Faurbye 1960; Chien and Cole 1973; Mehta et al. 1977; Jus et al. 1979; Levine et al. 1980; Branchey et al. 1981; Gibson 1981; Smith et al. 1981; Gardos et al. 1983). However, it is difficult to compare these results because different data collection and analysis procedures were used. In studies of long-term outcome, many of the initial patients were no longer available for evaluation at follow-up. Also, there was no way of assessing the effects of intervening treatment which might influence the outcome. Where treatment and symptom data are available, findings are usually limited to short- or intermediate-term follow-up of 2 years or less.

The preferred methodological approach is to assess patients over a long period of time while controlling neuroleptic dosage and monitoring TD and psychiatric status. Without these serial measures, misleading information may develop. For example, TD may initially appear to increase when drug dosage is decreased, because symptoms are unmasked. These unmasked symptoms may gradually improve, however, which is an important observation that would be missed without long-term follow-up. Similarly, TD symptoms may decrease when drug dosage is increased, because symptoms are suppressed. It would also be inaccurate to conclude that TD is improving. A 1-year follow-up report on TD (Barron and McCreadie 1983) illustrates this complex problem. The prevalence rate of TD decreased from 31% to 27%. But the true change in TD prevalence is clouded by the observation that many of these patients had an increase in neuroleptic dosage over the year – a factor known to suppress TD. On the other hand, the annual incidence rate of new cases of TD was 3%. Thus a single observation at one point in time is difficult to interpret.

A balanced clinical perspective must accommodate the practical reality that most psychotic patients cannot indefinitely remain without medication. The challenge is to develop a strategy that will successfully manage two potentially chronic illnesses: psychosis on the one hand, and TD on the other. Treatment interventions for one disorder will undoubtedly have an impact on the other.

To provide additional information on this subject, we retrospectively evaluated changes in TD and mental status over a 5-year period in patients who were closely monitored with a well-defined treatment plan (see algorithm, Fig. 1).

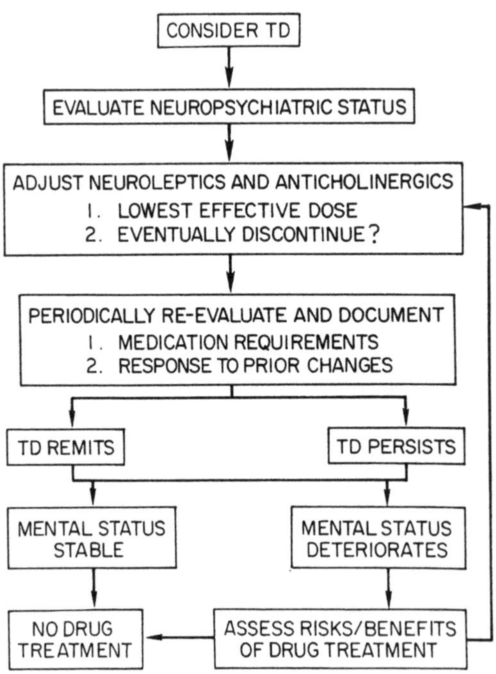

Fig. 1. An algorithm for managing tardive dyskinesia (reprinted by permission of the publisher from Figure 1, page 184, Chapter 12 in Guidelines for the Use of Psychotropic Drugs: A Clinical Handbook edited by Harvey C. Stancer, Paul E. Garfinkel and Vivian M. Rakoff. Spectrum Publications, Inc.: Jamaica, New York, 1984)

Three clinical questions were addressed:

1. What is the long-term outcome of TD if neuroleptics are discontinued or decreased?
2. What is the effect on mental status when drug treatment is altered?
3. Is there an acceptable trade-off between controlling psychosis and managing TD?

2 Methods

Patients. Twenty-seven patients (12 female, 15 male; average age, 53.2 years; range, 30–77 years) were evaluated over 5 years. Average length of illness was 11.4 years (range, 2–26 years). Additional patient characteristics are described in Table 1.

Medications. Patients were maintained with the neuroleptic they were receiving, which included all classes of these drugs. Medication adjustments were made as clinically required in accordance with the protocol described below. Neuroleptic doses are reported as CPZ equivalents (Baldessarini 1977).

Design and Evaluation. Patients were evaluated at the time of entry into the clinic with a thorough medical, psychiatric, and neurological examination. At each clinic visit thereafter, which varied from biweekly to every 3 months, the Ab-

Table 1. Patient characteristics

TD outcome	*n*	Mean age (years)	Mean duration of treatment (years)	CPZ equivalents (mg/day)		Psychiatric diagnosis	Relapse
				Initial	Final		
No drugs							
100%↓	3	48.3	8.7	300	0	1 schizophrenia	1/1
						1 affective	0/1
						1 dementia	1/1
>50%↓	5	67.1	11.6	330	0	5 affective	1/5[a]
<50%↓	2	59.5	3.0	200	0	2 affective	1/2[a]
Mean		59.9	9.0	293			
With drugs							
>50%↓	9	46.4	12.6	398	239	5 schizophrenia	5/5
						3 schizoaffective	3/3[b]
						1 neurosis	0/1
<50%↓	6	58.1	13.7	285	200	4 schizophrenia	4/4
						1 schizoaffective	1/1[b]
						1 neurosis	0/1
Mean		51.1	13.0	353	223		
High doses	2	35.0	10.9	750	1675	2 schizophrenia	2/2

[a] Lithium
[b] Lithium + neuroleptic

normal Involuntary Movement Scale (AIMS) (Guy 1976) was completed. The required treatment approach included the following:

1. Reduce drug dosage by 10%–25%.
2. Reassess and monitor outcome of dosage change for 1–3 months.
3. Continue drug dosage reduction by 10%–25%, if possible.
4. Increase drug dosage to lowest effective level if psychosis exacerbates.

Data Analysis. Data presented are from the time of entry into the project and at 6 and 12 months, followed by reassessments at 2, 3, 4, and 5 years. The total AIMS score for items 1–7 was used to determine mean group scores. Data are presented as percent changes in mean group AIMS scores from the baseline mean score at the time of entry. Relapse of psychosis was defined as exacerbation of symptoms requiring hospitalization, or an increase in neuroleptic drug dose.

3 Results

Over the 5-year treatment period, two different patterns of outcome emerged (Table 1). Ten patients discontinued drugs; 17 required continued medication, 15 of whom received maintenance doses below 600 mg/day CPZ equivalents, whereas the remaining two required doses of 1350 mg/day and 2000 mg/day CPZ equivalents. The mean total AIMS scores (severity) for both groups (with and without drugs) were similar, ranging from 10.1 to 11.9. Research criteria for TD (Schooler and Kane 1982) of at least two scores of 2 (mild) or one score of 3 (moderate) on individual items were used. The majority of patients had mild to moderate TD.

The ten patients who discontinued neuroleptic drugs were divided into two groups: rapid and slow improvers. The slow improver group was further divided into those patients who had greater or lesser than 50% improvement in TD (Table 1, Fig. 2). Two of the three patients who rapidly improved had TD resolve by the end of the first year, and the third patient had the symptoms resolve in the second year. The group with 50% or more change improved 68% over 5 years. The remaining patients showed little improvement in the first 2 years, but did improve by 17% over 5 years (Fig. 2).

In the group continuing treatment improvement was steady, reaching 76% at 5 years. A subgroup continuing treatment showed little or no change, with only 12% overall improvement (Fig. 2). None of the patients in this group had symptoms worsen. The two other patients receiving much higher neuroleptic doses of 1350 and 2000 mg/day CPZ equivalents had TD increase by 25% and decrease by 13%, respectively. Drug dosage at the beginning and end of the 5 years did not correlate with the eventual outcome of TD.

In both groups, with the exception of the rapid improvers, the trend identifying the eventual outcome was not evident until the 1- or 2-year assessment. In addition to the rapid improvers, one patient receiving no drugs had symptoms completely resolve in year 3. For those continuing with drugs, TD resolution occurred in one patient at the end of the first year, in two patients during the third year, and in another in the fifth year.

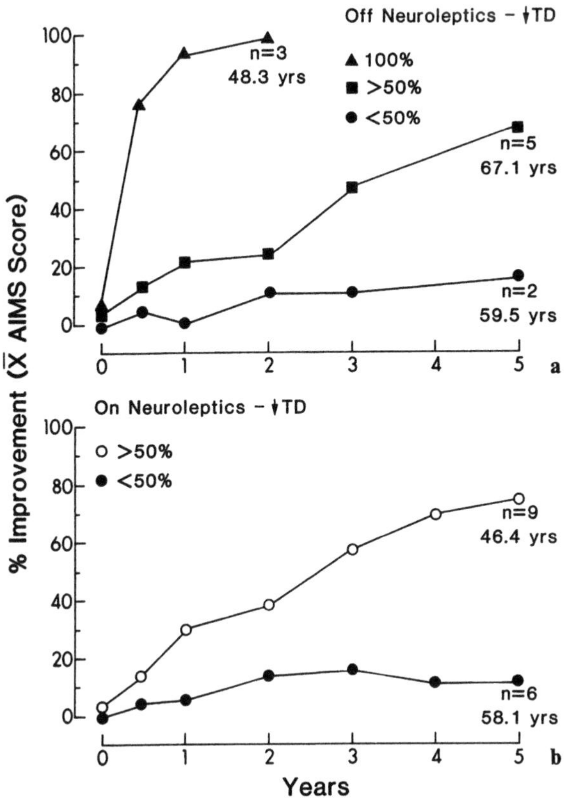

Fig. 2a, b. Improvement in tardive dyskinesia in patients **a** discontinuing and **b** continuing with neuroleptics (< 600 mg/day CPZ equivalents)

Age was inversely associated with degree of improvement. Rapid improvers receiving no drugs were considerably younger than those improving slowly but steadily (48.3 vs 67.1 years). However, age did not correlate with the final outcome of TD in the slowly improving group off drugs. The group continuing with drugs also showed an inverse correlation between age and improvement. Those improving by 76% were 46.4 years old on average; the group with 12% improvement, 58.1 years old.

Psychiatric symptoms primarily determined drug treatment status (Table 1). The majority of patients discontinuing neuroleptics had affective disorders. Two patients required additional pharmacotherapy with lithium. There was no change in TD when lithium was used. The group continuing with drugs did so because of exacerbating psychotic symptoms from schizophrenia or schizoaffective illness. Lithium was added to the neuroleptic treatment in four patients, but did not influence TD scores. In neither the group with nor that without drug treatment did the length of prior treatment correlate with outcome of TD. The two patients requiring the higher neuroleptic doses of 1350 and 2000 mg/day CPZ equivalents were 33- and 37-year-old men, both with schizophrenia.

4 Discussion

This 5-year outcome study shows that TD can be successfully managed while severe mental illness is adequately treated. Though the treatment plan of decreasing drug doses to the lowest effective levels has been repeatedly encouraged on the basis of common sense (Ayd 1977; Casey 1978; Baldessarini et al. 1980; Casey and Gerlach 1984), few data have been available to support or refuse this recommendation. The results of this study confirm that such an approach is rational and can be successful. Overall, TD improved or stabilized. Only in the exceptional case did TD worsen. Age was the most important factor influencing prognosis; younger patients improved more than older patients. The time course for adequate evaluation of the eventual remission rate of TD is much longer than has been widely recognized. Finally, the proposal that the majority of hyperkinetic dyskinesias are an integral part of or a sequela to chronic psychosis (Crow et al. 1982; Owens et al. 1982) is not compatible with the resolution or improvement of TD.

Reversibility of TD has been noted since the initial report of this disorder, but irreversibility has been more commonly emphasized and is widely believed to be the expected outcome. This study re-emphasizes the potential for a favorable outcome since the majority of patients improved 50% or more over 5 years. In 8 of 27 patients (29.6%) TD resolved; in only 1 (3.7%) did symptoms increase. Similarly, in other studies in which neuroleptics were discontinued the principal pattern was stabilization or gradual improvement of TD (Schönecker 1957; Uhrbrand and Faurbye 1960; Paulson 1968; Moline 1975; Yagi et al. 1976; Quitkin et al. 1977; Itoh and Yagi 1979; Jeste et al. 1979; Jus et al. 1979; Gardos and Cole 1980; Levine et al. 1980; Seeman 1981; Wegner and Kane 1982; Gardos et al. 1983). The range of improvement across these studies varies widely, from 0 to 92%, and depends on multiple factors including patient age and length of follow-up. A few patients will improve rapidly (Moline 1975; Gardos and Cole 1980), but the majority must be followed much longer to observe symptom changes.

In a few studies in which drugs were discontinued, TD appeared to increase in some patients as symptoms were unmasked before eventual improvement was observed (Carpenter et al. 1980; Branchey et al. 1981; Seeman 1981). Increased TD more than 1 year after drug discontinuation has been reported, but the temporal relationship between changes in treatment and symptoms could not be assessed (Crane 1971; Smith et al. 1981; Barnes et al. 1983).

Since the majority of psychotic patients eventually relapse without drug treatment, it is important to clarify the outcome of TD when neuroleptic therapy must be continued. The critical issue is to establish the minimum effective dose in patients with chronic psychosis responsive to drug treatment. This study and others suggest that the maintenance neuroleptic dose can be lower than is commonly recognized. When doses (reserpine and/or haloperidol) were tapered in 62 patients with TD, symptoms resolved in 23, improved in 26, and were unchanged in 13 over 4 years (Jus et al. 1979). In another study, patients with schizophrenia were adequately maintained over a 4- to 5-month period with one-quarter to one-eighth of their original neuroleptic dose, with only a modest, nonsignificant increase in TD (Branchey et al. 1981). However, when neuroleptics were discontinued, the majority of patients relapsed and TD was further unmasked. In patients who discontinued neuroleptics at early signs of TD, but who subsequently received episodic drug treatment during psychotic episodes, TD resolved or improved to a minimal and stable level over 3–5 years (Wegner and Kane 1982).

The observation that TD may improve while psychosis is controlled with continuing neuroleptic treatment supports the proposal that different thresholds or mechanisms of action may underlie the antipsychotic and neurological effects of neuroleptics. Low to moderate doses of neuroleptics (less than 600 mg/day CPZ equivalents) make it possible to control psychosis in the majority of patients while still allowing TD to improve or stabilize. The relative risk in this setting may be that the resolution of TD will be slowed down or impaired due to the presence of neuroleptic drugs, whereas improvement might be more rapid without drug treatment.

This is not to suggest that TD cannot get worse. Certainly it can. One patient of the 27 in this study had symptoms increase during the third year of treatment while receiving a higher than average dose of 1350 mg/day CPZ equivalents. In another follow-up study over 3 years, which re-evaluated approximately 50% of the original cohort, the point prevalence of orofacial dyskinesia increased from 39% to 47%. This change was due to a 22% increase in new cases and a 14% remission rate (Barnes et al. 1983).

The time course for defining the outcome of TD may need reconsideration. Most of the patients in this study showed minimal changes at 6 months, and only modest signs of amelioration at the end of 1 year (except for the rapid improvers receiving no drugs). The trend of gradual improvement was confirmed in the second through fifth years. Thus it is premature to conclude that TD is irreversible after only 6 or 12 months. Just as it may take a long time for TD to develop, it may also take an extended period of time for TD to resolve or stabilize. A careful distinction must be made between TD that is "persisting" though slowly improving, and TD that is "irreversible." Even the most severe and persistent cases of TD may eventually improve.

Age is the factor most consistently correlated with the outcome of TD. Younger patients improve the most, and older patients improve the least (Jeste et al. 1979; Smith and Baldessarini 1980; Seeman 1981; Smith et al. 1981). The findings of this study are consistent with earlier observations. The age differences between the groups receiving and not receiving drugs in this study raise a caveat for interpreting these and other results. Though more improvement (> 50%) was seen in those continuing with drugs than in those receiving no medication (76% vs 68%), this may be accounted for by the relative youthfulness of the drug group (46.4 vs 67.1).

Early detection has been suggested as an important variable in the reversibility of TD. When drug dosages were adjusted downward at the first signs of TD, most patients improved (Quitkin et al. 1977; Gardos and Cole 1982). It is too early to know whether this outcome will occur in all patients or whether the course of improvement is primarily seen in younger patients.

In any trade-off balancing the benefits and risks of neuroleptic medications, the strategy is to manage two potentially chronic syndromes: psychosis and TD. In contrast to earlier reports that approximately 50% of patients receiving maintenance neuroleptics could successfully discontinue drugs without relapse (Gardos and Cole 1976), the results of this study and others in chronic schizophrenia have shown that 80%–100% eventually relapse (Carpenter et al. 1980). Patients with affective disorders had substantially lower rates of psychotic relapse and were managed with lithium while being spared re-exposure to neuroleptics. The possibility that patients with affective disorders are more susceptible to TD further emphasizes the importance of proper psychiatric diagnosis and treatment (Casey 1984).

In summary, this 5-year outcome study of TD gives reason for cautious optimism. Neuroleptic drugs, particularly in low doses, can be effectively used in chronic psychosis without the feared inescapable aggravation of TD. The assumptions that TD inevitably increases in the presence of neuroleptics and that TD is primarily irreversible were not verified and must be reconsidered. Though there are many areas requiring further research, competing needs for controlling psychosis and managing TD can be developed into successful strategies for long-term neuroleptic use.

References

Ayd FJ (1977) Ethical and legal dilemmas posed by tardive dyskinesia. Int Drug Ther Newsletter 12:29–36

Baldessarini RJ (1977) Chemotherapy in psychiatry. Harvard University Press, Cambridge, pp 12–56

Baldessarini RJ, Cole JO, Davis JM, Simpson G, Tarsy D, Gardos G, Preskorn SH (1980) Tardive dyskinesia; a task force report. American Psychiatric Association, Washington DC

Barnes TRE, Kidger T, Gore SM (1983) Tardive dyskinesia: a 3-year follow-up study. Psychol Med 13:71–81

Barron ET, McCreadie RG (1983) One-year follow-up of tardive dyskinesia. Br J Psychiatry 143:423–424

Branchey MH, Branchey LB, Richardson MA (1981) Effects of neuroleptic adjustment on clinical condition and tardive dyskinesia in schizophrenic patients. Am J Psychiatry 138:608–612

Carpenter WT, Rey AC, Stephens JH (1980) Covert dyskinesia in ambulatory schizophrenia. Lancet 2:212–213

Casey DE (1978) Managing tardive dyskinesia. J Clin Psychiatry 39:748–753

Casey DE (1984) Tardive dyskinesia and affective disorders. In: Gardos G, Casey DE (eds) Tardive dyskinesia and affective disorders. American Psychiatric Association, Washington DC, pp 1–20

Casey DE, Gerlach J (1984) Tardive dyskinesia: management and new treatment. In: Stancer HC, Garfinkel PE, Rakoff VM (eds) Guidelines for the use of psychotropic drugs. Spectrum, New York, pp 183–203

Chien CP, Cole JO (1973) Eighteen-months follow-up of tardive dyskinesia treated with various catecholamine-related agents. Psychopharmacol Bull 9:38

Crane GE (1971) Persistence of neurological symptoms due to neuroleptic drugs. Am J Psychiatry 127:1407–1410

Crow TJ, Cross AJ, Johnstone EC, Owen F, Owens DG, Waddington JL (1982) Abnormal involuntary movements in schizophrenia: are they related to the disease process or its treatment? Are they associated with changes in dopamine receptors? J Clin Psychopharmacol 2:336–340

Gardos G, Cole JO (1976) Maintenance antipsychotic therapy: is the cure worse than the disease? Am J Psychiatry 133:32–36

Gardos G, Cole JO (1980) Overview: public health issues in tardive dyskinesia. Am J Psychiatry 137:776–781

Gardos G, Cole JO (1982) Early dyskinesia: course, outcome, and prognosis. Proc Ann Meet Am Psychiatr Assoc 68 D:171
Gardos G, Perenyi A, Cole JO, Samu I, Kallos M (1983) Tardive dyskinesia: changes after three years. J Clin Psychopharmacol 3:315–318
Gibson AC (1981) Incidence of tardive dyskinesia in patients receiving depot neuroleptic injection. Acta Psychiatr Scand [Suppl] 63:111–116
Guy W (1976) ECDEU assessment manual for psychopharmacology. US department of health, education, and welfare. US Government Printing Office, Washington DC, pp 534–537
Itoh H, Yagi G (1979) Reversibilitiy of tardive dyskinesia. Folia Psychiatr Neurol Jpn 33:43–54
Jeste DV, Potkin SG, Sinha S, Feder S, Wyatt RJ (1979) Tardive dyskinesia-reversible and persistent. Arch Gen Psychiatry 36:585–590
Jus A, Jus K, Fontaine P (1979) Long-term treatment of tardive dyskinesia. J Clin Psychiatry 40:72–77
Levine J, Schooler N, Severe J, Escobar J, Gelenberg A, Mandel M, Sovner R, Steinbook R (1980) Discontinuation of oral and depot fluphenazine in schizophrenic patients after one year of continuous medication: a controlled study. In: Cattabeni F, Racagni G, Spano PF, Costa E (eds) Long-term effects of neuroleptics. Adv Biochem Psychopharmacol 24:483–493
Mehta D, Mehta S, Mathew P (1977) Tardive dyskinesia in psychogeriatric patients: a five-year follow-up. J Am Geriatr Soc 25:545–547
Moline RA (1975) Atypical tardive dyskinesia. Am J Psychiatry 132:534–535
Owens DGC, Johnstone EC, Frith CD (1982) Spontaneous involuntary disorders of movement. Arch Gen Psychiatry 39:452–461
Paulson GW (1968) "Permanent" or complex dyskinesias in the aged. Geriatrics 23:105–110
Pyke J, Seeman MV (1981) Neuroleptic-free intervals in the treatment of schizophrenia. Am J Psychiatry 138:1620–1621
Quitkin F, Rifkin A, Gochfeld L, Klein DF (1977) Tardive dyskinesia: are first signs reversible? Am J Psychiatry 134:84–87
Schönecker M (1957) Ein eigentümliches Syndrom im oralen Bereich bei Megaphenapplikation. Nervenarzt 28:35
Schooler NR, Kane JM (1982) Research diagnoses for tardive dyskinesia. Arch Gen Psychiatry 39:486–487
Seeman MV (1981) Tardive dyskinesia: two-year recovery. Compr Psychiatry 22:189–192
Sigwald J, Bouttier D, Raymondeaud C (1959) Quatre cas de dyskinesie faciobucco-linguo-masticatrice a l'evolution prolongee secondaire a un traitement par les neuroleptiques. Rev Neurol 100:751–755
Smith JM, Baldessarini RJ (1980) Changes in prevalence, severity and recovery in tardive dyskinesia with age. Arch Gen Psychiatry 37:1368–1373
Smith JM, Burke MP, Moon CO (1981) Long-term changes in AIMS ratings and their relation to medication history. Psychopharmacol Bull 17:120–121
Uhrbrand L, Faurbye A (1960) Reversible and irreversible dyskinesia after treatment with perphenazine, chlorpromazine, reserpine and electroconvulsive therapy. Psychopharmacologia 1:408–418
Wegner JT, Kane JM (1982) Follow-up study on the reversibility of tardive dyskinesia. Am J Psychiatry 139:368–369
Yagi G, Ogita K, Ohtsuka N, Itoh H, Miura S (1976) Persistent dyskinesia after long-term treatment with neuroleptics in Japan. Keio J Med 25:27–35

Pathophysiological Mechanisms Underlying Tardive Dyskinesia

J. Gerlach[1]

Contents

Abstract 98
1 Introduction 98
2 Classification of Extrapyramidal Symptoms 99
3 Relationship Between Initial and Tardive Dyskinesia 99
4 Pathophysiological Mechanisms Underlying Tardive Dyskinesia 101
References 103

Abstract

Movement abnormalities in neuroleptic-treated, psychiatric patients are classified as (a) initial syndromes, including dystonia, parkinsonism, and hyperkinetic abnormalities such as initial dyskinesia (ID) and akathisia, all of which are related to the neuroleptic dose and can be considered as overdose phenomena; (b) tardive syndromes, mainly the classic tardive dyskinesia (TD) syndrome, more seldom tardive akathisia and tardive dystonia, which may all develop or aggravate after withdrawal of neuroleptic treatment; and (c) age-related, spontaneous dyskinesia, akathisia, and dystonia, and schizophrenia-related, hyperkinetic, often stereotyped, movements and restlessness. ID and TD can occur simultaneously, and may depend, at least partially, on identical mechanisms.

The pathophysiology of TD is still not clear, and the traditional dopamine (DA) hypersensitivity model seems inadequate. Animal experiments suggest that blockade of some DA receptors in the brain (e.g., in ventromedian striatum) may counteract hyperkinesia and produce parkinsonism, while a concomitant blockade of other similar receptors in other brain regions (e.g., in anterodorsal striatum) may aggravate hyperkinetic movements. This offers an explanation for the concomitant occurrence of parkinsonism and hyperkinetic movement abnormalities (ID and akathisia) relatively early in a neuroleptic treatment, and may also contribute to the understanding of the pathophysiology of TD. It is concluded that pathophysiologically TD is a heterogeneous syndrome depending on a subtle balance between several neurotransmitters in the brain, including DA receptor blockade and hypersensitivity of DA and GABA receptors.

1 Introduction

The aims of this paper are (a) to present a classification of extrapyramidal movement disturbances in neuroleptic-treated psychiatric patients; (b) to discuss the relationship between initial and tardive extrapyramidal phenomena; and (c) to propose a new hypothesis concerning the pathophysiology underlying tardive dyskinesia (TD).

1 Sct. Hans Mental Hospital, Department AEH, DK-4000 Roskilde, Denmark

Dyskinesia – Research and Treatment
(Psychopharmacology Supplementum 2)
Editors: Casey, Chase, Christensen, Gerlach

2 Classification of Extrapyramidal Symptoms

Extrapyramidal syndromes in neuroleptic-treated, psychotic patients have been classified as follows (Gerlach and Korsgaard 1981, 1983).

1. *Initial extrapyramidal syndromes.* This group consists of dystonia (acute or prolonged), parkinsonism (acute or prolonged), and hyperkinetic movement abnormalities [initial dyskinesia (ID) and akathisia]. These symptoms may occur separately or in combination, and they have been directly related to the antidopaminergic treatment; an increased dose appears to aggravate the symptoms, whereas a decreased dose usually reduces them. Thus, they may be considered as overdose phenomena. Following withdrawal of the neuroleptic treatment they resolve quickly in some cases, but in others they are prolonged and diminish slowly over several months and in a few can apparently be irreversible.
2. *Tardive extrapyramidal syndromes.* This group of syndromes develops during or following prolonged neuroleptic treatment and consists mainly of the classic TD syndrome. In some cases, tardive akathisia (indistinguishable from the above-mentioned initial akathisia) and tardive dystonia may occur (Fahn 1983). These syndromes are usually regarded as withdrawal-like phenomena.
3. *Age- and disease-related syndromes.* Dystonia, parkinsonism, and hyperkinesia all occur in elderly, untreated people. The spontaneous (senile) oral dyskinesia cannot be distinguished from TD in elderly patients, just as parkinsonism in elderly patients cannot be distinguished from neuroleptic-induced parkinsonism. Senile dystonia and akathisia are relatively rare phenomena, although they have been described in a few cases. It is an old observation that schizophrenic symptomatology may include various types of hyperkinetic, stereotyped movements and restlessness, which can look exactly like the neuroleptic-produced movements. Schizophrenic akinesia and catatonic symptoms may similarly resemble parkinsonian and dystonic symptoms.

3 Relationship Between Initial and Tardive Dyskinesia

From the above classification it should be noted that almost identical neurological symptoms (dystonia, parkinsonism, and hyperkinetic disturbances) can occur as a result of (a) neuroleptic treatment, (b) withdrawal of such treatment, and (c) old age and/or the psychotic process. This complicates research (e.g., prevalence studies) and treatment in TD. On the other hand, this observation may contribute to our understanding of the pathophysiological mechanisms underlying the syndromes.

Traditionally, initial and tardive extrapyramidal syndromes are regarded as partly opposite movement disturbances, the initial syndromes depending on dopamine (DA) hypofunction, the tardive on a DA hyperfunction. This view appears to be too simple. The following examples of overlapping and coincidental occurrence of initial and tardive symptoms might lead to a more comprehensive understanding of the relationship between the early and late extrapyramidal side-effects.

ID are TD-like movements that develop in about 10% of neuroleptic-treated patients, usually relatively early in the course of the treatment but in some cases after several years' treatment (Casey et al. 1981; Gerlach and Korsgaard 1981). The syndrome has most often been seen in young patients and has a widespread and varied localization including the extremities and the trunk, whereas TD preferentially occurs in elderly patients and is confined to the oral region. This apparently different localization of ID and TD may, however, be a result of the different age of these patients, and not of the stage in the treatment course (early – late). Thus, it is well known that hyperkinetic movements, including withdrawal TD in younger patients, are mainly confined to the extremities, whereas a rising tendency to oral preponderance of hyperkinesia is seen with increasing age, both for TD and for L-dopa-induced hyperkinesia in Parkinson's disease (Gerlach and Korsgaard 1983). In some cases, however, ID occurs solely in the oral region, and in such cases it is impossible to distinguish it from TD. Even a combined pre- and postsynaptic antidopaminergic treatment with pimozide and tetrabenazine may induce such a syndrome. This observation indicates that hyperkinetic movements may be directly related to an antidopaminergic treatment.

Anticholinergic treatment usually aggravates TD (Casey et al. 1981; Gerlach 1979), at least partly due to the antiparkinsonian effect of such treatment. No consistent effects of anticholinergics have been found in ID. Often, but not always, ID is associated with elements of dystonia, parkinsonism or, particularly, akathisia, and in such cases anticholinergic drugs can probably indirectly reduce ID.

It used to be thought that ID and TD could be distinguished by discontinuation of the neuroleptic treatment (Gerlach and Korsgaard 1983) after which TD would temporarily become worse and later diminish, while ID would resolve relatively quickly. However, recent observations (unpublished) suggest that in some cases ID diminishes slowly over months or remains irreversible, like TD. This means that ID and TD can be indistinguishable and may be one and the same phenomenon. If these results can be confirmed it might be necessary to change the terminology.

This overlap between or coincidental occurrence of initial and tardive extrapyramidal syndromes poses the clinician an insoluble problem. The hyperkinetic movements may be very severe and disturbing, but any antidopaminergic treatment may aggravate the symptoms and perhaps add a severe akathisia. Such a case is briefly described below.

Case History

A 66-year-old man was treated with diazepam 5–20 mg daily for about 5 years, up to the age of 60. He suffered from nervousness and depression, but had never had psychotic symptoms. The benzodiazepine treatment was changed to thioridazine 150–200 mg/day for 2 months, and later levomepromazine 100 mg/day for 1 year. During the following year he received flupenthixol 1.5–3.0 mg/day together with levomepromazine 50 mg and metakvalon 400 mg for the night. Gradually, he became more restless, and at 62 years old he developed oral dyskinesia, 2–3 months after discontinuation of flupenthixol and during treatment with levomepromazine 75 mg/day and metakvalon 400 mg for the night. Following treatment with tetrabenazine increasing from 37.5 mg/day to 200 mg/day, the TD diminished but akathisia increased, together with an overwhelming feeling of distress. Therefore tetrabenazine had to be discontinued. After 2 1/2 years his oral movements were so intensive that from time to time he broke a tooth. All types of antidopaminergic treatment, even 4–8 mg perphenazine and 12.5 mg tetrabenazine, aggravated his akathisia and produced stereotyped movements of the hands and facial hyperkinesia. He now receives clozapine 150 mg/day, diazepam 30 mg/day, and mekvalon 400 mg for the night. He is still severely disturbed by akathisia as well as oral dyskinesia.

The conclusion from these clinical observations appears to be that initial and tardive extrapyramidal symptoms, especially akathisia, ID, and TD are closely related symptoms, often overlapping and sometimes phenomenologically indistinguishable. This suggests that the underlying pathogenetic mechanisms may be partly the same.

4 Pathophysiological Mechanisms Underlying Tardive Dyskinesia

Traditional neuroleptics block postsynaptic DA receptors, leading to an increased acetylcholine turnover. Clinically, this appears to be related to parkinsonism. During long-term neuroleptic treatment, various phenomena of adaptation occur: The DA receptor blockade leads to a dopaminergic hypersensitivity, which can be shown by an increased behavioral response to DA agonists; this hypersensitivity appears to be associated with an increased number of DA receptors, together with a decrease in the acetylcholine turnover and probably other compensatory reactions beyond the DA receptors (Jenner and Marsden 1983; Seeman 1980).

During the past 15 years, the development of TD has been related to the increased DA receptor sensitivity. However, several observations suggest that there is no clear correlation between TD and DA hypersensitivity:

1. Parkinsonism and TD can occur simultaneously, in different regions or in the same region.
2. In some cases, ID and TD may be indistinguishable, both phenomenologically and pharmacologically.
3. During long-term, stable, decreased, or increased neuroleptic treatment, TD may decrease (Casey and Toennissen 1983), in contrast to neuroleptic-induced DA hypersensitivity (Jenner and Marsden 1983).
4. TD in psychiatric patients shows only slight deterioration or none at all during treatment with DA agonists such as L-dopa (Gerlach and Casey 1980), in contrast to the animal hypersensitivity model. Only in patients with a concomitant idiopathic parkinsonism does L-dopa clearly aggravate/precipitate TD, at least partly by counteracting the parkinsonism (Klawans and McKendall 1971).
5. Endocrinological studies do not suggest any increased DA sensitivity in TD patients, but rather the opposite (Ettigi et al. 1976; Tamminga et al. 1977).
6. Cross et al. (this volume) found no increased number of DA receptors in postmortem brains from patients with TD compared with patients without TD.
7. During neuroleptic treatment, there is no correlation between the time course of development of DA hypersensitivity in animals and TD in patients. For example, the DA hypersensitivity in animals develops in all cases and after one

single dose (Christensen 1981), whereas TD develops in only some patients and only after treatment for some months/years.
8. Some antidopaminergic neuroleptics, such as the thioxanthenes, have an inherent D-1 antagonistic effect which appears to be able to prevent DA hypersensitivity (Christensen et al., this volume). However, clinical experience, although uncontrolled, and case reports do not suggest any difference between neuroleptics with and without D-1 components with respect to TD-inducing effect.

These observations indicate that the DA hypersensitivity theory cannot fully explain the pathophysiology of TD. Therefore, other possibilities should be considered.

During recent years, the knowledge about various neurotransmitters and their interactions in the brain has increased rapidly (Jenner and Marsden 1983; Seeman 1980; Scheel-Krüger and Arnt, this volume). One of the most interesting aspects in relation to TD is the observation of distinct types of DA receptors and GABA neurons. Thus, it has been shown that neuroleptics injected into the ventromedian part of the striatum can antagonize apomorphine-induced gnawing, while neuroleptics injected into the anterodorsal part aggravate the same movements (Scheel-Krüger and Arnt, this volume). A similar differentiation has been found for different GABA neurons in the striatum: one type (from the anterior part of the striatum to the globus pallidus, lateral segment) is inhibited by DA, while another type (from the posterior part of the striatum to zona reticulata of substantia nigra and to globus pallidus, median segment) is stimulated by DA (Scheel-Krüger and Arnt, this volume). This means that neuroleptics disinhibit the GABA neurons projecting to the lateral segment of globus pallidus, while they inhibit the GABA neurons projecting to substantia nigra and medial globus pallidus. From animal studies using intracerebral injection technique it is known that increased GABA activity in lateral globus pallidus induces parkinsonism in animals, while the decreased GABA function in the medial segment and in substantia nigra seems to be associated with hyperkinetic movements (Scheel-Krüger and Arnt, this volume). The last observation mentioned is in agreement with that of a decreased glutamic acid decarboxylase activity in substantia nigra and in the median pallidal segment in postmortem brains from Cebus monkeys with persistent dyskinesias (Häggström 1984).

These observations clearly suggest that a DA receptor blockade has distinct behavioral effects depending on the localization of the DA receptors in the brain. Blockade of some DA receptors leads to hyperkinetic disturbances, while blockade of others results in decreased mobility.

From a clinical point of view, these observations indicate that neuroleptic drugs might be able to induce hyperkinetic movement disturbances including akathisia, ID and TD, and at the same time, parkinsonism and dystonia. In most cases, parkinsonism and/or sedation may suppress the hyperkinetic movements at the initial stage of the treatment. Later, when tolerance has developed to parkinsonism and sedation, the hyperkinetic movements may become manifest.

The pathogenetic implication of these considerations may be that ID and TD do not have to be considered as distinct entities. It may be that both result from

DA receptor blockade, merely of DA receptors sited at different points in the brain. In some cases the parkinsonism may be dominating and long standing, in other cases the hyperkinesia.

This new hypothesis does not disregard the traditional DA hypersensitivity theory. TD is probably a heterogeneous syndrome which depends on a multitude of pathogenetic mechanisms. It turns on a subtle balance between various neurotransmitters and the sensitivity of receptors of different type and localization. Furthermore, an unknown predisposition for TD is a necessary prerequisite for development of the syndrome. The DA hypersensitivity may still play a role and lower the threshold for manifestation of dyskinetic disturbances.

The question of the pathophysiology of TD is far from solved. However, the biochemical background for various movement abnormalities has expanded enormously, and postmortem brain studies in human and monkey organs (Häggström 1984) have contributed to a clarification. From a clinical point of view, the major objective is still prevention of the syndrome, and in this respect attempts to find new antipsychotics with little or no antidopaminergic effect appear to be the most promising.

References

Casey DE, Toenniessen LM (1983) Neuroleptic treatment in tardive dyskinesia: Can it be developed into a clinical strategy for long-term treatment? In: Ban TA, Pichot P, Pöldinger LW (eds) Modern problems of pharmacopsychiatry. Karger, Basel, pp 65–79

Casey DE, Gerlach J, Korsgaard S (1981) Clinical pharmacological approaches to evaluating tardive dyskinesia. In: Usdin E, Dahl S, Gram LF, Lingjaerde O (eds) Clinical pharmacology in psychiatry: neuroleptic and antidepressant research. MacMillan, London, pp 369–382

Christensen AV (1981) Dopamine hyperactivity. Effects of neuroleptics alone and in combination with GABA agonists. In: Perris C, Struwe G, Jansson B (eds) Biological psychiatry. Elsevier, Amsterdam, pp 828–832

Ettigi P, Nair NPV, Lal S, Cervantes P, Guyda H (1976) Effect of apomorphine on growth hormone and prolactin secretion in schizophrenic patients, with or without oral dyskinesia, withdrawn from chronic neuroleptic therapy. J Neurol Neurosurg Psychiatry 39:870–876

Fahn S (1983) Treatment of tardive dyskinesia: use of dopamine-depleting agents. Clin Neuropharmacol 6:151–157

Gerlach J (1979) Tardive dyskinesia. Dan Med Bull 26:209–245

Gerlach J, Casey DE (1983) Dopamine agonists in clinical research for new tardive dyskinesia treatments. Mod Probl Pharmacopsychiatry 21:97–110

Gerlach J, Korsgaard S (1981) Classification and prevalence of neuroleptic-induced hyperkinetic movement disorder. In: Perris C, Struwe G, Jansson B (eds) Biological psychiatry. Elsevier, Amsterdam, pp 844–851

Gerlach J, Korsgaard S (1983) Classification of abnormal involuntary movements in psychiatric patients. Neuropsychiatr Clin 2:201–208

Häggström J-E (1984) Neuroleptic-induced persistent dyskinesia. Behavioral and biochemical studies. Reprocentralen HSC, Uppsala Universitet, Uppsala

Jenner P, Marsden CD (1983) Neuroleptics and tardive dyskinesia. In: Coyle JT, Enna SJ (eds) Neuroleptics: neurochemical, behavioral, and clinical perspectives. Raven, New York, pp 223–253

Klawans H, McKendall RR (1971) Observations on the effect of levodopa on tardive lingual-facial-buccal dyskinesia. J Neurol Sci 14:189–192

Seeman P (1980) Brain dopamine receptors. Pharmacol Rev 32:229–313

Tamminga CA, Smith RC, Pandey G, Frohman LA, Davis JM (1977) A neuroendocrine study of supersensitivity in tardive dyskinesia. Arch Gen Psychiatry 34:1199–1203

Chemical and Structural Changes in the Brain in Patients with Movement Disorder

A. J. Cross, T. J. Crow, I. N. Ferrier, J. A. Johnson, E. C. Johnstone,
F. Owen, D. G. C. Owens, and M. Poulter [1]

Contents

Abstract 104
1 Introduction 104
2 Effects of Neuroleptic Treatment on Dopaminergic Function in Man 105
3 Dopaminergic Function and Dyskinesia in Schizophrenics 107
4 Chemical Correlates of Structural Changes in Schizophrenics with Movement Disorder 108
5 Conclusions 109
References 109

Abstract

Neurochemical indices of dopaminergic function were assessed in basal ganglia of post-mortem brains of control subjects and schizophrenic patients who had been rated in life for the presence of movement disorder and neuroleptic intake. In schizophrenics who had been treated chronically with high doses of neuroleptics, concentrations of dopamine D2 receptors were significantly increased above controls, whereas dopamine D1 receptors and dopamine metabolism were unchanged. Increased D2 receptors were also observed in basal ganglia of drug-free patients. Concentrations of dopamine D1 and D2 receptors in schizophrenics with movement disorder were not significantly different to those in schizophrenics without movement disorder. Moreover, no relationship was found between dopamine receptor levels and the severity of movement disorder. Concentrations of the dopamine metabolite homovanillic acid were increased in the putamen and nucleus accumbens in a small number of patients with movement disorder compared with controls or patients without movement disorder. No changes were observed in markers of cholinergic and GABA-containing neurones. The present findings are not consistent with a "dopamine receptor hypersensitivity" concept of movement disorder in schizophrenia.

1 Introduction

The syndrome of abnormal involuntary movements frequently associated with schizophrenia has become generally known as tardive dyskinesia. This terminology presupposes an aetiologic association with neuroleptic administration, and it is widely held that these abnormal involuntary movements are a side-effect of chronic neuroleptic treatment. It has been argued that the responsiveness of such abnormal movements to pharmacological manipulations is consistent with an increased activity of brain dopaminergic mechanisms (Tarsy and Baldessarini 1977; Marsden and Jenner 1980). By analogy with the changes in dopaminergic

1 Division of Psychiatry, Clinical Research Centre, Watford Road, Harrow, Middlesex HA1 3UI, England

Dyskinesia – Research and Treatment
(Psychopharmacology Supplementum 2)
Editors: Casey, Chase, Christensen, Gerlach

function observed in experimental animals after chronic neuroleptic administration, it has been suggested that tardive dyskinesia might be associated with an increased responsiveness of postsynaptic dopamine receptors. The evidence supporting such a concept is entirely circumstantial, however, and moreover, a straightforward relationship between abnormal movements in schizophrenia and prior neuroleptic treatment has recently been questioned (Brandon et al. 1971; Owens et al. 1982). It has been suggested that the dyskinesia may be associated with the disease process rather than its treatment (Owens et al. 1982) and that the dyskinesia may constitute one of several disabilities associated with the "defect state" or type II syndrome (Crow et al. 1983).

Our studies of neurochemical parameters in postmortem brains of schizophrenics have led us to collect a large series of samples in which we have studied dopaminergic function. Included in this sample are a group of patients who were clinically assessed during life for the presence and severity of movement disorder (Owens et al. 1982). A second group of patients whose drug histories have been reliably assessed have also been studied. The availability of these groups of samples has enabled us to critically examine two areas of relevance to tardive dyskinesia. First, the neurochemical effects of chronic neuroleptic treatment in schizophrenics have been studied by comparison with neuroleptic-free patients and also controls. Secondly, such neurochemical parameters can be compared in relation to the presence of abnormal involuntary movements.

In these groups of patients we studied dopaminergic function by measuring the concentrations of dopamine and its metabolites (Cross and Joseph 1981). Dopamine receptors were quantified with the aid of ligand-binding techniques, dopamine D1 receptors being assessed with ^{3}H-piflutixol as ligand (Cross and Rossor 1983) and D2 receptors with ^{3}H-spiperone (Owen et al. 1978). As it has been suggested that the dyskinesia of schizophrenia as part of the type II syndrome may be associated with structural changes in the brain (Owens et al. 1982), we also examined a number of other neurochemical markers. Thus, the concentrations of γ-aminobutyric acid (GABA) and the activity of choline acetyltransferase (CAT) were used as markers of GABA- and acetylcholine-containing neurones, respectively. In addition, the concentrations of several neuropeptides were studied in relation to the presence of movement disorder.

2 Effects of Neuroleptic Treatment on Dopaminergic Function in Man

The concentrations of dopamine and its metabolites dihydroxyphenylacetic acid (DOPAC) and homovanillic acid (HVA) in basal ganglia areas of post-mortem brains of controls and schizophrenics are shown in Table 1. In agreement with other studies (Bacopoulos et al. 1979; Crow et al. 1978), no increase in the basal ganglia concentration of HVA was observed in schizophrenics after chronic neuroleptic intake, and HVA concentrations were not increased in the total schizophrenic group compared with controls.

The results of an analysis of ^{3}H-spiperone binding to dopamine D2 receptors against drug state are presented in Table 2. In both the putamen and nucleus

Table 1. Dopamine and HVA concentrations[a] in schizophrenics and relationship to drug status

	Dopamine	HVA
Putamen		
Control ($n = 10$)	16.7 ± 2.6	45.0 ± 3.8
Drug free ($n = 4$)	16.8 ± 5.5	56.4 ± 13.0
Drug treated ($n = 7$)	15.0 ± 2.9	50.8 ± 5.9
N. accumbens		
Control ($n = 7$)	11.4 ± 3.1	56.2 ± 3.8
Drug free ($n = 4$)	12.3 ± 0.5	56.7 ± 10.7
Drug treated ($n = 6$)	16.9 ± 3.1	57.3 ± 6.1
S. nigra		
Control ($n = 11$)	2.6 ± 0.7	30.8 ± 4.5
Drug free ($n = 3$)	3.9 ± 1.0	41.0 ± 11.8
Drug treated ($n = 6$)	3.7 ± 0.9	42.5 ± 6.2

[a] Dopamine and HVA concentrations were determined by HPLC (Cross and Joseph 1981). Values are expressed as ng/mg protein mean ± SEM

Table 2. Neuroleptic treatment and ^{3}H-spiperone binding[a] in human striatum

		Controls	Drug-free patients	Drug-treated patients
Schizophrenia	Putamen	208 ± 11 (39)	324 ± 75 (7)[c]	419 ± 34 (23)[c]
	Accumbens	181 ± 15 (33)	305 ± 76 (5)[b]	318 ± 36 (16)[c]
Huntington's chorea	Caudate	—	73 ± 8 (8)	87 ± 10 (15)
Senile dementia	Putamen	—	90 ± 9 (10)	89 ± 12 (10)

[a] Figures given for ^{3}H-spiperone binding in schizophrenics are maximum binding values determined from saturation analysis. Values in Huntington's chorea and senile dementia samples were determined at 0.8 nM ^{3}H-spiperone. Values are mean fmol ligand bound/mg protein ± SEM; the number of samples is given in parentheses in each case

[b] $P < 0.02$

[c] $P < 0.01$

accumbens of drug-treated schizophrenics the number of ^{3}H-spiperone-binding sites was increased above controls, reaching 100% in putamen. In patients who, as far as could be determined, were neuroleptic-free, the increase in ^{3}H-spiperone binding was less pronounced than in the drug-treated group, but was nonetheless significantly elevated above controls. Two further groups of patients were studied in a similar way. In a group of Huntington's chorea patients who had been treated with neuroleptic drugs, ^{3}H-spiperone binding in caudate nucleus was not significantly elevated in comparison with a group of drug-free subjects. Whilst there is considerable striatal degeneration in Huntington's chorea, similar degeneration induced in rats by kainic acid treatment had no effect on the development of dopamine-receptor hypersensitivity (Owen et al. 1980). Striatal degeneration in senile dementia is minimal, but yet again chronic neuroleptic treatment did not significantly elevate ^{3}H-spiperone binding in the putamen (Table 2). These results are consistent with a recent report that neuroleptic treatment increases striatal dopamine D2 receptors only marginally in Parkinson's disease patients (Bokobza et al. 1984; but see Rinne 1982).

From these data it appears that the increase in D2 receptors in response to neuroleptic treatment in nonschizophrenic subjects is small. It is interesting to compare the magnitude of the increase in D2 receptors in schizophrenics (= 100% of control) with that of other neuroleptic-treated patients, and neuroleptic-treated experimental animals, where D2 receptor increases vary between 30% and 60% above controls (Muller and Seeman 1978; Owen et al. 1980). The increase in dopamine receptors observed in schizophrenic patients with a history of chronic neuroleptic intake is thus considerably greater than would be expected from other data. In a smaller number of patients, dopamine D1 receptors quantitated with ^{3}H-piflutixol as ligand were within the control range in neuroleptic-free and neuroleptic-treated schizophrenics (data not shown).

3 Dopaminergic Function and Dyskinesia in Schizophrenics

The concentrations of dopamine and its metabolites DOPAC and HVA were unchanged in the putamen, nucleus accumbens, and substantia nigra of schizophrenics (Table 3). When analysed on the basis of presence or absence of movement disorder, schizophrenics with movement disorder had significantly higher concentrations of HVA in putamen and nucleus accumens compared with controls. This effect was not seen in the substantia nigra (Table 3). The concentrations of dopamine and the minor metabolite DOPAC were unchanged in all brain regions studied.

Dopamine D2 receptors assessed as the binding of ^{3}H-spiperone were increased in the total schizophrenic group compared with controls. There were no differences in D2 receptors between patients with and without movement disor-

Table 3. Dopamine and its metabolites in schizophrenics[a]

	Dopamine	DOPAC	HVA
Putamen			
Control ($n = 12$)	16.7 ± 2.4	3.0 ± 0.3	45.0 ± 3.5
AIMs present ($n = 7$)	14.4 ± 3.4	5.1 ± 1.3	64.5 ± 5.4[c]
AIMs absent ($n = 7$)	20.7 ± 5.2	3.8 ± 2.0	42.1 ± 3.9
N. accumbens			
Control ($n = 7$)	11.4 ± 3.1	3.6 ± 0.7	56.2 ± 3.8
AIMs present ($n = 5$)	16.3 ± 3.4	3.7 ± 0.8	105 ± 25[b]
AIMs absent ($n = 5$)	13.1 ± 0.7	3.8 ± 1.4	65 ± 15
S. nigra			
Control ($n = 11$)	2.6 ± 0.7	—	30.8 ± 1.6
AIMs present ($n = 6$)	3.5 ± 0.5	—	47.6 ± 6.3
AIMs absent ($n = 5$)	4.4 ± 1.0	—	47.0 ± 8.2

[a] Values are ng/mg protein, mean ± SEM
[b] $P < 0.05$
[c] $P < 0.01$ vs controls

Table 4. Dopamine receptors[a] and movement disorder in schizophrenics

	Control	Schizophrenics with AIMs	Schizophrenics without AIMs
Dopamine D1 receptors			
Putamen	458 ± 33 (11)	403 ± 48 (6)	432 ± 69 (6)
N. accumbens	327 ± 36 (7)	441 ± 72 (8)	372 ± 65 (5)
S. nigra	120 ± 9 (11)	88 ± 19 (6)	122 ± 42 (4)
Dopamine D2 receptors			
Putamen	128 ± 10 (11)	280 ± 20 (7)	250 ± 11 (7)
N. accumbens	107 ± 16 (5)	171 ± 17 (6)	216 ± 30 (5)

[a] Dopamine D1 receptors were determined with the aid of 1.5 n*M* ^{3}H-piflutixol and D2 receptors with 1.2 n*M* ^{3}H-spiperone as described previously (Cross and Rossor 1983). Values are fmol ligand bound/mg protein, mean ± SEM; number of samples is given in parentheses in each case

der, in any of the brain regions studied (Table 4). As shown in an earlier study (Cross et al. 1981), dopamine D1 receptors were within the control range in the total schizophrenic group, and again were unrelated to the presence of movement disorder (Table 4).

4 Chemical Correlates of Structural Changes in Schizophrenics with Movement Disorder

We have assessed the integrity of a number of neurochemical markers known to be associated with specific groups of neurones in the basal ganglia. The concentrations of GABA, a reliable post-mortem marker of GABA neurones, were lower in the caudate nucleus of patients with movement disorder than of patients without movement disorder (Table 5). This difference, however, was due to an increase in GABA concentrations in schizophrenics without movement disorder compared with controls. GABA concentrations were unchanged in both groups in all other brain regions studied (Table 5). Choline acetyltransferase, the marker

Table 5. GABA concentrations[a] and movement disorder in schizophrenics

Brain region	Controls ($n = 21-48$)	Schizophrenics with AIMs ($n = 11$)	Schizophrenics without AIMs ($n = 9$)
Caudate nucleus	33.4 ± 2.2	32.9 ± 4.0[b]	59.2 ± 9.0[c]
Lateral globus pallidus	53.5 ± 4.5	60.0 ± 9.9	63.4 ± 7.6
Medial globus pallidus	44.7 ± 2.7	48.5 ± 4.5	49.0 ± 3.9
Nucleus accumbens	33.0 ± 1.8	31.5 ± 4.3	31.4 ± 3.4
Substantia nigra	30.8 ± 1.9	36.2 ± 3.8	45.7 ± 5.3

[a] GABA concentration were determined by a radioreceptor assay; values are expressed as 0,7 nmol/mg protein, mean ± SEM
[b] $P < 0.05$ vs schizophrenic with AIMs
[c] $P < 0.01$ vs controls

enzyme of cholinergic neurones, was no different in schizophrenics than in controls, and was unrelated to the presence of movement disorder. Similar results were obtained for high-affinity ligand binding to GABA and muscarinic cholinergic receptors (data not shown). In the same series of post-mortem brains the neuropeptides cholecystokinin, substance P, neurotensin, somatostatin, and vasoactive intestinal polypeptide were measured as markers of peptidergic neurones. No consistent relationship between peptide concentrations and movement disorder was found (Ferrier et al, unpublished observations).

5 Conclusions

The post-mortem studies described in the present report clearly demonstrate that schizophrenics who have received prolonged treatment with high doses of neuroleptics have increased numbers of dopamine D2 receptor in basal ganglia compared with controls or drug-free schizophrenics. It should be noted, however, that D2 receptors in drug-free schizophrenics are also significantly elevated above controls. Furthermore, no causal relationship between increased dopamine D2 receptors in schizophrenics and prior neuroleptic treatment can be assumed, as the patients were not randomly allocated to treatment groups. No association was observed between the presence of dyskinesia and dopamine D1 or D2 receptors in several basal ganglia regions of brains from schizophrenics. Moreover, in those patients with abnormal involuntary movements no relationship was observed between either D1 or D2 receptors and the severity of movement disorder. These results confirm and extend our previous studies of dopamine receptors in movement disorder (Crow et al. 1983).

In agreement with previous studies (Bacapoulos et al. 1979; Crow et al. 1978), dopamine metabolism in basal ganglia of schizophrenics was unaffected by chronic neuroleptic intake. The concentrations of HVA were selectively elevated in putamen and nucleus accumbens of those schizophrenics with dyskinesia: this effect was not seen in substantia nigra. These differences in HVA concentrations are unlikely to be due to differences in CSF clearance of acids or in MAO activity, as DOPAC (and 5HIAA, data not shown) concentrations were unchanged. Such increased HVA concentrations may therefore reflect increased release and metabolism of dopamine in those patients with dyskinesia. It should be stressed that the number of samples studied was small; nonetheless, the relevance of increased dopamine metabolism to the presence of dyskinesia warrants further study.

No relationships were found between markers of GABA-, acetylcholine-, and peptide-containing neurones and the presence of dyskinesia. Thus neurochemical correlates of structural brain changes in dyskinetic patients remain to be determined.

References

Bacopoulos NC, Spokes EG, Bird ED, Roth RH (1979) Antipsychotic drug action in schizophrenic patients: effect on cortical dopamine metabolism after long-term treatment. Science 205:1405–1407

Bokobza B, Ruberg M, Scatton B, Javoy-Agid F, Agid Y (1984) ^{3}H-spiperone binding, dopamine and HVA concentrations in Parkinson's disease and supranuclear palsy. Eur J Pharmacol 99:167–175

Brandon S, McClelland HA, Protheroe C (1971) A study of facial dyskinesia in a mental hospital population. Br J Psychiatry 118:171–184

Cross AJ, Joseph MH (1981) The concurrent estimation of the major monoamine metabolites in human and non-human primate brain by HPLC with fluorescence and electrochemical detection. Life Sci 28:499–505

Cross AJ, Rossor M (1983) Dopamine D1 and D2 receptors in Huntington's disease. Eur J Pharmacol 88:223–229

Cross AJ, Crow TJ, Owen F (1981) ^{3}H-flupenthixol binding in the brains of schizophrenics: evidence for a selective increase of dopamine D2 receptors. Psychopharmacology 74:122–124

Crow TJ, Baker HF, Cross AJ, Joseph MH, Lofthouse R, Longden A, Owen F, Riley GJ, Glover V, Killpack W, Dahlstrom S (1978) Monoamines in chronic schizophrenia. Br J Psychiatry 134:249–256

Crow TJ, Owens DGC, Johnstone EC, Cross AJ, Owen F (1983) Does tardive dyskinesia exist? Mod Probl Pharmacopsychiatry 21:206–219

Marsden CD, Jenner P (1980) The pathophysiology of extrapyramidal side effects of neuroleptic drugs. Psychol Med 10:55–72

Muller P, Seeman P (1978) Dopaminergic supersensitivity after neuroleptics: time course and specificity. Psychopharmacology 60:1–11

Owen F, Cross AJ, Crow TJ, Longden A, Poulter M, Riley GJ (1978) Increased dopamine-receptor sensitivity in schizophrenia. Lancet II:223–226

Owen F, Cross AJ, Waddington JL, Poulter M, Gamble SJ, Crow TJ (1980) Dopamine-mediated behavior and ^{3}H-spiperone binding to striatal membranes in rats after nine months haloperidol administration. Life Sci 26:55–59

Owens DGC, Johnstone EC, Frith CD (1982) Spontaneous involuntary disorders of movement in neuroleptic treated and untreated chronic schizophrenics – prevalence, severity and distributions. Arch Gen Psychiatry 39:452–461

Rinne UK (1982) Brain dopamine receptors in Parkinson's disease. In: Marsden CD, Fahn S (eds) Movement disorders. Butterworth, London, pp 59–74

Tarsy D, Baldessarini RJ (1977) The pathophysiologic basis of tardive dyskinesia. Biol Psychiatry 12:431–450

Medical Treatment of Dystonia

H. Pakkenberg and B. Pedersen [1]

Contents

Abstract 111
1 Introduction 111
2 Dystonia Musculorum Deformans and Segmental Dystonia 112
3 Focal Dystonia 114
3.1 Meige's Syndrome 114
3.2 Torticollis 116
3.3 Dystonic Dysphonia 116
References 116

Abstract

We review dystonia treatment results since 1981, including our own findings. Anticholinergics are still the most effective drugs, but less than 50% of patients continue with treatment. The authors recommend a combination of an anticholinergic, a benzodiazepine, and another drug (an antidopaminergic, carbamazepine, or fluperlapine) for the treatment of dystonia.

1 Introduction

Many papers on the treatment of dystonia begin by emphasizing the difficulties, especially the many failures. However, dystonia is so troublesome for many patients that the many trials necessitated are justified in the search for an effective treatment. When more than a slight measure of relief is afforded the inevitable side-effects are acceptable to many patients. Patients with slight dystonia should not be treated, as the side-effects of the drugs will be more unpleasant than the disease (Marsden and Fahn 1982).

In several types of dyskinesia diagnosis is difficult. Many patients are treated for several years by non-neurologists (e.g., the Tourette syndrome for 8 years; Pakkenberg et al. 1982) before the correct diagnosis is made. The most common misdiagnosis is hysteria but, as emphasized by Marsden and Fahn (1982), hysterical movement disorders are very rare. Were this fact better known to most psychiatrists, many patients would have been helped earlier.

As Marsden reviewed the treatment of dystonia in 1981, only later papers will be mentioned here.

1 Department of Neurology, Hvidovre University Hospital, DK-2650 Hvidovre, Denmark

Dyskinesia – Research and Treatment
(Psychopharmacology Supplementum 2)
Editors: Casey, Chase, Christensen, Gerlach

2 Dystonia Musculorum Deformans and Segmental Dystonia

Although the drugs used in generalized and in focal dystonia are the same, there are some differences of effect in the different groups.

Anticholinergics are still the most widely used drugs, especially trihexyphenidyl. There is no "maximum dose"; the dose should be increased to the point of optimal effect or unacceptable side-effects. Fahn (1983 a, b) used increasing doses of trihexyphenidyl in the treatment of 11 children and 13 adults with generalized dystonia; 8 of the 11 children and 6 of the 13 adults improved significantly. Of 10 children and 12 adults with segmental dystonia, 6 children and 5 adults improved. Since 1979, the author has used ethopropazine for all adults. The average daily dose of trihexyphenidyl was about 40 mg, and that of ethopropazine about 350 mg. Side-effects were the major factor limiting dose increase in adults, but not in children.

Burke and Fahn (1983) made a double-blind evaluation of trihexyphenidyl. Eleven patients entered the trial, and six were evaluated. All six improved, five of whom were patients with generalized dystonia. The dose was 30 mg/day.

Tardive dyskinesias have been known for decades (Faurbye et al. 1964). Burke et al. (1982) described 42 patients with tardive dystonia following psychopharmacological treatment. They emphazise that it is not a separate entity, but a special type of tardive dyskinesia, which usually starts years after, but may appear within only a few days of commencement of psychopharmacological treatment. Clinically, the picture is like idiopathic torsion dystonia or secondary dystonia (torticollis, blepharospasm, Meige's syndrome). Tetrabenazine (68% improved) and anticholinergics (39% improved) were of benefit.

Another interesting special type is myoclonic dystonia. Obeso et al. (1983) examined 14 patients with a combination of myoclonia and dystonia, and found that in most cases the same muscles were involved in myoclonus and dystonia. Other types of dyskinesias were often suspected. The myoclonia were thought to originate from a subcortical focus. Several drugs were used for the combined symptoms, but with little success.

Our Own Experience. As Table 1 shows, our four patients with generalized dystonia were all treated with three drugs. If one drug was discontinued the patient's status deteriorated to a greater or lesser extent, especially in patient 3. In patient 4, fluperlapine has stabilized the improvement obtained with the other two drugs (trihexyphenidyl, clonazepam). Our impression is that it is often necessary, in the treatment of these two groups of dystonia, to use two or three drugs to ensure a lasting effect. A possible explanation might be that, to obtain a lasting improvement, more than one mechanism of the neurotransmitter effect must be affected (Fog and Pakkenberg 1970), because many single drugs produce short-term effects. Three of the four patients are still taking a benzodiazepine preparation, which is often a useful supplement to an anticholinergic.

Table 1. Results[a] of treatment in patients with generalized (G) or segmental dystonia

Patient no.	Age	Duration	Distribution	Treatment (mg/day)										Treatment now
				Trihexyphenidyl	Tetrabenazine	Pimozide	Diazepam	Clonazepam	Valproate	Carbamazepine	Fluperlapin	Dopa	Other drugs	
1	30	25	G				++ 20						Baclofen 100	Baclofen 100; diazepam 20
2	22	10	G	++ 30	0 150	0 3	0 15	+ 12	+ 1800	0 rash		0 600		Tetrabenazine 75; trihexyphen 45; clonazepam 12
3	52	10	G		++ 75	++ 3		+ 4						Clonazepam, pimozide, tetrabenazine
4	11	5	G	(++) 35						(++) 750	+ 100			Trihexyphen 35; fluperlapin 100; carbamazepin 750
5	14	4	Feet	++ 50						+ 800		0 190		Trihexyphen 50
6	38	4	Hands, neck	0 35		0 75		0 6				0 750		0
7	48	4	Hands	(+++) 25	(+++) 37		(++) 15	(+++) 1.5			++ 30			Trihexyphen 30; clonazepam 5; fluperlapin 60

[a] +, slight improvement; ++, moderate improvement; +++, free of symptoms; ( ), transitory effect

3 Focal Dystonia

3.1 Meige's Syndrome

Since Marsden (1976) described 39 patients with Brueghel's syndrome, interest in this peculiar condition has increased. Tolosa (1981) described 17 patients, and a family history of dystonia, a high rate of depression, and dystonia in other regions of the body were frequently found. Spontaneous improvements would occur for some years; other neurological abnormalities suggesting basal ganglia dysfunction were common.

Jankovic and Ford (1983) collated 100 patients with this syndrome. In their sample, 61 patients had the complete syndrome and 60 had neck or generalized dystonia together with the orofacial symptoms; 21 patients had spasmodic dysphonia. Essential tremor and other movement disorders were often seen in Meige's syndrome, and an organic cause was suspected.

Some improvement was seen in 69% of the treated patients, and in 22% the improvement was marked. Tetrabenazine, lithium, and trihexyphenidyl were most useful for dystonia, and clonazepam for blepharospasm.

The effectiveness of three anticholinergic drugs, with somewhat differing central actions, was tested in adult-onset focal dystonias (Lang et al. 1982). An acute study was performed with atropine, benztropine, and chlorpheniramine, given IV to 20 patients with various forms of idiopathic focal or segmental adult-onset dystonia. None of the three drugs significantly improved the six patients with Meige's syndrome. In a retrospective study with chronic PO administration, 4 of 25 patients with Meige's syndrome improved, and 3 patients deteriorated. Tanner et al. (1982) found that 6 patients studied acutely during scopolamine treatment improved. Of 13 patients, 12 were treated with benztropine or trihexyphenidyl for several months and 10 improved for 3–12 months while 2 responded for less than 3 months. It is concluded that Meige's syndrome is pharmacologically similar to other dystonic syndromes and that central cholinergic antagonism is more consistently of benefit than is an influence on dopaminergic systems. However, following experiments with L-dopa, benztropine, and deanol in two patients, Casey (1980) suggested that cholinergic agents were less efficient than dopaminergic drugs. Marsden et al. (1983) comment on these ideas by emphasizing that their own experiences do not allow them to conclude that manipulation with any of the two neurotransmitter systems will give a *consistent* response. Meige's syndrome has been described by Weiner and Nausieda (1982) in two patients with Parkinson's disease who were treated for 1 and 2 years with L-dopa/carbidopa. These authors think that the dystonia is a result of altered dopaminergic mechanisms in the parkinsonian brain. Stahl and Berger (1982) studied eight patients by administering agonists and antagonists of acetylcholine and dopamine. Seven patients receiving physostigmine deteriorated; six patients receiving anticholinergic agents improved; and five of eight patients treated with bromocriptine improved. They concluded that an imbalance between the dopamine and acetylcholine systems may explain the dystonia in some patients.

Nutt et al. (1983) found that of seven patients in an open study three improved, but in a double-blind study of five patients treated with tridihexethyl

Table 2. Results[a] of treatment in patients with Meige's syndrome (M), torticollis (T), or focal dystonia

Patient no.	Age	Duration	Distribution	Treatment (mg/day)									
				Trihexyphenidyl	Tetrabenazine	Pimozide	Diazepam	Clonazepam	Carbamazepine	Tiapride	Dopa	Other drugs	Treatment now
8	49	3	M					+ + + 6					Clonazepam 6
9	75	16	M + legs	0 20	(+) 75	(+) 3		0 9					Trihexyphen 15; clonazepam 4
10	59	9	M	0 30	0 75	0 4	0 60		0	0 900	0 600	Propanolol 80 (+) Deanol 0	Clonazepam 6
11	66	3	M	(+ +) 20	+ 50	(+ + +) 3				+ + 400	(+ + +) 750		Tiapride 100
12	69	8	T	(+ +) 30		0 12	0 15		0 600			Amitriptyline 75 0	0
13	60	13	T		0 75	0 9	0 40			0 600			0
14	40	4	T		0 37	0 3				0 600		Amantadine 200 0	Biofeedback
15	34	2	T	0 30	0 150	0 6					0 300		0
16	29	4	T		0 75						+ 600		Biofeedback
17	55	2	Writer's cramp + tremor								0 750	Propanolol 30 0	Propanolol 160
18	23	11	Tongue dystonia during speech		0 75	0 6							

[a] +, slight improvement; + +, moderate improvement; + + +, free of symptoms; ( ), transitory effect

chloride or trihexyphenidyl, no significant improvement was found. Finally, Gollomp et al. (1983), in 43 Meige's syndrome patients, found significant effect of different drugs in 21 patients (8/23 with haloperidol, 7/18 with tetra benazine, and 4/9 with anticholinergics).

Knowledge of the pathology of dystonia is still limited. However, in a case of Meige's syndrome, Altrocchi and Forno (1983) found changes in the dorsal halves of the caudate and putamen, with an uneven loss of nerve cells accompanied by severe gliosis and narrowing of the fiber tracts giving a mosaic appearance. The only previous pathological study (Garcia-Albea et al. 1981) of a patient with Meige's syndrome revealed no abnormality in the basal ganglia or elsewhere. The new case, therefore, is especially interesting, although more cases must be examined before any conclusions can be drawn.

Our Own Experience. Our unsystematic trials in four patients demonstrate the confusion once again. Some drugs give excellent short-term results, but only one patient has remained symptom-free. One patient with severe symptoms improved dramatically with amitriptyline, but within a week the syndrome had reappeared. Still, we find it worthwhile to try the long list of drugs that may have an effect, because socially the disease is a severe handicap.

3.2 Torticollis

Only a limited number of patients with torticollis have been evaluated since 1981. Lang et al. (1982) did not find any significant effect of anticholinergics in an acute study of 9 patients, while 9/38 patients in a chronic study showed some improvement. Fahn (1983 a) reported that 6 of 16 patients improved in a long-term study with anticholinergics.

Our Own Experience. Of five patients with torticollis one responded to trihexyphenidyl, but no other drug had any convincing effect. Two patients are currently undergoing biofeedback treatment. This type of dystonia is one of the most difficult for which to provide relief.

3.3 Dystonic Dysphonia

Marsden (1981) mentions this rare type of dystonia. He does not find medical treatment efficient, but unilateral section of one recurrent laryngeal nerve can improve speech. We have only observed one patient with dystonic protrusion of the tongue on speech; neither tetrabenzine nor pimozide was effective.

References

Altrocchi PH, Forno LS (1983) Spontaneous oral-facial dyskinesia: Neuropathology of a case. Neurology 33:802–805

Burke R, Fahn S (1983) Double-blind evaluation of trihexyphenidyl in dystonia. In: Fahn S, Calne D, Shoulson I (eds) Experimental therapeutics of movement disorders. Raven, New York, pp 189–192

Burke RE, Fahn S, Jankovic J, Marsden CD, Lang AE, Gollomp S, Ilson J (1982) Tardive dystonia and inappropriate use of neuroleptic drugs. Lancet I:1299
Casey DE (1980) Pharmacology of blepharospasm-oromandibular dystonia syndrome. Neurology 30:690–695
Fahn S (1983a) High-dosage anticholinergic therapy in dystonia. In: Fahn S, Calne D, Shoulson I (eds) Experimental therapeutics of movement disorders. Raven, New York, pp 177–188
Fahn S (1983b) High dosage anticholinergic therapy in dystonia. Neurology 33:1255–1261
Faurbye A, Rasch PJ, Bender Petersen P, Brandborg G, Pakkenberg H (1964) Neurological symptoms in pharmacotherapy of psychosis. Acta Psychiatry Scand 40:10–27
Fog R, Pakkenberg H (1970) Combined nitoman-pimozide treatment of Huntington's chorea and other hyperkinetic syndromes. Acta Neurol Scand 46:249–251
Garcia-Albea E, Franch O, Munoz D, Recoy JR (1981) Brueghel's syndrome, report of a case with postmortem studies. J Neurol Neurosurg Psychiatry 44:437–440
Gollomp SM, Fahn S, Bush R, Recher A, Ilson J (1983) Therapeutic trial in Meige's syndrome. In: Fahn S, Calne D, Shoulson I (eds) Experimental therapeutics of movement disorders. Raven, New York, pp 207–214
Jankovic J, Ford J (1983) Blepharospasm and orofacialcervical dystonia: clinical and pharmacological findings in 100 patients. Ann Neurol 13:402–411
Lang AE, Sheehy MP, Marsden CD (1982) Anticholinergics in adult-onset focal dystonia. J Can Sci Neurol 9:313–319
Marsden CD (1976) Blepharospasm-oromandibular dystonia syndrome (Brueghel's syndrome). J Neurol Neurosurg Psychiatry 37:1204–1209
Marsden CD (1981) Treatment of torsion dystonia. In: Barbeau A (ed) Disorders of movement. MTP Press, Lancaster, pp 81–104
Marsden CD, Fahn S (1982) Problems in dyskinesias. In: Marsden CD, Fahn S (eds) Movement disorders. Butterworth, London, pp 191–195
Marsden CD, Lang AE, Sheehy MP (1983) Pharmacology of cranial dystonia. Neurology 33:1100–1101
Nutt JG, Hammerstad JP, Carter JH, DeGarmo P (1983) Meige's syndrome: treatment with trihexiphenidyl. Adv Neurol 37:201–205
Obeso JA, Rothwell JC, Lange AE, Marsden CD (1983) Myoclonic dystonia. Neurology 33:825–830
Pakkenberg B, Regeur L, Fog R, Pakkenberg H (1982) Gilles de la Tourette's syndrom. Ugeskr Læger 144:3078–3080
Stahl SM, Berger PA (1982) Bromocriptine, physostigmine, and neurotransmitter mechanisms in the dystonias. Neurology 32:889–892
Tanner CM, Glantz RH, Klawans HL (1982) Meige's disease: acute and chronic cholinergic effects. Neurology 32:783–784
Tolosa ES (1981) Clinical features of Meige's disease. Arch Neurol 38:147–151
Weiner WJ, Nausieda PA (1982) Meige's syndrome during long-term dopaminergic therapy in Parkinson's disease. Arch Neurol 39:451–452

The Effect of Dopamine Antagonists in Spontaneous and Tardive Dyskinesia

R. Fog[1]

Contents

Abstract 118
1 Introduction 118
2 Therapeutic Effect of DA Antagonists 118
3 Side-Effects 119
4 Future Treatment Strategies 120
References 120

Abstract

Dopamine antagonists are effective in suppressing hyperkinetic symptoms in patients with tardive dyskinesia, spontaneous oral dyskinesia, Huntington's chorea, and Gilles de la Tourette's syndrome. These neuroleptics have no curative effect upon the conditions and may even aggravate symptoms in the long term. In many cases a single neuroleptic drug may lose its effect. A more lasting effect may be obtained by combining drugs with pre- and postsynaptic antidopamine effects.

1 Introduction

The etiology and the pathogenesis of the various hyperkinetic syndromes are still unknown. Although it must be considered a fact that neuroleptic drugs can induce tardive dyskinesia, it is necessary to proceed with a certain native caution in those (few) patients who develop this syndrome. In Huntington's chorea there is a known genetic factor and in Gilles de la Tourette's syndrome "minimal brain damage" can be demonstrated in some cases. Still, there are some "spontaneous" dyskinesias such as the bucco-lingual masticatory syndrome seen in old age.

This paper will deal with the results of antidopaminergic treatment of tardive dyskinesia, spontaneous oral dyskinesia, Gilles de la Tourette's syndrome, and Huntington's chorea.

2 Therapeutic Effect of DA Antagonists

The treatment of hyperkinesias with DA antagonists is theoretically based upon the dopamine hypothesis of movement disorders developed by Carlsson et al. (1967). These workers suggested a relative overactivity of dopamine in the basal

1 Laboratory of Psychopharmacology, Saint Hans Mental Hospital, DK-4000 Roskilde, Denmark

Dyskinesia – Research and Treatment
(Psychopharmacology Supplementum 2)
Editors: Casey, Chase, Christensen, Gerlach

ganglia in hyperkinetic syndromes such as Huntington's chorea and a relatively reduced dopamine activity in hypokinetic syndromes such as parkinsonism. The questions of a change in dopamine metabolism, content, sensitivity, or number of receptors have still not been solved, but it is an unquestionable fact that DA-antagonistic drugs have a beneficial effect upon hyperkinetic symptoms. However, they have no curative effects upon the disease and in some cases (at least hypothetically) may even worsen the symptoms in the long term.

Tetrabenazine was one of the first neuroleptic drugs to be used in hyperkinetic syndromes (Brandrup 1961). It has a presynaptic antidopamine effect because of its inhibiting effect upon dopamine storage in the nerve terminals. In clinical use tetrabenazine has fewer side-effects than reserpine (Fog and Pakkenberg 1980b).

Neuroleptic drugs with a postsynaptic blocking effect upon dopamine have also been widely used against hyperkinesias. Their clinical profile in different syndromes are slightly different (Stahl and Berger 1982); but as a general rule "specific" neuroleptics from the low-dose range (such as haloperidol and pimozide, which seem to have a special affinity for striatal dopamine) are more effective than sedative high-dose drugs (such as thioridazine and clozapine, which seem to have more affinity for limbic dopamine).

In many cases the clinical effect upon the hyperkinetic symptoms diminishes after weeks or months (Fog and Pakkenberg 1980) if only one neuroleptic drug is used. In some cases the effect totally disappears, and an increased dose will then only give a short-lasting effect, and in many cases also induce side-effects.

A combination treatment with neuroleptic drugs having different (i.e., presynaptic and postsynaptic) antidopamine properties (e.g., tetrabenazine plus pimozide) has a more lasting effect and fewer side-effects, because both drugs can be given in lower doses. The effect was better in Huntington's chorea than in tardive dyskinesia (Fog and Pakkenberg 1980b). In spontaneous oral dyskinesia the effect of the combination was best upon pure oral symptoms (Fog and Pakkenberg 1980b). In Gilles de la Tourette's syndrome this treatment was very effective in about 70% of the cases (Pakkenberg et al. 1982).

Combinations of presynaptically acting drugs (reserpine, α-methyltyrosine, tetrabenazine) have also been used (Fahn 1983) against tardive dyskinesia with rather good results.

All known neuroleptic drugs have antidopamine effects. The choice of drug should depend upon the patient's mental state: a sedative "side-effect" might be desirable in an aggressive schizophrenic patient with tardive dyskinesia, but might aggravate a confusional state in a senile patient with a spontaneous oral dyskinesia, and inhibit learning in a child with Gilles de la Tourette's syndrome.

3 Side-Effects

All neuroleptic drugs (except clozapine) can induce tardive dyskinesia, even in low doses and even in young individuals. It should be emphasized again that these drugs merely suppress hyperkinetic symptoms, and that they may aggravate the condition in the long term. The smallest possible dose should therefore be used over the shortest possible time.

In Gilles de la Tourette's syndrome it is rather easy to evaluate the side-effects of neuroleptic treatment, because these patients are not psychiatrically ill. Apart from the motor inhibition (parkinsonism) induced by a too high dose, the most common side-effects are withdrawal, anhedonia, sadness, and reduced intellectual performance (Bruun 1982).

In animal studies a neurotoxic effect upon neurons in the basal ganglia has been demonstrated (Fog and Pakkenberg 1980a) and these findings may be related to irreversible tardive dyskinesia in clinical practice or to tardive Tourette syndrome (Fog et al. 1982).

4 Future Treatment Strategies

In the basal ganglia there is a balance between dopaminergic and cholinergic mechanisms. Instead of blocking dopamine it might be useful to stimulate acetylcholine. Until now such trials have not been very successful (Chien 1980).

Dopamine might also be antagonized in substantia nigra with GABAergic drugs, but so far drugs with a specific action upon these structures have not been available (Gerlach et al. 1980).

These types of investigations, and also trials of peptide interaction with brain dopamine, are dealt with by Casey and Tamminga et al. (this volume).

A very interesting trial concerning dopamine receptor sensitivity modification has been performed by Alpert et al. (1983), who treated patients with tardive dyskinesia with dopamine agonists (L-dopa) for 1 or 2 months. A slight expectable exacerbation of symptoms was observed during treatment, but when L-dopa was stopped a marked improvement was seen in about half the patients. The same procedure has also been used in the treatment of patients with Gilles de la Tourette's syndrome (Friedhoff 1982) and improvements were seen.

These experiments may lead to better treatments for the patients, but also to a better understanding of the brain mechanisms behind hyperkinetic syndromes.

References

Alpert M, Friedhoff AJ, Diamond F (1983) Use of dopamine receptor agonists to reduce dopamine receptor number as treatment for tardive dyskinesia. In: Fahn S, Calne DB, Shoulson I (eds) Experimental therapeutics of movement disorders. Raven, New York, pp 253–266

Brandrup E (1961) Tetrabenazine treatment in persisting dyskinesia caused by psychopharmaca. Am J Psychiatry 118:551–552

Bruun RD (1982) Dysphoric phenomena associated with haloperidol treatment of Tourette syndrome. In: Friedhoff AJ, Chase TN (eds) Gilles de la Tourette syndrome. Raven, New York, pp 433–436

Carlsson A, Lundquist M, Magnusson T (1967) 3,4-dehydroxyphenalanine and 5-hydroxtryptophan as reserpine antagonists. Nature 180:1200

Chien CP (1980) Tardive dyskinesia: controlled studies of several therapeutic agents. In: Fann WE, Smith RC, Davis JM, Domino EF (eds) Tardive dyskinesia. Spectrum, New York, pp 429–469

Fahn S (1983) Long-term treatment of tardive dyskinesia with presynaptically acting dopamine-depleting agents. In: Fahn S, Calne DB, Shoulson I (eds) Experimental therapeutics of movement disorders. Raven, New York, pp 267–276

Fog R, Pakkenberg H (1980a) Anatomical and metabolic changes after long and short-term treatment with perphenazine in rats. In: Fann WE, Smith RC, Davis JM, Domino EF (eds) Tardive dyskinesia. Spectrum, New York, pp 89–93

Fog R, Pakkenberg H (1980b) Combination treatment of choreiform and dyskinetic syndromes with tetrabenazine and pimozide. In: Fann WE, Smith RC, Davis JM, Domino EF (eds) Tardive dyskinesia. Spectrum, New York, pp 507–510

Fog R, Pakkenberg H, Regeur L, Pakkenberg B (1982) "Tardive" Tourette syndrome in relation to long-term neuroleptic treatment of multiple tics. In: Friedhoff AJ, Chase TN (eds) Gilles de la Tourette syndrome. Raven, New York, pp 419–421

Friedhoff AJ (1982) Receptor maturation in pathogenesis and treatment of Tourette syndrome. In: Friedhoff AJ, Chase TN (eds) Gilles de la Tourette syndrome. Raven, New York, pp 133–140

Gerlach J, Kristjansen P, Rye T (1980) Effect of haloperidol, haloperidol + biperiden, thioridazine, clozapine, alpha-methyl-p-tyrosine, and baclofen on tardive dyskinesia. In: Fann WE, Smith RC, Davis JM, Domino EF (eds) Tardive dyskinesia. Spectrum, New York, pp 497–506

Pakkenberg H, Regeur L, Fog R, Pakkenberg B (1982) A follow-up study of 12 patients with Tourette syndrome. Acta Neurol Scand 65:234–235

Stahl SM, Berger PA (1982) Cholinergic and dopaminergic mechanisms in Tourette syndrome. In: Friedhoff AJ, Chase TN (eds) Gilles de la Tourette syndrome. Raven, New York, pp 141–150

GABA Dysfunction in the Pathophysiology of Tardive Dyskinesia

C. A. Tamminga, G. K. Thaker, and T. N. Chase [1]

Contents

Abstract 122
1 Introduction 122
2 Dopamine System 123
3 GABA System 123
4 Conclusions 125
References 126

Abstract

Pharmacologic treatments which diminish central dopaminergic transmission improve symptoms of tardive dyskinesia (TD). These clinical data, supported by results from animal model studies, have provided a basis for the dopamine (DA) receptor hypersensitivity hypothesis of TD. Since its initial formulation, however, knowledge of the multiple effects of prolonged neuroleptic administration in mammalian CNS has greatly expanded. Clinical and animal model studies carried out independently now both suggest that GABA-mediated neuronal tracts of the basal ganglia are important, perhaps pivotal, in TD. Thus, we would extend the DA hypothesis of TD to include the idea that neuroleptic-induced DA receptor hypersensitivity in striatum results in GABA system hypofunction in striatal projection areas in those individuals who develop TD.

1 Introduction

Strategies for the rational development of effective pharmacologic treatments for tardive dyskinesia (TD) depend on a clear understanding of the pathophysiologic mechanisms. Although TD is most often associated with chronic neuroleptic administration, precisely how these drugs induce hyperkinetic symptoms remains a matter of conjecture. Nevertheless, studies of animal models, which now rather convincingly replicate the human disorder, have provided a number of important insights. In general, these preclinical studies support the dopamine (DA) receptor hypersensitivity hypothesis of TD (Klawans and Rubovits 1974; Tarsy and Baldessarini 1973). According to this theory, TD symptoms reflect an enhancement of DA-mediated neural transmission due to a neuroleptic-stimulated proliferation and sensitization of the postsynaptic DA receptors. Incontrovertible evidence now supports the occurrence of enhanced sensitivity of central DA recep-

1 Maryland Psychiatric Research Center, University of Maryland, Baltimore, MD 21228, USA and the Experimental Therapeutics Branch, National Institute of Neurological and Communicative Disorders and Stroke, Bethesda, MD 20205, USA

Dyskinesia – Research and Treatment
(Psychopharmacology Supplementum 2)
Editors: Casey, Chase, Christensen, Gerlach

tors following chronic neuroleptic exposure in the experimental animal (Cattabeni et al. 1980; Burt et al. 1977; Clow et al. 1978). Furthermore, the clinical pharmacology of TD is compatible with the DA hypersensitivity hypothesis (Chase and Tamminga 1980).

2 Dopamine System

Drugs which diminish DA-mediated transmission by any mechanism improve TD. Those compounds which act centrally to block postsynaptic DA receptors reduce dyskinetic symptoms; indeed, these drugs constitute one of the most effective and widely used approaches to the treatment of severe hyperkinetic symptoms (see the chapter by R. Fog in this volume). Conversely, neuroleptic withdrawal is well known to exacerbate or precipitate dyskinesia. While the use of neuroleptics to treat TD has heretofore been discouraged, recent evidence calls this into question. Little or no progression of symptoms has been noted with ongoing neuroleptic treatment in individuals with the disorder (Casey and Toenniessen 1983). Thus, although these findings will require further confirmation, neuroleptic treatment for TD could become a recommended approach. In addition, other pharmacologic strategies exist, which reduce DA system activity in man and are effective in ameliorating TD. Reserpine improves dyskinetic symptoms, although side-effects often complicate its use. Low-dose DA agonist treatment, directed at DA autoreceptor stimulation, diminishes DA synthesis and release in the experimental animal (Walters and Roth 1976) and possibly also in man (Cutler et al. 1982). The administration of DA agonists, such as apomorphine and piribedil, reduces TD (Smith et al. 1977; Carroll et al. 1977; Tamminga 1979b; Offermeier and Rooyen 1983). Furthermore, preliminary evidence now suggests that the orally active aporphine DA agonist, *n*-propylnorapomorphine, may also suppress hyperkinesis in TD patients (Tamminga and Thaker 1984). Since no truly selective presynaptic DA agonists have yet come to clinical trial, the safety and efficacy of these agents for the symptomatic relief of TD remain to be established.

3 GABA System

The DA hypothesis for TD, despite the support of animal model and clinical pharmacologic studies, no longer seems entirely sufficient to explain the pathogenesis of this disorder. First, characteristics of DA receptor binding in postmortem tissue do not differ between groups of dyskinetic and nondyskinetic schizophrenics all of whom have had long-term neuroleptic exposure. Second, whereas chronic neuroleptic treatment in the experimental animal characteristically produces alterations in DA receptors (Jenner, this volume), TD occurs in only a limited number of neuroleptic-treated individuals; at most, 35%–50% of these patients manifest overt or masked TD (see the chapter by J. M. Kane et al. in this volume; Carpenter et al. 1982), whereas presumably all may have hypersensitive DA receptors (Cross et al. 1983). The discrepancy between the theoretical and actual prevalence implies the existence of an additional factor(s) contributing to the expression of the syndrome. Since TD occurs most often in the elderly, especially in those with antecedent brain dysfunction such as schizophrenia (Kane, this volume), host factors must be considered in any comprehensive theory of pathogenesis. In addition, however, since chronic neuroleptic exposure alters a number of neural systems within the basal ganglia, any one of these could potentially be involved in the pathogenesis of TD.

An expansion of the DA hypersensitivity hypothesis for TD might propose that an interrelated series of changes occur in the basal ganglia with neuroleptic treatment, beginning with DA-receptor blockade in striatum, and extending to secondary biochemical and functional changes in striatal projection areas. Whether the presence of secondary and/or tertiary neural effects discriminates for TD is at present unknown, but evidence does suggest this possibility. Numerous studies have identified alterations in the GABA-mediated striatal efferent projections after chronic neuroleptic administration. Sensitivity of the GABA receptor in substantia nigra is increased with chronic treatment (Gale and Casu 1981), as is the electrophysiologic response of substantia nigra, pars reticulata (SNR) neurons to GABA-ergic stimulation (Waszczak et al. 1980). The substantia nigra, pars reticulata has become identified as a major relay point and processing area for motor information within the basal ganglia. This structure receives a prominent GABA-mediated pathway from the striatum and sends GABA-containing neuronal tracts to premotor areas of the thalamus, tectum, and reticular formation (Beckstead and Frankfurter 1982; Graybiel and Ragsdale 1979), and thus could be pivotal for modifying extrapyramidal motor function (see the chapter by J. Scheel-Krüger and J. Arnt in this volume). However, the regulation of nigral neuronal activity is complex. In the SNR, DA is able to directly modulate GABA-mediated neural actions at a DA receptor, an effect suggesting a role in the nigra for the dendritic release of dopamine (Waszczak and Walters 1983). Furthermore, electrophysiologic evidence suggests that the inhibitory potency of the GABA-mediated striatonigral pathway increases in animals having hypersensitive DA receptors. Specifically, IV administration of apomorphine to an untreated rat produces a mixed firing response in SNR neurons; in contrast, the administration of apomorphine to animals pretreated with 6-hydroxydopamine results in a uniform inhibition of nigra cell firing (Waszczak et al. 1984). In light of these observations, the finding by Gunne (1983) that levels of glutamic acid decarboxylase (GAD) are depleted in the SNR of neuroleptic-treated monkeys who develop dyskinesias but not in similarly treated nondyskinetic monkeys, may be important.

Indeed, clinical pharmacologic data are consistent with the idea that changes in GABA content or its metabolism in basal ganglia nuclei may differentiate between neuroleptic-treated individuals with and without TD, all of whom purportedly have characteristic DA receptor changes. Drugs which are effective GABA agonists in humans, especially when tested in otherwise drug-free individuals, appear to improve TD. Muscimol, perhaps the most specific and potent direct-acting receptor agonist, has been observed to reduce dyskinetic symptoms by over 45% (Table 1). γ-Acetylenic GABA, a GABA transaminase inhibitor, and THIP, which is active at the GABA receptor, reportedly have some but

Table 1. Effect of muscimol on TD. (Tamminga et al. 1979a)

Hour	Percent of baseline score (mean ± SEM)			
	1	2	3	4
Muscimol (9 mg)	74 ± 1.2	55 ± 8	56 ± 10	60 ± 1.5
Placebo	99 ± 2	96 ± 1.3	92 ± 12	115 ± 13

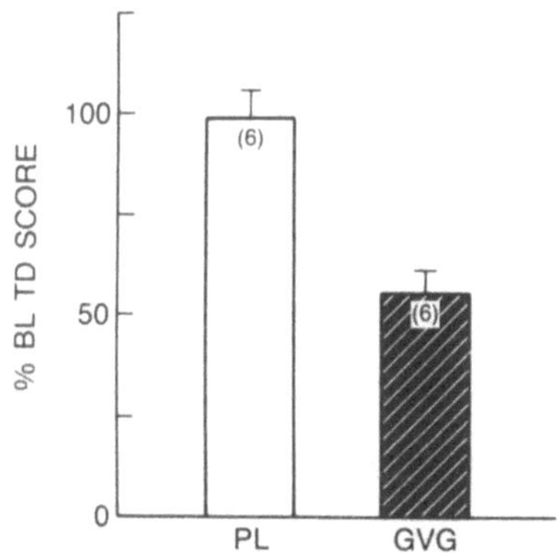

Fig. 1. The effect of oral administration of GVG at a dose of 30υ0 mg daily for 3 weeks, compared with a double-blind, matched, random-assignment placebo period. Seven patients have been included in this study group. Dyskinesia scores dropped significantly from baseline with drug treatment compared with placebo, and returned to baseline with terminal placebo treatment. No alterations in mental status occurred with GVG treatment. (Tamminga et al. 1983)

limited antidyskinetic efficacy (Casey et al. 1980; Korsgaard et al. 1982), although these results may have been influenced by the co-administration of the GABA agonists with neuroleptics. On the other hand, in several recent clinical trials in neuroleptic-treated patients, progabide has been observed to have a significant antidyskinetic activity (see the chapter by P. L. Morselli et al. in this volume).

Initial results obtained with the indirect-acting GABA agonist γ-vinyl-GABA (GVG) lend further support to a significant antidyskinetic action of GABA stimulation. This GABA transaminase inhibitor at a dose of 3 g daily, while elevating CSF GABA levels 2- to 3-fold, diminishes dyskinesias in neuroleptic-free schizophrenics by nearly 48 % (Fig. 1). Preliminary data with THIP administration suggest it has a less potent but still significant antidyskinetic action. In an ongoing attempt to test a more widely available and potentially less toxic treatment, clonazepam in now being evaluated for antidyskinetic efficacy, based on the rationale that benzodiazepines potentiate the action of endogenous GABA. Although the drug's sedative properties complicate the interpretation of antidyskinetic efficacy, we have found clonazepam to suppress symptoms by 29 % in two subjects with TD.

4 Conclusions

These clinical data confirm previous observations of the therapeutic potential of both DA antagonist and GABA agonist treatment in tardive dyskinesia. The hypothesis of a GABA depletion or GABA neuronal dysfunction in the substantia nigra, pars reticulata as a consequence of chronic neuroleptic treatment is consistent with these data. There is an emerging consensus that chronic neuroleptic treatment produces a cascade of receptor and neuronal alterations within the basal ganglia. Conceivably, neuroleptics induce TD by initially altering DA receptor hypersensitivity in striatum and thereafter reducing GABA system function in substantia nigra, pars reticulata. Correcting either defect in symptomatic patients may be responsible for altering the disease manifestations. Additional biochemical and physiologic studies in patients with and without dyskinetic symptoms will be necessary to develop this theory further.

References

Beckstead RM, Frankfurter A (1982) The distribution and some morphological features of substantia-nigra neurons that project to the thalamus, superior colliculus and pedunculopontine nucleus in the monkey. Neuroscience 7:2377–2388

Burt DR, Creese J, Snyder SH (1977) Antischizophrenic drugs. Chronic treatment elevates dopamine receptor binding in brain. Science 196:326–328

Carpenter WT Jr, Rey AC, Stephens JH (1982) Further remarks on covert dyskinesia in ambulatory schizophrenia. Lancet I:1421

Carroll BJ, Curtis CC, Kokmen E (1977) Paradoxical response to dopamine agonists in tardive dyskinesia. Am J Psychiatry 134:785–789

Casey DE, Toenniessen LM (1983) Neuroleptic treatment in tardive dyskinesia: can it be developed into a clinical strategy for long-term treatment? In: Bannet J, Belmaker RH (eds) New directions in tardive dyskinesia research. Karger, Basel, pp 65–79

Casey D, Gerlach J, Magelund G, Christensen T (1980). Gamma-acetylenic GABA in tardive dyskinesia. Arch Gen Psychiatry 37:1376–1379

Cattabeni F, Racagni G, Spano PE, Costa E (1980) Long term effects of neuroleptics. Raven, New York

Chase TN, Tamminga CA (1980) Pharmacologic studies of tardive dyskinesia. Adv Biochem Psychopharm 24:457–462

Clow A, Jenner P, Marsden CD (1978) An experimental model of tardive dyskinesias. Life Sci 23:421–423

Cross AJ, Crow TJ, Ferrier IN, Johnstone EC, MacCreadie RM, Owen F, Owens DGC, Poulter M (1983) Dopamine receptor changes in schizophrenia in relation to the disease process and movement disorder. J Neural Transm 18:265–272

Cutler NR, Jeste DV, Karoum F, Wyatt RJ (1982) Low dose apomorphine reduces serum homovanillic acid concentration in schizophrenic patients. Life Sci 30:753–756

Gale K, Casu M (1981) Dynamic utilization of GABA in substantia nigra: regulation by dopamine and GABA in the striatum, and its clinical and behavioral implications. Mol Cell Biochem 39:369–405

Graybiel AM, Ragsdale CW (1979) Fiber connections of the basal ganglia. In: Cuenod M, Kreutzberg GW, Bloom FE (eds) Progress in brain research, vol 51. Elsevier, Amsterdam, pp 239–283

Gunne L (1983) Presentation at 5th international catecholamine symposium, Gothenburg, 15 June 1983

Klawans H, Rubovits R (1974) Effect of cholinergic and anticholinergic agents in tardive dyskinesia. J Neurol Neurosurg Psychiatry 27:941–947

Korsgaard S, Casey D, Gerlach J, Hetmar O, Kalden B, Mikkelsen L (1982) The effect of tetrahydroisoxazolo-pyridinol (THIP) in tardive dyskinesia. Arch Gen Psychiatry 39:1017–1021

Offermeier J, Rooyen JM (1983) Dopamine inhibitory and excitatory systems in tardive dyskinesia. In: Bannet J, Belmaker RH (eds) New directions in tardive dyskinesia research. Karger, Basel, pp 124–142

Smith RC, Tamminga CA, Haraszti J, Pandey GN, Davis JM (1977) Effects of dopamine agonists in tardive dyskinesia. Am J Psychiatry 134:763–768

Tamminga CA, Thaker GK (1983) Dopamine and GABA treatments in tardive dyskinesia. Presented at the 5th international catecholamine symposium, Gothenburg, 15 June 1983
Tamminga CA, Crayton JW, Chase TN (1979a) Improvement in tardive dyskinesia after muscimol therapy. Arch Gen Psychiatry 36:595–598
Tamminga CA, Schaffer MH, Chase TN (1979b) Ergot derivatives in the treatment of psychotic and hyperkinetic disorders. In: Fuxe K, Calne DB (eds) Dopaminergic ergot derivatives and motor function. Pergamon, Oxford, pp 349–360
Tamminga CA, Thaker GK, Ferraro TN, Hare TA (1983) GABA agonist treatment improves tardive dyskinesia. Lancet II:97–98
Tarsy D, Baldessarini RJ (1973) Pharmacologically-induced behavioral super-sensitivity to apomorphine. Nature 245:262–263
Walters JR, Roth RH (1976) Dopaminergic neurons: An in vivo system for measuring drug interaction with presynaptic receptors. Naunyn-Schmiedebergs Arch Pharmacol 296:5–14
Waszczak BL, Walters JR (1983) Dopamine modulation of the effects of gamma aminobutyric acid on substantia nigra pars reticulata neurons. Science 220:218–221
Waszczak BL, Eng N, Walters JR (1980) Effects of muscimol and picrotoxin on single unit activity of substantia neurons. Brain Res 188:185–197
Waszczak BL, Le EK, Tamminga CA, Walters JR (1984) Effect of dopamine system activation on substantia nigra pars reticulata output neurons: variable single unit responses in normal rats and inhibition in 6-hydroxydopamine lesioned rats. J Neurosci (to be published)

Clinical Activity of GABA Agonists in Neuroleptic- and L-Dopa-Induced Dyskinesia

P. L. Morselli, V. Fournier, L. Bossi, and B. Musch [1]

Contents

Abstract 128
1 Introduction 128
2 Studies of Progabide 130
2.1 Effect of Progabide in Neuroleptic-Induced Dyskinesia 130
2.2 Effect of Progabide in L-Dopa-Induced Dyskinesia 132
3 Discussion 133
References 135

Abstract

It is well known that the therapeutic effect of neuroleptics is counterbalanced by the property of these drugs to induce serious neurological side-effects mainly represented by tardive dyskinesia. Several reports indicate that at the experimental level GABA agonists interact with dopamine neurons with effects on behavior, stereotyped and dyskinetic movements induced by either lesions or dopamine agonists. This action on dopamine-related events provides a basis for a possible therapeutic action of GABA agonists in dyskinesia. Previous results with the GABA agonists muscimol and THIP in tardive dyskinesia have not been encouraging.

The present paper deals with clinical results obtained with the new GABA agonist progabide both in neuroleptic-induced dyskinesia and in L-dopa-induced dyskinesia from five studies conducted on a total of 57 patients. Twenty-nine patients suffering from neuroleptic-induced dyskinesia have been treated in three studies (two open, one double-blind cross over) with progabide at doses from 900 to 2400 mg/day; clinical evaluation and EMG testing are in favor of a therapeutic effect of progabide on dyskinesia. Twenty-eight patients with L-dopa dyskinesia have been studied in two double blind trials. At variance with studies in tardive dyskinesia progabide was not effective in this kind of dyskinesia but an increase in the "on" time has been observed in both studies.

Attempts to treat tardive dyskinesia with various pharmacological tools are reviewed and discussed, showing that at present no established effective treatment exists for this frequent complication of neuroleptic use. The possible mechanism of action of progabide in dyskinesia is discussed in the light of its pharmacological properties. These results suggest that progabide can be useful in the treatment of neuroleptic-induced dyskinesia.

1 Introduction

The introduction of neuroleptics into clinical practice in 1952 was a milestone in the treatment of psychiatric disorders. Unfortunately, the positive therapeutic effect of neuroleptics is counterbalanced by their property of inducing serious

1 LERS SYNTHELABO, Department of Clinical Research, 58 rue de la Glacière, F-75013 Paris, France

Dyskinesia – Research and Treatment
(Psychopharmacology Supplementum 2)
Editors: Casey, Chase, Christensen, Gerlach

neurological side-effects, which represent a limiting factor, sometimes insoluble, in their clinical use. The single side-effect that has caused most concern in recent years is tardive dyskinesia.

Tardive dyskinesia is defined as a syndrome consisting of abnormal stereotyped involuntary movements, usually of choreoathetoid type, principally affecting the mouth, face, limbs, and trunk, which occur relatively late in the course of neuroleptic treatment (Jeste and Wyatt 1982). Dyskinesia has also been reported as a side-effect of short-term and long-term treatment with a number of different drugs, such as metoclopramide, amantadine, amphetamine, L-dopa and MAO inhibitors.

The syndrome induced by metoclopramide, amphetamine, and amantadine is generally acute and self-limiting, while that induced by L-dopa is persistent and closely resembles that caused by neuroleptics.

Tardive dyskinesia was described in the late 1950s after the observation of other extrapyramidal reactions to neuroleptics (acute dystonias, akathisia, parkinsonism) (Sigwald et al. 1959; Uhrbrand and Faurbye 1960). Although some authors suggest that tardive dyskinesia may be related to the primary disorder, it is generally accepted that neuroleptic-induced tardive dyskinesia is a separate clinical entity and that its prevalence has been increasing over the past 20 years.

Several reports indicate that on the experimental level, GABA agonists interact with dopamine neurons, with effects on behavior, stereotyped and dyskinetic movements induced by either lesions or dopamine agonists (Bartholini et al. 1979a, 1979b; Scatton et al. 1982; Lloyd et al., this volume, 1980; Christensen and Hyttel 1981; Christensen et al. 1979).

At low doses, muscimol, THIP, and progabide potentiate apomorphine or methylphenidate stereotypies and antagonize haloperidol-induced catalepsy (Worms and Lloyd 1978, 1980).

Conversely, at higher doses all three GABA agonists inhibit apomorphine or L-dopa-induced stereotypies and/or dyskinetic movements (Lloyd et al. 1980, 1981, 1983). Muscimol and progabide have been shown to block the hypersensitivity to apomorphine and the tolerance to neuroleptic-induced catalepsy that follows repeated neuroleptic administration.

The data have been reviewed and discussed at length by Lloyd et al. (this volume) and Scatton et al. (this volume). These actions on dopamine-related events provide a basis and a rationale for a possible therapeutic action of GABA agonists in dyskinesia.

The available data on the activity of GABA agonists other than progabide in movement disorders, and more specifically on dyskinesia, are very scarce, and to the best of the authors' knowledge, are limited to two papers (Tamminga et al. 1979; Korsgaard et al. 1982).

Muscimol, at the dose of 5–9 mg/day, may have a positive action on neuroleptic-induced choreiform movements according to Tamminga et al. (1979), but apparently exacerbates extrapyramidal symptoms in patients suffering from drug-induced parkinsonism. A similar negative effect of THIP on drug-induced parkinsonism was observed (Korsgaard et al. 1982), but without any effect on dyskinetic movements. From these first two reports on the possible therapeutic action of GABA agonists on drug-induced dyskinesias, results do not really appear encouraging. However, we know that in the case of muscimol most of the effects observed in animals and humans after 1 or 2 hours are mostly due to metabolites, which may have an opposite action (Lloyd and Morselli 1982; Morselli and Lloyd 1983). THIP's spectrum of activity in man is quite different from that of progabide (Morselli and Lloyd 1983).

For these reasons we thought it would be interesting to evaluate the activity of progabide in two types of patient populations, viz. patients suffering from (a) neuroleptic-induced dyskinesia and (b) L-dopa-induced dyskinesia.

So far, the results appear to be encouraging (Morselli et al. 1980; Bathien et al. 1982), suggesting that within the new class of the GABA agonists the compounds may display major differences in therapeutic activity though having a similar spectrum at the experimental level. The available data on the effects of progabide in human dyskinesia are reviewed below.

2 Studies of Progabide

The available data on progabide refer to five studies (two open and three double blind) conducted in a total of 57 patients (19 in open and 38 in double blind studies) suffering from either neuroleptic-induced or L-dopa-induced dyskinesia (Tab. 1).

2.1 Effect of Progabide in Neuroleptic-Induced Dyskinesia

2.2.1 Open Studies

In the two open studies (conducted in collaboration with Dr. Rondot and Dr. Sevestre of St Anne Hospital, Paris) 19 patients suffering from neuroleptic-

Table 1. Clinical studies with progabide in neuroleptic- and L-dopa-induced dyskinesia

Study	Indication	No. of Patients	Duration of treatment (weeks)	Progabide daily dose (mg)	Results
Open (Rondot–Sevestre)	Tardive dyskinesia	19	6–10	1200–2400	Excellent or good therapeutic response in 15 patients; EMG improved in 14 patients
Double-blind (Bathien)	Tardive dyskinesia	10	6	900–1200	Simpson's Scale score reduced ($P < 0.05$) after progabide; EMG improved in 5 patients
Double-blind (Ziegler–Rondot)	L-dopa-induced dyskinesia	13	12	8–20 mg/kg	Global improvement of parkinsonian symptoms; increased on time: no effect on dyskinesia
Double-blind (Yahr–Bergmann)	L-dopa-induced dyskinesia	15	2	25 mg/kg	Increased on time: reduced severity of off state; no effect on dyskinesia

induced dyskinesias were studied. Progabide was administered for 6–10 weeks at doses of 1200–2400 mg/day. Inclusion criteria were based on the presence of orofacial, axial, and limb dyskinesias that appeared after the introduction of neuroleptic treatment and manifested continuously for at least 1 month. Neuroleptic treatment, when present, was kept constant and no anticholinergic drugs were permitted.

The evaluation was based on a visual analog scale and/or the Simpson Scale for the scoring of dyskinesia; an electrophysiological examination based on EMG recordings of abnormal movements, the polysynaptic sural test and the piribedil test; and a global clinical judgement at the end of the observation period.

Patients were 13 men and 6 women 26–76 years of age. Seventeen suffered from orofacial limb dyskinesia and two from dystonia. Six were receiving no neuroleptics and thirteen, maintenance neuroleptic. Dyskinesia had been present for 1–20 years.

At the end of the treatment, results were considered excellent in eight cases (4 of them having achieved total remission of dyskinesia) and good in seven cases. Two patients dropped out because of side-effects and two were judged as "nonresponders." In the eleven patients treated for up to 10 weeks the score on the Simpson Scale was significantly reduced ($P < 0.001$) at the various study intervals and at the end of the treatment (Fig. 1).

The EMG showed a normal response in two out of three tests in 14 of the 17 patients, who completed the treatment, confirming the clinical results.

2.1.2 Double-Blind Studies

The above-mentioned results were verified in a subsequent double-blind crossover study against placebo, where progabide was again administered for 6 weeks at doses ranging from 900 to 1200 mg/day. The criteria for inclusion and evaluation were as in the open study. The population studied consisted of ten patients (three women and seven men) 32–74 years of age with orofacial limb dyskinesias.

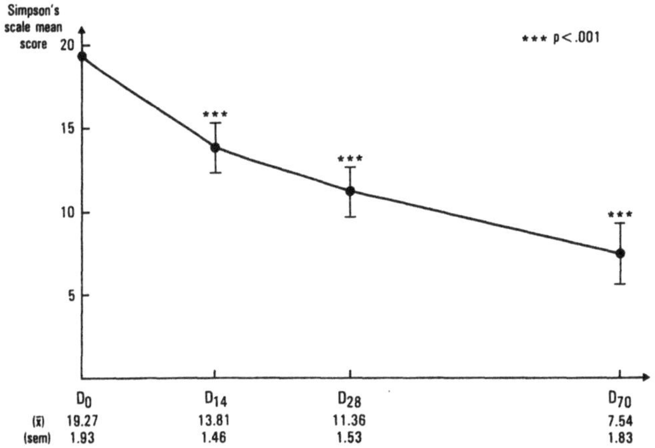

Fig. 1. Course of the mean score on the Simpson scale in an open study with progabide in patients ($n = 11$) suffering from tardive dyskinesia. (Sevestre et al. 1982)

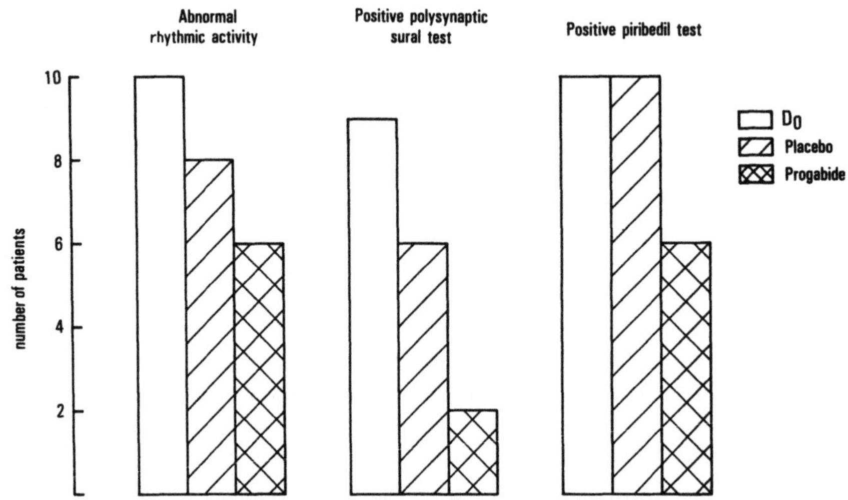

Fig. 2. EMG evaluation of the effects of progabide in a double-blind study against placebo ii patients ($n = 10$) suffering from tardive dyskinesia

Five of the ten patients showed a significant improvement with progabide and only two after placebo. The total score (Simpson Scale) was significantly ($P < 0.05$) lower with progabide than with placebo. The EMG showed a significant improvement in five cases out of ten with progabide and in none with placebo (Fig. 2).

This controlled study confirms the positive effect of progabide observed in the open studies.

On the whole, the three studies, involving a total of 29 patients, suggest that progabide can exert a significant therapeutic action in neuroleptic-induced dyskinesias.

2.2 Effect of Progabide in L-Dopa-Induced Dyskinesia

The possible therapeutic activity of progabide in L-dopa-induced dyskinesia has been evaluated in two double-blind studies involving a total of 28 patients. In the first preliminary study, run in parallel groups against placebo and conducted in collaboration with Dr. Ziegler and Dr. Rondot of St. Anne Hospital, Paris, 13 patients (4 women and 9 men) entered the study, but 3 had to be dropped because of poor compliance. Progabide doses ranged from 8 to 20 mg/day. Treatment duration was 12 weeks.

The clinical assessment included scoring of parkinsonism symptoms on a four-point scale (from absent to severe; scoring of severity of abnormal involuntary movements on the same four-point scale; duration of the "on" time; the global clinical impression at the end of treatment. The "on" time means the period during which L-dopa displays its therapeutic effect; the "off" state is the period when parkinsonian symptoms reappear notwithstanding the fact that the patient is on L-dopa treatment. "On-off phenomenon" is the alternating succession of the two events during the day in a patient on L-dopa treatment.

Four patients received progabide and six, placebo. In three out of four patients receiving progabide a global improvement of parkinsonian symptoms was evident, while no changes were observed with placebo.

A significant increase ($P < 0.05$) of the on time was noticed in the progabide group. However, no modification of dyskinesia could be detected in either group.

In the second study, conducted by Dr. Yahr and collaborators, 15 parkinsonian patients (10 women and 5 men) were treated with progabide at 25 mg/kg per day and placebo according to a crossover design with two 2-week periods.

Progabide appeared to affect the clinical expression of the "on-off" phenomenon by significantly reducing ($P < 0.001$) the severity of the off state and significantly increasing ($P < 0.001$) the daily on time (Bergman et al. 1984).

In contrast, no positive effects on dyskinesia were observed, which in some cases actually worsened.

3 Discussion

In the clinical literature, the prevalence of tardive dyskinesia among chronically ill psychiatric patients ranges from 0.5% to 56% with an overall weighted mean prevalence of 17.6% in reliable studies. In L-dopa-treated patients the reported prevalence ranges from 40% to 80% (Jeste and Wyatt 1982).

With reference to the epidemiologic relationship between neuroleptic treatment and tardive dyskinesia, it seems that the timing and daily amount of neuroleptic administered may be more important than the total amount of the drug that a patient receives (Goetz et al. 1982). From the diagnostic point of view, which is particularly important in designing clinical trials, three features seem to be essential:

1. The duration of dyskinesia (presence for at least 3 weeks)
2. The duration of neuroleptic treatment (at least 3 months without a break)
3. The temporal relationship between the appearance of dyskinesia and neuroleptic treatment (appearance during treatment or within a few weeks from neuroleptic withdrawal).

Several pharmacological and other treatments have been proposed or used in tardive dyskinesia. Although the study of their efficacy has contributed to the better understanding of the neurochemistry of the disorder, they have all failed, so far, to unearth "the" treatment for tardive dyskinesia.

Neuroleptics have been shown to produce a significant improvement of tardive dyskinesia, which however, usually leads to recurrence of dyskinesia and may even make it irreversible. Drug-free periods are recommended by some Health Authorities, but their clinical usefulness does not seem unequivocally proven. On the contrary, a slow but progressive reduction in neuroleptic doses may be advantageous (Jus et al. 1979).

Compounds such as oxypertine, methyl-dopa, bromocriptine, and methyl-*p*-tyrosine have been found to be useful in about 50% of patients with tardive dyskinesia, but this effect has been observed only in short-term studies (Freeman and Soni 1980; Gerlach 1977; Tamminga and Chase 1980). Available data do not support the use of cholinergic agents, such as deanol (Davis et al. 1977), or of dopaminergic drugs, which can even aggravate dyskinetic movements and psychotic symptoms (Lambert et al. 1978; Tarsy and Bralower 1977; Alpert and Friedhoff 1980).

In contrast, physostigmine has proved to be effective in several studies, but safety problems limit its clinical use (Davis et al. 1975; Tamminga et al. 1977). Anticholinergic drugs are also of little use, and they can aggravate the syndrome. A huge number of miscellaneous drugs, such as pyridoxine, lithium, estrogens, tryptophan, propranolol, and diphenylhydantoin, have been tried, as have non-drug treatments, but the results are far from convincing (Jeste and Wyatt 1982).

The reported data on progabide suggest that GABA agonists have a therapeutic action in neuroleptic-induced dyskinesia. These data, though preliminary, do permit some comments. Unlike muscimol and THIP, progabide appears to have a genuine therapeutic activity in neuroleptic-induced dyskinesia. While the difference with respect to muscimol can be explained on the basis of possible toxic metabolites of the latter drug, no obvious explanations are available for the differences from THIP. In L-dopa-induced dyskinesia, progabide does not appear to have any therapeutic activity on abnormal movements but the drug significantly extends the on period.

Three possible mechanisms have been proposed for the action of progabide in neuroleptic-induced dyskinesia:

1. Reduction of the dopamine neuronal activity due to an inhibitory action of progabide on both cell bodies and terminals of dopamine neurons (Scatton et al. 1982)
2. An antidopaminergic action exerted distal to the dopamine receptors and evidenced by the antagonism by progabide of the apomorphine-induced stereotypies in the rat (Worms et al. 1982)
3. Reduction by progabide of the neuroleptic-induced enhancement of dopamine receptor density (Scatton et al. this volume).

In the case of L-dopa-induced dyskinesia in Parkinson's disease, the apparent lack of action of GABA agonists is unexplained. In fact, while the impaired nigrostriatal system may not fully respond to the inhibitory action of GABA agonists there are clear indications that progabide antagonizes:

1) The dyskinesia induced by dopamine mimetics in monkeys with ventrotegmental lesions
2) The stereotyped movements induced in the rat by apomorphine
3) The turning behavior induced by dopamine mimetics in the rat bearing lesions of the substantia nigra following 6-OHDA (Lloyd et al. 1980, 1981, 1983).

The observed prolongation of the on period is also difficult to interpret. Possible explanations are increased L-dopa availability or alternatively, as suggested by Bergman et al. (1984), an action of the drug in the pars reticulata, an area subject to GABA regulation, with activation of GABA receptors, which in normally functioning brain is elicited by DA stimulation.

A further alternative explanation is the reduction in striatal cholinergic transmission induced by progabide, an action which in animals, at least, favors DA-mediated events (Scatton et al. 1982).

In conclusion, persisting abnormal movements can be debilitating, leading to psychic and social problems and having a negative effect on attempts at rehabilitation and on acceptance of the patients in the community. The loss of job skills and self-care skills resulting from tardive dyskinesia is undoubtedly a limiting factor in the use of neuroleptics, affecting the possibility of controlling the psychotic symptoms especially in long-term treatment. The possible availability of a new therapeutic class of drugs active in tardive dyskinesia appears very promising. Further efforts are needed for better definition of the therapeutic potential of GABA agonists through basic and clinical studies with the aim of providing tardive dyskinesia patients with an effective and safe treatment.

Acknowledgments. The authors thank Prof. Rondot, Prof. Sevestre, Dr. Bathien, and Dr. Ziegler (Ste-Anne Hospital, Paris and Esquirol Hospital, Charenton), Prof. Yahr and Dr. Bergman for their valued collaboration, and Prof. G. Bartholini (L.E.R.S. Synthelabo, Paris) for stimulating discussion of the manuscript.

References

Alpert M, Friedhoff AJ (1980) Clinical application of receptor modification. In: Fann WE, Smith RC, Davis JM (eds) Tardive dyskinesia: research and treatment. Medical and Scientific Books, New York

Bathien N, Sevestre P, Rondot P, Morselli PL, Van Landeghem V (1982) The effect of progabide, a specific GABAergic agonist, on neuroleptic-induced tardive dyskinesia – a result of a pilot study. In: Collegium Internationale Neuro-Psychopharmacologicum (eds) 13th C.I.N.P., abstracts, vol III, Jerusalem

Bartholini G, Lloyd KG, Worms P, Constantinidis J, Tissot R (1979a) GABA and GABA-ergic medication: relation to striatal dopamine function and parkinsonism. In: Poirier LJ, Sourkes TL, Bedard PJ (eds) Advances in neurology, vol 24. Raven, New York, pp 253–257

Bartholini G, Scatton B, Zivkovic B, Lloyd KG (1979b) On the mode of action of SL 76002, a new GABA receptor agonist. In: Krogsgaard-Larsen P, Scheel-Krüger J, Kofod H (eds) GABA neurotransmitters. Raven, New York, pp 326–339

Bergman KJ, Limongi JCP, Lowe YH, Mendoza MR, Yahr MD (1984) Potentiation of the "DOPA" effect in parkinsonism by a direct GABA receptor agonist. Lancet 10:559

Christensen AV, Hyttel J (1981) Prolonged treatment with the GABA agonist THIP increases dopamine receptor binding more than it changes dopaminergic behaviour in mice. Drug Develop Res 3

Christensen AV, Arnt J, Scheel-Krüger J (1979) Decreased antistereotypic effect of neuroleptics after additional treatment with a benzodiazepine, a GABA agonist or an anticholinergic compound. Life Sci 24:1395–1402

Davis KL, Berger PA, Hollister LE (1975) Choline for tardive dyskinesia. N Engl J Med 293:152

Davis KL, Berger PA, Hollister LE (1977) Deanol in tardive dyskinesia. Am J Psychiatry 134:807

Freeman H, Soni SD (1980) Oxypertine for tardive dyskinesia. Br J Psychiatry 137:522–523

Gerlach J (1977) Relationship between tardive dyskinesia, L-dopa-induced hyperkinesia and parkinsonism. Psychopharmacology 51:259–263

Goetz CG, Weiner WJ, Nausieda PA, Klawans HL (1982) Tardive dyskinesia: pharmacology and clinical implications. Clin Neuropharmacol 5, 1:3–22

Jeste DV, Wyatt RJ (1982) Understanding and treating tardive dyskinesia. Guilford, London

Jus A, Jus K, Fontaine P (1979) Long-term treatment of tardive dyskinesia. J Clin Psychiatry 40:72–77

Korsgaard S, Casey DE, Gerlach J, Hetmar O, Kaldan B, Mikkelsen LB (1982) The effect of tetrahydroisoxazolopyridinol (THIP) in tardive dyskinesia. Arch Gen Psychiatry 39:1017–1021

Lambert PA, Wolff P, DeManimy B (1978) Le dimethylaminoethanol dans le traitement des dyskinésies tardives induites par les neuroleptiques. Ann Méd Psychol 136:625–629

Lloyd KG, Morselli PL (1982) Potential anticonvulsants, GABA receptor agonists. In: Woodbury DM, Penry JK, Pippenger CE (eds) Antiepileptic drugs. Raven, New York, pp 839–858

Lloyd KG, Worms P, Zivkovic B, Scatton B, Bartholini G (1980) Interaction of GABA mimetics with nigro-striatal dopamine neurons. Brain Res Bull 5 [Suppl 2]:439–445

Lloyd KG, Broekkamp CLE, Cathala F, Worms P, Goldstein M, Asano T (1981) Animal models for prediction and prevention of dyskinesias induced by dopaminergic drugs. In: Corsini GU, Gessa Gl (eds) Apomorphine and other dopaminomimetics. Raven, New York, pp 123–135 (Clinical pharmacology, vol 2)

Lloyd KG, Broekkamp R, Worms P (1983) Involvement of GABA neurons in the induction and reversal of dopamine receptor related dyskinesia. In: Zbinden G, Cuomo V, Racagni G, Weiss B (eds) Application of behavioral pharmacology and toxicology. Raven, New York, pp 203–215

Morselli PL, Lloyd KG (1983) Clinical pharmacology of GABA agonists. In: Enna S (ed) GABA receptors. Humana, Clifton, pp 305–336

Morselli PL, Bossi L, Henry JF, Zarifian E, Bartholini G (1980) On the therapeutic action of SL 76002, a new-GABA-mimetic agent: preliminary observations in neuropsychiatric disorders. Brain Res Bull 5 [Suppl 2]:411–414

Scatton B, Bartholini G (1981) γ-Aminobutyric acid (GABA) receptor stimulation. IV: Effect of progabide (SL 76002) and other GABAergic agents on acetylcholine turnover in rat brain areas. J Pharmacol Exp Ther 220:689–695

Scatton B, Zivkovic B, Dedek J, Lloyd KJ, Constandinidis J, Tissot R, Bartholini G (1982) γ-Aminobutyric acid (GABA) receptor stimulation. III. Effect of progabide (SL 76002) on norepinephrine, dopamine and 5-hydroxytryptamine turnover in rat brain areas. J Pharmacol Exp Ther 220:678–688

Sevestre P, Rondot P, Bathien N, Morselli PL, Van Landeghem V (1982) The effect of progabide, a specific GABAergic agonist, on neuroleptic-induced tardive dyskinesia – result of a pilot study. In: Collegium Internationale Neuro-Psychopharmacologicum (eds) 13th C.I.N.P., abstracts vol II, Jerusalem

Sigwald J, Banthee D, Raymondeaud C, Piot C (1959) Quatre cas de dyskinesia facio-bucco-linguo-masticatrice à l'évolution prolongée secondaire à un traitement par les neuroleptiques. Rev Neurol 100:751–755

Tamminga CA, Chase TN (1980) Bromocriptine and CF 25-397 in the treatment of tardive dyskinesia. Arch Neurol 37:204–205

Tamminga CA, Smith RC, Eriksen SE (1977) Cholinergic influences in tardive dyskinesia. Am J Psychiatry 134:769–774

Tamminga CA, Crayton JW, Chase TN (1979) Improvement in tardive dyskinesia after muscimol therapy. Arch Gen Psychiatry 36:595–598

Tarsy D, Bralower M (1977) Deanol acetamidobenzoate treatment in choreiform movement disorders. Arch Neurol 34:756–758

Uhrbrand L, Faurbye A (1960) Reversible and irreversible dyskinesia after treatment with perphenazine, chlorpromazine, reserpine, E.C.T. therapy. Psychopharmacologia 1:408–418

Worms P, Lloyd KG (1978) Influence of GABA-agonist and antagonists on neuroleptic-induced catalepsy in rats. Life Sci 23:475–478

Worms P, Lloyd KG (1980) Biphasic effect of direct, but not indirect, GABA mimetics and antagonists on haloperidol-induced catalepsy. Arch Pharmacol 311:179–184

Worms P, Depoorter H, Durand A, Morselli PL, Lloyd KG, Bartholini G (1982) γ-Aminobutyric acid (GABA) receptor stimulation. I. Neuropharmacological profiles of progabide (SL 76002) and SL 75102, with emphasis on their anticonvulsant spectra. J Pharmacol Exp Ther 220:660–671

Tardive Dyskinesia: Nondopaminergic Treatment Approaches [1]

D. E. Casey [2]

Contents

Abstract 137
1 Introduction 137
2 Acetylcholine 138
2.1 Cholinergic Agonists 138
2.2 Anticholinergics 138
3 GABA 139
4 Serotonin 140
5 Lithium 140
6 Neuropeptides 140
7 Adrenergics 140
8 Miscellaneous 141
9 Conclusion 141
References 142

Abstract

The continuing concern about tardive dyskinesia (TD) has stimulated a broad search for therapies for this disorder. Since neuroleptic drugs are thought to be the etiological agents, acting presumably through dopamine receptor blockade, nondopaminergic drugs have been the focus of recent study. However, no uniformly safe and effective drug treatment has been identified. Augmentation of cholinergic function is theoretically attractive, but further research is needed to develop practical and effective compounds. GABA drugs do not consistently suppress TD. The effect of benzodiazepines in TD is unclear, but these agents may be of some temporary benefit in patients with distressing symptoms. Lithium, serotonergic compounds, and numerous neuropeptides all fail to have any consistent effect in TD. Early reports of benefit with α- and β-noradrenergic agents are interesting but require further study. Many other drug types have been tried without benefit. For the majority of patients, it may be best to give no drug treatment. Any drug that is capable of suppressing TD may aggravate the disorder in the long term. The potential for a spontaneous gradual remission of TD is an argument in favor of a patient, nonaggressive, and cautiously optimistic approach to this disorder.

1 Introduction

Treatment of tardive dyskinesia (TD) has proven to be a difficult challenge. No drug treatments have been shown to be both safe and effective over extended treatment periods. Though neuroleptic drugs very effectively suppress TD, these

1 The research described in this paper was funded in part by the Veterans Administration Career Development Award and Merit Review Program and by grant no. 36657 from NIMH
2 Psychiatry Service, Veterans Administration Medical Center, Portland, OR 97207, USA

Dyskinesia – Research and Treatment
(Psychopharmacology Supplementum 2)
Editors: Casey, Chase, Christensen, Gerlach

compounds are not recommended for masking symptoms, because they are thought to be the causative agents. The possibility exists that with continued neuroleptic use TD may be increasingly aggravated, though this outcome has seldom been observed (Casey and Toenniessen 1983). The reverse approach of treating TD with dopamine agonists is theoretically attractive, but has not been very effective in the clinical setting.

The drugs mentioned below include agents that are designed to manipulate acetylcholinergic, GABA-ergic, serotonergic, neuropeptide, and noradrenergic influences of the basal ganglia. Some compounds with unknown mechanisms of action and/or no clear basis for a therapeutic approach are also noted.

2 Acetylcholine

2.1 Cholinergic Agonists

The rationale for increasing cholinergic influence is to counterbalance the purported relative excess of dopamine underlying TD. The attempt is to reestablish the reciprocal dopamine-acetylcholine balance in the basal ganglia. Physostigmine, an acetylcholine esterase inhibitor, usually decreases TD, but can have variable effects in a minority of patients in whom symptoms increase (Casey and Gerlach 1984). The use of this compound is also limited because it must be given IV, has a short half-life, and has undesirable effects of sedation, dizziness, nausea, and vomiting. Arecoline, a cholinergic agonist, had inconsistent effects in TD (Nutt et al. 1979).

Augmentation of cholinergic function via precursor loading has received considerable attention. The initial optimistic results with deanol were not supported by later findings (Casey 1977). Choline moderately reduced TD in some patients (Davis et al. 1976; Growdon et al. 1977), but side-effects limit the widespread use of this compound. Lecithin also moderately suppressed TD in some patients (Gelenberg et al. 1979; Jackson et al. 1979). The use of lecithin is limited by the relative unavailability of pure compound and the requirement of administering large quantities, which may lead to excessive weight gain.

2.2 Anticholinergics

These agents temporarily increase or have no effect on TD. Combination of anticholinergics with neuroleptics may also inhibit the antihyperkinetic effect of neuroleptics (Gerlach and Simmelsgaard 1978). In a few reports, anticholinergic agents have reduced rather than aggravated TD (Gerlach et al. 1974; Casey and Denney 1977; Moore and Bowers 1980). It is not clear whether this paradoxical response is identifying a subgroup of patients with TD, or whether these infrequently reported cases of anticholinergic-induced improvement represent patients with the seldom recognized syndrome of initial hyperkinesia (the symptoms of which mimic TD but are more properly classified as acute extrapyramidal symptoms because they improve with antiparkinson therapy) (Gerlach 1979). A review of anticholinergic drugs in 14 TD studies with 177 patients noted an improvement rate of 7.3 % (Jeste and Wyatt 1982). The same review of the effects of cholinergic drugs in 68 studies of 379 patients with TD revealed that 47 % of the patients improved in open studies, and 30 % improved in double-blind trials (Jeste and Wyatt 1982).

3 GABA

The rationale for testing GABA drugs in TD comes from the findings that GABA influences may have an inhibitory effect on dopamine-mediated functions. Enhancement of GABA function by inhibiting the breakdown enzyme GABA transaminase has been a strategy with a few compounds. γ-Acetylenic-GABA significantly reduced TD (Casey et al. 1980). This compound had a significantly greater antihyperkinetic effect in older patients taking neuroleptic drugs, suggesting that increased GABA influences may reduce TD by indirect effect on dopaminergic mechanisms. γ-Vinyl-GABA, another GABA transaminase inhibitor, also decreased TD (Tell et al. 1981; Casey et al. 1983; Korsgaard et al. 1983; Tamminga et al. 1983). The patients benefiting the most with decreased TD had the greatest increases in parkinsonism (Casey et al. 1983; Korsgaard et al. 1983).

Sodium valproate may also inhibit GABA transaminase, though this effect is unclear. After the initial positive report with this compound (Linnoila et al. 1976), much less encouraging reports appeared (Casey and Hammerstad 1979). As with the other GABA transaminase inhibitors, valproate was more effective in suppressing TD when combined with a neuroleptic (Nair et al. 1980).

GABA agonists have also been evaluated. Muscimol, a compound occurring naturally in mushrooms, decreased TD in a short-term study, but this experimental agent has psychotomimetic effects (Tamminga et al. 1979). Another experimental GABA agonist, THIP, had no significant effect in TD (Korsgaard et al. 1982).

Baclofen, a structural analog of GABA with unclear effects on GABA mechanisms, moderately suppressed TD. As with GABA-T inhibitors, this drug potentiated the neuroleptic antihyperkinetic effects, increased existing drug-induced parkinsonism, and was less effective in patients not receiving neuroleptics (Korsgaard 1976; Gerlach et al. 1978; Nair et al. 1980).

Benzodiazepines may also enhance GABA function by potentiating GABA mechanisms. Though these agents were among the first to be used in TD, they have not been systematically studied. Diazepam has both reduced (Jus et al. 1974; Singh et al. 1980) and aggravated TD (Rosenbaum and de la Fuente 1979). Clonazepam, a benzodiazepine that may also affect serotonin, was as effective as phenobarbital in reducing TD (Bobruff et al. 1981). The question as to whether antihyperkinetic effects with benzodiazepines occur through specific or nonspecific sedative effects remains to be answered. In a review of 19 studies with GABA agents involving 204 patients with TD, 58 % improved in open studies and 42.6 % improved in double-blind evaluations (Jeste and Wyatt 1982).

4 Serotonin

Serotonergic agents have been postulated as potentially therapeutic on the basis of serotonergic input to the basal ganglia and the clinical observation that tryptophan and pyridoxine caused a rapid deterioration in patients with Parkinson's disease. Treatment with tryptophan and 5-hydroxytryptophan has not consistently reduced TD (Prange et al. 1973; Jus et al. 1974; Nasrallah et al. 1982). The opposite approach with cyproheptadine, a purported central nervous system serotonin antagonist, yielded mixed results (Goldman 1976; Gardos and Cole 1978).

5 Lithium

The purported ability of lithium to decrease amine release is the theoretical rationale for the use of this drug in hyperkinetic disorders. Though the initial studies were encouraging, later double-blind evaluations showed no benefit or improvement only in selected patients (Yassa and Ananth 1980). A similar conclusion was reached in a review of ten studies involving 90 patients with TD, where only 27% improved (Jeste and Wyatt 1982). Lithium has been shown to prevent the development of neuroleptic-induced dopamine receptor proliferation in rodents (Pert et al. 1978). Though it has been suggested that a combination of lithium plus neuroleptic treatment in clinical practice would reduce the risk of TD, this hypothesis has not been tested.

6 Neuropeptides

The high concentration of enkephalins in the basal ganglia and the proposal that peptides may function as neurotransmitters support the rationale for testing these compounds in TD. The synthetic met-enkephalin analog FK 33-824 significantly reduced TD but this effect was of minimal clinical significance. Morphine also had a nonspecific suppressant effect on TD. Naloxone, an opiate antagonist, had no consistent effect (Bjørndal et al. 1980). The nonopiate peptide fragment, des-tyr-gamma-endorphin, also had no effect on TD (Casey et al. 1981). Vasopressin was similarly without effect in TD (Korsgaard et al. 1981).

7 Adrenergics

Drugs that influence adrenergic receptor subtypes have been tried in TD on an empirical basis. The β-receptor antagonist propranolol showed either suppression (Bacher and Lewis 1980; Kulik and Wilbur 1980) or no benefit (Perenyi and Farkas 1983). The role of propranolol in movement disorders is unclear, as it effectively reduces essential tremor and may also reduce neuroleptic-induced parkinsonism (Kulik and Wilbur 1980) and akathisia (Lipinski et al. 1984). Clonidine, an α-adrenergic agonist, reduced both TD and psychotic symptoms in two patients (Freedman et al. 1980). Obviously these reports require substantially more study to clarify whether the noradrenergic system has specific or nonspecific effects in TD.

8 Miscellaneous

Many other medications have been used to treat TD. Estrogen, which may have a weak dopamine antagonist effect, produced conflicting results of benefit or no change (Villeneuve et al. 1980; Koller et al. 1982). Pyridoxine (vitamin B6) had no consistent effects (Crane et al. 1970; DeVeaugh-Geiss and Manion 1978). Fusaric acid, a dopamine β-hydroxylase inhibitor that decreases norepinephrine, reduced TD, but this has not been subsequently re-evaluated (Viukari and Linnoila 1977). Manganese has been tried on the basis that neuroleptic drugs chelate manganese, thus theoretically producing a deficit. While the results with manganese were quite promising with reference to suppression of TD, they require further evaluation before this approach can be recommended (Kunin 1976). Barbiturates (Bobruff et al. 1981) and phenytoin (Jus et al. 1974) also suppressed TD. Hydergine and papaverine, both of which may have weak dopamine antagonist activity, may suppress TD (Gardos et al. 1976; Gomez 1977; Rastogi et al. 1982). Melanocyte-stimulating hormone release-inhibiting factor 1 (MIF-1) has also produced mixed results in TD (Ehrensing et al. 1977).

9 Conclusion

The continuing concern about TD has stimulated a wide interest in potential pharmacological therapies for this disorder. Despite a broad spectrum of interest and effort, to date no uniformly safe and effective treatment has been identified. Though the concept of augmenting cholinergic function via precursor loading is theoretically attractive, further research is needed to develop practical and effective compounds. GABA drugs do not have a primary antidyskinetic effect on TD. Though the role of benzodiazepines in TD is unclear, these compounds may be palliative for some patients who have distressing symptoms. Lithium, serotonergic compounds, and numerous neuropeptides all fail to exert any substantial effect in TD. Noradrenergic influences in TD are interesting and may lead to potential advancements in treatment if the preliminary results with drugs that affect α- and β-receptors are verified in further studies. A broad array of other types of drugs has produced inconsistent results.

What are we to prescribe for patients with TD? For the majority of patients, it may be best to give no drug treatment. The possibility that TD will gradually resolve provides some reason to hope for a reversible course. Though there is understandable enthusiasm to suppress TD symptoms, it may be that any drugs which are capable of suppressing TD are in the long-term also capable of aggravating the disorder. In cases requiring some degree of symptom suppression, drugs with minimum liability and possible benefit, such as benzodiazepines or the adrenergic agents, could be tried. Only in the exceptional case of severely limiting or life-threatening TD should neuroleptics be used solely to treat TD. On the other hand, if psychosis is present and responsive to treatment, the lowest effective neuroleptic dose is clearly justified.

References

Bacher NM, Lewis HA (1980) Low-dose propranolol in tardive dyskinesia. Am J Psychiatry 137:495–497

Bjørndal N, Casey DE, Gerlach J (1980) Enkephalin, morphine, and naloxone in tardive dyskinesia. Psychopharmacology 69:133–136

Bobruff A, Gardos G, Tarsy D, Rapkin RM, Cole JO, Moore P (1981) Clonazepam and phenobarbital in tardive dyskinesia. Am J Psychiatry 138:189–193

Casey DE (1977) Deanol in the management of involuntary movement disorders: a review. Dis Nerv Syst 38 (Section 2):7–15

Casey DE, Denney D (1977) Pharmacological characterization of tardive dyskinesia. Psychopharmacology 54:1–8

Casey DE, Gerlach J (1984) Tardive dyskinesia: management and new treatment. In: Stancer HC, Garfinkel PE, Rakoff VM (eds) Guidelines for the use of psychotropic drugs. Spectrum, New York, pp 183–203

Casey DE, Hammerstad JP (1979) Sodium valproate in tardive dyskinesia. J Clin Psychiatry 40:483–485

Casey DE, Toenniessen LM (1983) Neuroleptic treatment in tardive dyskinesia: can it be developed into a clinical strategy for long-term treatment? In: Bannet J, Belmaker RH (eds) New directions in tardive dyskinesia research. Mod Probl Pharmacopsychiatry 21:65–79

Casey DE, Gerlach J, Magelund G, Rosted Christensen T (1980) Gamma-acetylenic GABA in tardive dyskinesia. Arch Gen Psychiatry 37:1376–1379

Casey DE, Korsgaard S, Gerlach J (1981) Des-tyrosine-gamma-endorphin in tardive dyskinesia. In: Perris C, Struwe G, Jansson B (eds) Biological psychiatry 1981. Elsevier, New York, pp 402–404 (Developments in psychiatry, vol 5)

Casey DE, Korsgaard S, Gerlach J (1983) Tardive dyskinesia: the effect of gamma-vinyl GABA. Proc Ann Meet Am Psychiatr Assoc NR54

Crane GE, Turek IS, Kurland AA (1970) Failure of pyridoxine to reduce drug-induced dyskinesias. J Neurol Neurosurg Psychiatry 33:511–512

Davis KL, Hollister LE, Barchas JD, Berger PA (1976) Choline in tardive dyskinesia and Huntington's disease. Life Sci 19:1507–1516

DeVeaugh-Geiss J, Manion L (1978) High-dose pyridoxine in tardive dyskinesia. J Clin Psychiatry 39:573–575

Ehrensing RH, Kastin AJ, Larsons PF, Bishop GA (1977) Melanocyte-stimulating-hormone release-inhibiting factor-I and tardive dyskinesia. Dis Nerv Syst 38:303–307

Freedman R, Bell J, Kirch D (1980) Clonidine therapy for coexisting psychosis and tardive dyskinesia. Am J Psychiatry 137:629–630

Gardos G, Cole JO (1978) Pilot study of cyproheptadine (periactin) in TD. Psychopharmacol Bull 14:18–20

Gardos G, Cole JO, Sniffen C (1976) An evaluation of papaverine in tardive dyskinesia. J Clin Pharmacol 16:304–310

Gelenberg AJ, Doller-Wojcik JC, Growdon JH (1979) Choline and lecithin in the treatment of tardive dyskinesia: preliminary results from a pilot study. Am J Psychiatry 136:772–776

Gerlach J (1979) Tardive dyskinesia. Dan Med Bull 26:209–245

Gerlach J, Simmelsgaard H (1978) Tardive dyskinesia during and following treatment with haloperidol, haloperidol + biperiden, thioridazine, and clozapine. Psychopharmacology 59:105–112

Gerlach J, Reisby N, Randrup A (1974) Dopaminergic hypersensitivity and cholinergic hypofunction in the pathophysiology of tardive dyskinesia. Psychopharmacologia 34:21–35

Gerlach J, Rye T, Kristjansen P (1978) Effect of baclofen on tardive dyskinesia. Psychopharmacology 56:145–151

Goldman D (1976) Treatment of phenothiazine-induced dyskinesia. Psychopharmacology 47:271–272
Gomez E (1977) Clinical observations in the treatment of tardive dyskinesia with dihydrogenated ergot alkaloids (hydergine), preliminary findings. Psychiatr J Univ Ottawa 2:67–71
Growdon JH, Hirsch MJ, Wurtman RJ, Wiener W (1977) Oral choline administration to patients with tardive dyskinesia. N Engl J Med 297:524–527
Jackson IV, Nuttall EA, Ibe IO, Perez-Cruet J (1979) Treatment of tardive dyskinesia with lecithin. Am J Psychiatry 136:1458–1460
Jeste DV, Wyatt RJ (1982) Therapeutic strategies against tardive dyskinesia. Arch Gen Psychiatry 39:803–816
Jus K, Jus A, Gautier J, Villeneuve A, Pires P, Pineau R, Villeneuve R (1974) Studies on the action of certain pharmacological agents on tardive dyskinesia and on the rabbit syndrome. Int J Clin Pharmacol 9:138–145
Koller WC, Barr A, Biary N (1982) Estrogen treatment of dyskinetic disorders. Neurology 32:547–549
Korsgaard S (1976) Baclofen (lioresal) in the treatment of neuroleptic-induced tardive dyskinesia. Acta Psychiatr Scand 54:17–24
Korsgaard S, Casey DE, Damgaard Pedersen NE, Jørgensen A, Gerlach J (1981) Vasopressin in anergic schizophrenia. A cross-over study with lysine-8-vasopressin and placebo. Psychopharmacology 74:379–382
Korsgaard S, Casey DE, Gerlach J, Hetmar O, Kaldan B, Mikkelsen LB (1982) The effect of tetrahydroisoxazolopyridinol (THIP) in tardive dyskinesia. Arch Gen Psychiatry 39:1017–1021
Korsgaard S, Casey DE, Gerlach J (1983) Effect of gamma-vinyl GABA in tardive dyskinesia. Psychiatry Res 8:261–269
Kulik FA, Wilbur R (1980) Propranolol for tardive dyskinesia and extrapyramidal side effects (pseudoparkinsonism) from neuroleptics. Psychopharmacol Bull 16:18–19
Kunin RA (1976) Manganese and niacin in the treatment of drug-induced dyskinesias. Orthomolec Psychiatry 5:4–27
Linnoila M, Viukari M, Hietala O (1976) Effect of sodium valproate on tardive dyskinesia. Br J Psychiatry 129:114–119
Lipinski JF, Zubenko GS, Cohen BM, Barreira PJ (1984) Propranolol in the treatment of neuroleptic-induced akathisia. Am J Psychiatry 141:412–415
Moore DC, Bowers MB (1980) Identification of a subgroup of tardive dyskinesia patients by pharmacologic probes. Am J Psychiatry 137:1202–1205
Nair NPV, Lal S, Schwartz G, Thavundayil JX (1980) Effect of sodium valproate and baclofen in tardive dyskinesia: clinical and neuroendocrine studies. In: Cattabeni F, Racagni G, Spano PF, Costa E (eds) Long-term effects of neuroleptics. Biochem Psychopharmacol 24:437–441
Nasrallah HA, Smith RE, Dunner FJ, McCalley-Whitters M (1982) Serotonin precursor effects in tardive dyskinesia. Psychopharmacology 77:234–235
Nutt JG, Tamminga CA, Eisler T, Chase TN (1979) Clinical experience with a cholinergic agonist in hyperkinetic movement disorders. In: Barbeau A, Growdon JH, Wurtman RJ (eds) Choline and lecithin in brain disorders. Raven, New York pp 317–324 (Nutrition and the brain, vol 5)
Perenyi A, Farkas A (1983) Propranolol in the treatment of tardive dyskinesia. Biol Psychiatry 18:391–394
Pert A, Rosenblatt JE, Sivit C, Pert CB, Bunney WE Jr (1978) Long-term treatment with lithium prevents the development of dopamine receptor supersensitivity. Science 201:171–173
Prange AJ, Wilson IC, Morris CE, Hall CD (1973) Preliminary experience with tryptophan and lithium in the treatment of tardive dyskinesia. Psychopharmacol Bull 9:36–37
Rastogi SC, Blowers AJ, Gibson AC (1982) Co-dergocrine (hydergine) in the treatment of tardive dyskinesia. Psychol Med 12:427–429
Rosenbaum AH, de la Fuente JR (1979) Benzodiazepines and tardive dyskinesia. Lancet 2:900
Singh MM, Nasrallah HA, Lal H, Pitman RK, Becker RE, Kucharski T, Karkalas J, Fox R (1980) Treatment of tardive dyskinesia with diazepam: indirect evidence for the involvement of limbic, possibly GABA-ergic mechanisms. Brain Res Bull [Suppl 2] 5:673–680

Tamminga CA, Crayton JW, Chase TN (1979) Improvement in tardive dyskinesia after muscimol therapy. Arch Gen Psychiatry 36:595–598

Tamminga CA, Thaker GK, Ferrano TN, Hare TA (1983) GABA agonist treatment improves tardive dyskinesia. Lancet 8341:97–98

Tell GP, Schechter PJ, Koch-Weser J (1981) Effects of gamma-vinyl GABA. N Engl J Med 305:581–582

Villeneuve A, Cazejust T, Cote M (1980) Estrogens in tardive dyskinesia in male psychiatric patients. Neuropsychobiology 6:145–151

Viukari M, Linnoila M (1977) Effect of fusaric acid on tardive dyskinesia and mental state in psychogeriatric patients. Acta Psychiatr Scand 56:57–61

Yassa R, Ananth J (1980) Lithium carbonate in the treatment of movement disorders. Int Pharmacopsychiatry 15:301–308

Pathophysiology of L-Dopa-Induced Abnormal Involuntary Movements

Y. Agid, A.-M. Bonnet, M. Ruberg, and F. Javoy-Agid[1]

Contents

Abstract 145
1 Introduction 146
2 Which Neurotransmitters are Involved in L-Dopa-Induced AIMs? 146
2.1 Pharmacological Studies Supporting the DA Hypothesis 147
2.2 Clinical Studies in Support of the DA Hypothesis 149
3 Which Brain Structures are Involved in the Genesis of L-Dopa-Induced AIMs? . . 150
4 What Biochemical Mechanisms are Involved in the Pathophysiology of L-Dopa-Induced AIMs? 151
4.1 Role of Postsynaptic Dopamine Receptor Hypersensitivity 152
4.2 Role of Increased Activity of the Remaining Dopaminergic Neurons 153
4.3 Role of Accumulated Metabolites of L-Dopa? 154
4.4 Pathogenesis of Interdose and Onset and End-of-Dose Dyskinesias 155
References 156

Abstract

Among the various deficiencies in neurotransmitters and neuropeptides in the brains of patients with Parkinson's disease, the loss of dopamine (DA) is implicated in a major way in the occurrence of L-dopa-induced abnormal involuntary movements (AIMs). Whatever the clinical pattern, they are triggered by drugs which stimulate DA transmission and can be modified by DA agonists and antagonists. They occur when DOPA plasma concentrations, and thus central DA receptor stimulation, reach a critical level. They are observed in patients with severely damaged central DA neurons, but involvement of other neurotransmitter-containing cells cannot be excluded.

L-Dopa-induced AIMs have clinical and somatotopic characteristics, which vary from patient to patient. One might speculate that variable damage to DA neurons, associated or not with other neurotransmitter-containing cells in the affected brain structures, causes these differences in AIM patterns.

By analogy with behavioral experiments in animals, the hypersensitivity of DA receptors observed in the basal ganglia of parkinsonian patients post mortem might reasonably be considered to mediate L-dopa-induced AIMs. However, the role of various subtypes of DA receptors or of changes in DA metabolism in the cell bodies and dendrites (substantia nigra) or nerve terminals (striatolimbic areas) must also be considered. In brief, the features, topography, and timing of L-dopa-induced AIMs are dependent upon alterations of the functional expression of striatal DA output, which is not yet well understood.

---

1 Laboratoire de Médecine Expérimentale, CHU Pitié-Salpêtrière, and Clinique de Neurologie et Neuropsychologie, Hôpital de la Salpêtrière, Boulevard de l'Hôpital, F-75635 Paris Cedex 13, France

Dyskinesia – Research and Treatment
(Psychopharmacology Supplementum 2)
Editors: Casey, Chase, Christensen, Gerlach

1 Introduction

Abnormal involuntary movements (AIMs) constitute one of the most disabling dose-limiting effects of L-dopa and dopamine (DA) agonists in patients with Parkinson's disease. These movements may assume a variety of clinical patterns (Sigwald and Raymondeaud 1970; Marsden et al. 1982), which resemble tardive dyskinesias observed in patients treated with DA receptor-blocking agents (Klawans et al. 1975). Iatrogenic AIMs in humans are induced almost exclusively by drugs known to affect DA transmission, either by blockade or by overstimulation.

The clinical features and topography of L-dopa-induced dyskinesias are very similar to and sometimes indistinguishable from the tardive dyskinesias that complicate administration of neuroleptic drugs: (a) They affect the face, neck, and trunk, but also the limbs. Unlike tardive dyskinesias they are often asymmetric, and usually more severe on the side first affected by the disease (Mones et al. 1971). (b) Whether choreoathetoid or dystonic and ballistic they can either be extremely violent and disabling, or more like an accentuation of normal gestures and behaviors in man, sometimes mimicking the mannerisms observed in schizophrenic patients treated with neuroleptics.

Two main characteristics distinguish L-dopa-induced AIMs from tardive dyskinesias: (a) They are a transient phenomenon occurring when maximum relief of parkinsonian symptoms is obtained (Barbeau et al. 1971). Their duration never exceeds a few hours, and is a function of the pharmacokinetics of the triggering drug. (b) They are not observed in normal subjects given L-dopa (Mena et al. 1970). Abnormal movements have, however, been described in monkeys (Sassin et al. 1972) receiving high doses of the drug. Although L-dopa has occasionally been reported to induce dyskinesias in patients with dystonia and Wilson's disease (Barbeau et al. 1971; Yahr 1970), L-dopa-induced AIMs are almost exclusively observed in patients with Parkinson's disease, i.e., in subjects with known brain lesions (Escourolle et al. 1970), particularly of catecholaminergic neurons (Hornykiewicz 1966; Javoy-Agid et al. 1984a). Schizophrenic patients with tardive dyskinesias, in contrast, have no known neuropathological lesions. L-Dopa-induced AIMs in Parkinson's disease thus represent an heuristic model for study of the pathophysiology of dyskinesias, since correlations between clinical, pharmacological, morphological and biochemical data can be sought.

2 Which Neurotransmitters are Involved in L-Dopa-Induced AIMs?

Among the numerous biochemical abnormalities found in the brain of patients with Parkinson's disease post mortem (Table 1), the most prominent is massive degeneration of the nigrostriatal DA system (Hornykiewicz 1966; Bernheimer et al. 1973) and partial destruction of the mesocorticolimbic (Scatton et al. 1983; Javoy-Agid et al. 1984a) and hypothalamic (Javoy-Agid et al. 1984c) DA systems. The DA lesions are not generalized, however, since DA levels in the spinal cord seem normal (Scatton et al. 1983). The incidence of AIMs in parkinsonian patients with severe degeneration of the DA systems who are receiving long-term

Table 1. Biochemical neuropathy of Parkinson's disease

Degeneration of dopaminergic (DA) systems	Massive destruction of mesostriatal DA system Partial lesion of mesocorticolimbic and hypothalamic DA systems DA neurons in spinal cord not damaged?
Degeneration of other systems of neurons	Acetylcholine (lesion of substantia innominata) Noradrenaline (lesion of locus ceruleus) Serotonin (lesion of raphé nuclei) GABA-ergic neurons spared?
Degeneration or dysfunction of peptidergic systems	Met-enkephalin Leu-enkephalin CCK-8 Substance P Somatostatin (in demented patients)
Intact neuronal sytems	Histidine decarboxylase TRH Vasopressin VIP (cerebral cortex)

treatment with L-dopa and/or DA receptor-stimulating agents (bromocriptine) indicates that they are related to an alteration of DA transmission.

2.1 Pharmacological Studies Supporting the DA Hypothesis

Two types ("interdose" and "onset and end-of-dose" dyskinesias) of AIMs are observed after administration of a single dose of L-dopa (see below). Both types of dyskinesias are triggered and modulated by drugs known to interact with the DA transmission.

In patients with interdose (or "peak") dose dyskinesias, AIMs are observed when DOPA concentrations in the blood (an indirect index of central DA receptor stimulation) are at peak levels (Peaston and Bianchine 1970; Muenter and Tyce 1971; Lhermitte et al. 1977b), i.e., during the period of maximal relief of parkinsonian symptoms. After levodopa administration three phases can be distinguished (Fig. 1): (a) blood dopa levels are subliminal and the patient remains akinetic; (b) dopa levels reach a critical level leading to reduction in parkin-

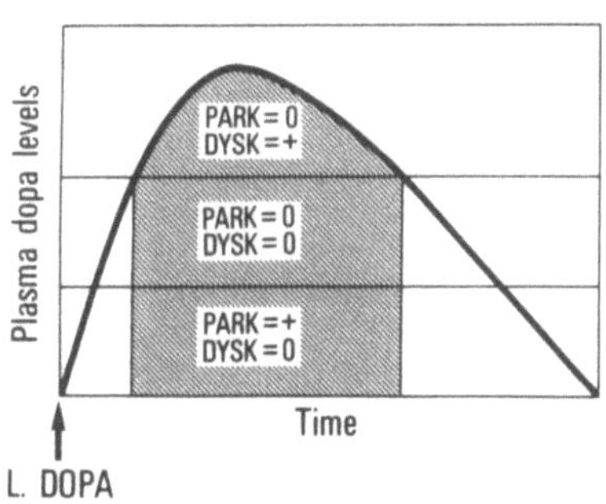

Fig. 1. Schematic representation of the occurrence of interdose dyskinesias in relation to plasma dopa levels after administration of a single dose of L-dopa. Duration of dyskinesias is represented by *hatched bars*. *PARK*, parkinsonian symptoms (0, absent; +, present); *DYSK*, dyskinesias (0, absent; +, present)

sonian disability; (c) when dopa concentrations increase further to peak concentrations a second threshold is reached beyond which interdose dyskinesias are observed. As these dyskinetic episodes regress parkinsonian signs become manifest again. The only way to avoid dyskinesias is to reduce stimulation of central DA receptors, i.e., by maintaining plasma dopa concentrations below the level at which AIMs occur but at a sufficient level to control parkinsonian symptoms. This can be achieved either by giving low doses of DA antagonists to patients (Klawans and Weiner 1974; Tarsy et al. 1975; Lhermitte et al. 1977c) or by reducing and fractionating the daily dose of medication (Barbeau 1976). Reduction of the dosage to avoid or attenuate interdose dyskinesias does in fact shorten the duration of clinical improvement, thus necessitating fractionation of the daily dose. Unfortunately, during the course of the disease the period during which the patient is clinically improved without dyskinesias is gradually reduced, so that the patient is either in a state of complete remission of parkinsonian movements, or in a state of disabling akinesia without AIMs. With time, the AIM phase expands to fill the whole period of clinical improvement ("on" period), with little variation in the pattern of the dyskinesias. These on-off phenomena accompanying the development of sudden AIMs might correspond to the progressive disappearance of the brain "buffer capacities" probably resulting from progressive degeneration of DA and other neuronal systems involved in the control of movement.

The pattern of onset and end-of-dose dyskinesias is entirely different. They account for less than 10% of all L-dopa-induced AIMs (Tolosa et al. 1975; Muenter et al. 1977; Lhermitte et al. 1977a) (Fig. 2). After administration of a single dose of L-dopa, the dyskinesias are not observed when dopa concentrations are low (i.e., when the patient is disabled) or when dopa levels are high (i.e., during the period of maximum relief), but precisely when dopa concentrations in the blood are increasing or decreasing. If stimulation of the DA receptor in the basal ganglia is directly related to plasma dopa concentration, this would mean that onset and end-of-dose dyskinesias are not dependent upon a subminimal or a maximal stimulation of DA receptors, but results from a partial stimulation of receptor sites occurring at a specific concentration of DA in the synapse, i.e., at the beginning and at the end of the action of the DA medication. The first phase of onset dyskinesias cannot be avoided, but end-of-dose dyskinesias can be delayed by administering a second dose of the drug earlier (Lhermitte et al. 1977b; Muenter et al. 1977; Lhermitte et al. 1978), to maintain plasma dopa

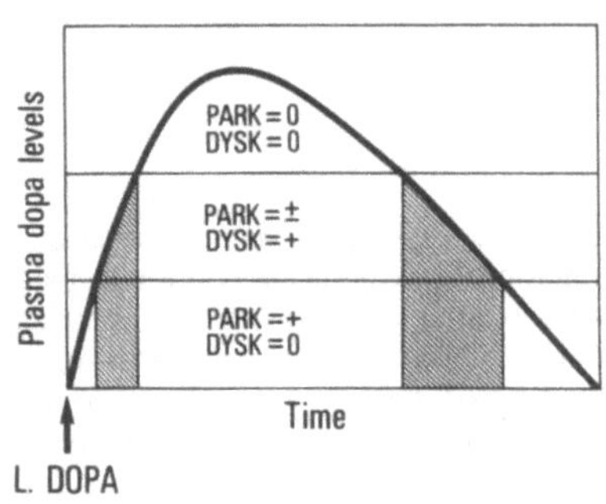

Fig. 2. Schematic representation of the occurrence of onset and end-of-dose dyskinesias in relation to plasma dopa levels after administration of a single dose of L-dopa. Duration of dyskinesias is represented by *hatched bars*. *PARK*, parkinsonian symptoms (0, absent; +, present); *DYSK*, dyskinesias (0, absent; +, present)

concentrations at a high enough level. Onset and end-of-dose dyskinesias can thus be partially relieved by increasing the doses of L-dopa. Unfortunately, it is difficult to increase the daily doses of L-dopa, because of its toxic side-effects. These biphasic dyskinesias can last for several hours when dopa levels remain at doses high enough to reduce central DA receptor stimulation and too low to provoke the return of the parkinsonian symptoms, or when a DA antagonist, such as tiapride, is administered (Lhermitte et al. 1977b).

Other drugs besides DA agonists and antagonists can modify the pattern of L-dopa-induced AIMs. Interdose dyskinesias have been described in patients treated with anticholinergic drugs (Fahn and David 1972). Ethybenztropine, a powerful cholinergic antagonist, has been shown to trigger onset and end-of-dose dyskinesias and to reduce their duration and severity (Kefalos and Agid, unpublished observation). To our knowledge, benzodiazepines are the only other class of drugs that can be used successfully in the routine treatment of L-dopa-induced AIMs. There is a certain lack of specificity, however, since many kinds of AIMs, whatever their cause, are ameliorated by benzodiazepines. Whether this is due to a specific action on the benzodiazepine receptor or to a sedative effect remains to be elucidated. Finally, from a pharmacological point of view, all types of drug-induced AIMs are almost exclusively provoked by L-dopa and/or DA agonists and modulated by drugs that either increase or decrease central DA transmission.

2.2 Clinical Studies in Support of the DA Hypothesis

L-Dopa-induced AIMs are not observed in normal subjects or in patients with degenerative lesions in the basal ganglia sparing DA neurons (Mena et al. 1970; Barbeau et al. 1971), but are seen in patients with severe central DA depletion. In Parkinson's disease there is much evidence that L-dopa-induced AIMs are observed mainly in patients with severe degeneration of the brain DA systems (Agid et al. 1979). In a prospective study concerning 148 patients with L-dopa-induced AIMs out of 279 patients with idiopathic Parkinson's disease, it was possible to draw the following conclusions. In parkinsonian patients prone to AIMs (a) age at onset was lower; (b) the first symptom was akinesia (slowness of movement) and not tremor; (c) patients who developed L-dopa-induced AIMs had improved to a greater extent after the first administration of L-dopa than patients who did not develop L-dopa-induced AIMs; (d) the main symptoms were akinesia and rigidity, which are typically DA-dependent symptoms; (e) there was a higher percentage of clinical improvement under long-term L-dopa treatment; (f) fluctuations of treatment were more frequent in patients with AIMs; and (g) the underlying parkinsonism was more disabling.

In brief, these AIMs were observed in patients with what might be called DA-dependent Parkinson's disease, i.e., in patients with severe central DA depletion.

This observation raises another question: why do only 60%–70% of parkinsonian patients develop L-dopa-induced AIMs? Two explanations can be proposed. (a) Patients with AIMs may have more severely degenerated DA systems. This is supported by the fact that the dyskinesias are observed mainly on the side first affected by the disease (Mones et al. 1971). (b) Dysfunction of other neuronal systems might also be involved. The fact that AIMs are reduced by contralateral thalamotomy and that they are not observed when lesions extend to other structures than the substantia nigra (e.g., the striatum in progressive supranuclear palsy) suggests that in addition to degeneration of DA neurons, other lesions may prevent the occurrence of AIMs, probably due to the disappearance of DA receptors (see below) and/or impairment of DA neuronal output.

In conclusion, L-dopa-induced AIMs seem to be dependent upon DA dysfunction for three main reasons: (a) They occur when dopa plasma levels (i.e., DA receptor stimulation) reach a critical level; (b) they are produced by DA-receptor-stimulating agents and modified by drugs known to interfere with DA transmission; and (c) they are observed in patients with severe loss of DA neurons. However, nondopaminergic neurons may also be implicated.

3 Which Brain Structures are Involved in the Genesis of L-Dopa-Induced AIMs?

From a theoretical point of view, the variable localization of biochemical changes in the brains of individual patients may be responsible for the topography and for the clinical features of L-dopa-induced AIMs. (a) The localization of L-dopa-induced AIMs, whether they are observed in the oral area or in the extremities, is obviously related to impairment of neurotransmission in the structures known to control movement in the corresponding part of the body. This is probably why parkinsonian patients with predominantly unilateral signs have been reported to develop dyskinesias on the more severely affected side (Mones et al. 1971). (b) The clinical profile of AIMs may also result from physiological dysfunction in specific nuclei (or better, to topographically organized neuronal systems) in the basal ganglia. The resulting imbalance between normal and impaired neuronal activities may differ from one patient to another, resulting in different clinical patterns.

This physiological dysfunction could result either from an impairment in DA transmission or from an alteration in other biochemically defined neuronal systems, which might be responsible for a modification of the activity of input or output systems in the basal ganglia. It can be assumed that differences in the severity of the DA neuronal loss may result, depending on the structures, in the clinical variations in parkinsonism from patient to patient. Thus, besides the marked decrease of DA concentrations in the putamen (−95%) and caudate nucleus (−85%) (Bernheimer et al. 1973; Bokobza et al. 1984), Parkinson's disease is also characterized by a reduction in DA levels in other areas of the basal ganglia, i.e., the globus pallidus and the subthalamic nucleus. For example, a large DA deficiency in the subthalamic nucleus might be responsible for the appearance of a specific pattern of AIMs (or at least for a tendency to induce such a pattern), i.e., ballistic movements, characteristically observed after lesions of this structure (Blackwood and Corsellis 1976).

Other neurotransmitters may be implicated in the appearance of AIMs, especially since they are heterogeneously distributed in functionally different structures. This is clearly demonstrated in the striatal complex, where the content of various neurotransmitters and peptides is different in the putamen, caudate nucleus, and nucleus accumbens (Javoy-Agid et al. 1984a). For example, compared with the first two structures, the nucleus accumbens is rich in noradrenaline (Farley and Hornykiewicz 1976) and TRH (Javoy-Agid et al. 1983) and has lower concentrations of Leu-enkephalin (Taquet et al. 1983) and substance P (Mauborgne et al. 1983). Moreover, as exemplified in the human substantia nigra (Javoy-Agid et al. 1982a), the distribution of markers of different neuronal systems is heterogeneous within brain structures. The distinct patterns of distribution of neurotransmitters, which do not necessarily coincide, suggest that they exert a complex influence on the control of motor activity. The situation is even more complex in Parkinson's disease, where the depletion in neurotransmitters is variable within structures and from one structure to another (Javoy-Agid et al. 1982b). For instance, the biochemical anomalies found in the globus pallidus of Parkinson's disease patients are different from those of the caudate nucleus. In the globus pallidus there is a substantial (−70%) decrease in DA concentrations, and levels of other neurotransmitters and neuropeptides are also subnormal (Javoy-Agid et al. 1984b) (Met-enkephalin −60%; serotonin −50%; substance P −40%; Leu-enkephalin −30%; bombesine −15%), whereas pallidal neurons containing choline acetyltransferase, glutamate decarboxylase, histidine decarboxylase, neurotensine, TRH, and cholecystokinin-8 seem to be spared. Discrete biochemical dysfunctions and/or neuronal damage within a given structure involved in motor behavior may be responsible for the corresponding somatotopic extrapyramidal symptoms. Finally, since the decrease in neurotransmitters, and thus the degeneration of the corresponding neurons, is variable from one patient to another, it might be speculated that differences in the modulation of the DA neuronal input and/or output may interfere with the clinical expression of L-dopa-induced AIMs, thus giving rise to various patterns of dyskinesias in different patients.

4 What Biochemical Mechanisms are Involved in the Pathophysiology of L-Dopa-Induced AIMs?

The pathogenesis of L-dopa-induced AIMs in man remains inconclusive, so that any interpretation is necessarily speculative. For simplification, this question will be discussed without reference to the topography and the clinical features of AIMs, which have been shown to result mainly from the localization of neuronal damage, and will focus on the impairment of DA transmission. Although altered central DA transmission is certainly involved in predisposing patients to L-dopa-induced AIMs, it must not be forgotten that the dyskinesias are not observed in patients with no treatment (i.e., with reduced DA transmission) but only when they are overtreated with L-dopa and/or DA agonists (i.e., when stimulation of the DA receptors is excessive due to DA replacement therapy). A biochemical disequilibrium concerning pre- and postsynaptic elements of the DA synapses may be the mechanism underlying AIMs.

4.1 Role of Postsynaptic Dopamine Receptor Hypersensitivity

On the basis of pharmacological (Ungerstedt 1971), electrophysiological (Ohye et al. 1970), and biochemical (Creese et al. 1977; Feuerstein et al. 1981) data it has been suggested that the development of L-dopa-induced dyskinesias is related to hypersensitivity of the striatal DA receptors caused by prolonged denervation. Functional modification of the DA receptor is certainly not solely and directly responsible for the heterogeneous patterns of AIMs in patients. It is, however, a key element for understanding the pathophysiology of L-dopa-induced AIMs, since it is the essential mediator of antiparkinsonian therapy with DA agonists. DA receptors have been studied in the brains of patients with Parkinson's disease post mortem, but no clear consensus has as yet emerged as to the fate of DA receptors. The density of DA receptors labeled with spiperone and haloperidol has been reported to be higher than normal in the caudate nucleus, putamen, and nucleus accumbens (Lee et al. 1978; Rinne et al. 1980), no changes having been observed in the frontal and limbic cortex (Quik et al. 1979; Reisine et al. 1977). Receptor levels have also been reported to be subnormal in the caudate nucleus (Reisine et al. 1977) and substantia nigra (Quik et al. 1979). In L-dopa-treated patients the density of neuroleptic binding sites in the striatum has been found to be subnormal (Lee et al. 1978; Rinne et al. 1980), suggesting that long-term L-dopa medication eliminates this compensatory feature. The latter results have not been confirmed, however (Bokobza et al. 1984). In all these experiments, the labeled receptors were assumed to be located postsynaptically. The existence of DA autoreceptors may, however, partially or completely mask the hypersensitivity of postsynaptic receptors, all the more so since putative D3-type DA receptors, some of which are thought to be autoreceptors, have been reported to decrease in the striatum of parkinsonian patients (Lee et al. 1981). This may explain the apparent absence of increase in the density of ^{3}H-spiperone receptors recently found in the nucleus caudatus and nucleus accumbens in a large series of parkinsonian patients (Bokobza et al. 1984) (Fig. 3).

In patients with progressive supranuclear palsy (a parkinsonian syndrome also characterized by a massive central DA depletion), the 40%–50% reduction in the density of DA receptors observed in all DA brain structures (Fig. 3) may explain why L-dopa does not help these patients and why they do not develop

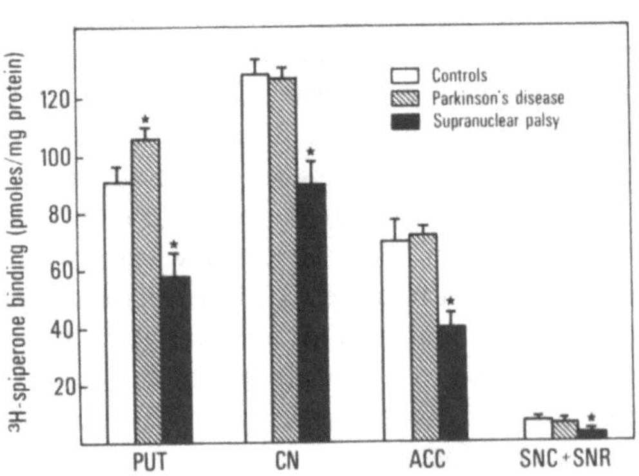

Fig. 3. Density of ^{3}H-spiperone binding sites in patients with Parkinson's disease and progressive supranuclear palsy. *PU*, putamen; *CN*, caudate nucleus; *ACC*, nucleus accumbens; *SNC-SNR*, substantia nigra, pars compacta-substantia nigra, pars reticulata; * significantly different from control patients ($P < 0.02$). (Bokobza et al. 1984)

AIMs. If parkinsonian patients receiving long-term L-dopa therapy have a reduced number of striatal DA receptors, this may explain why these patients are also free of AIMs. These observations thus strongly suggest that an abnormally high receptor density of ^{3}H-spiperone receptors is implicated in the occurrence of L-dopa-induced AIMs.

Dopamine-stimulated adenylate cyclase activity coupled with the DA D1 receptor has been reported to be decreased in the caudate nucleus of parkinsonian patients (Shibuya 1979; Riederer et al. 1978), but contradictory results have been obtained (Nagatsu et al. 1978) and the significance of this finding remains unclear. The role of D1 receptors in L-dopa-induced AIMs should not be underestimated, however, since activation of both D1 and D2 receptors seems to be necessary to restore normal locomotor behavior in reserpinized rats (Gershanik et al. 1983).

4.2 Role of Increased Activity of the Remaining Dopaminergic Neurons

In parkinsonian patients, evidence that the striatal HVA/DA ratio is shifted in favor of the metabolite was interpreted as a result of functional overactivity of the remaining nigrostriatal DA neurons (Bernheimer et al. 1973). This hypothesis was confirmed by animal experiments showing an increase in the synthesis and turnover of striatal DA after partial lesions of the nigrostriatal DA pathway (Agid et al. 1973). DA concentrations were found to be decreased more than HVA levels not only in the nerve terminal regions but also in the substantia nigra of patients (Fig. 4), suggesting that the increased liberation of DA also occurs at the level of cell bodies and dendrites of the remaining DA neurons.

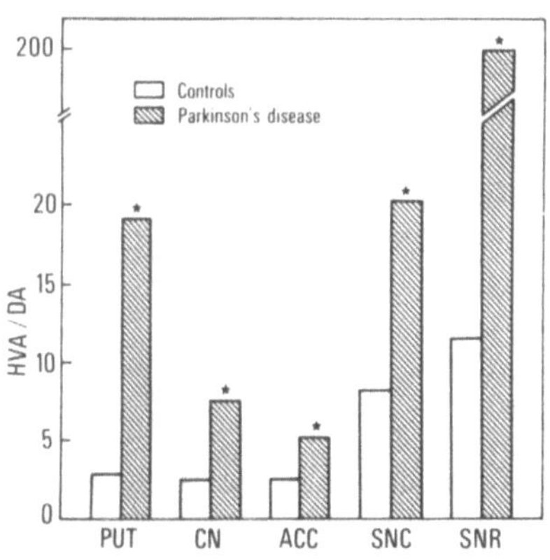

Fig. 4. Homovanillic acid/dopamine ratio (HVA/DA) in the brain of patients with Parkinson's disease. *PU*, putamen; *CN*, caudate nucleus; *ACC*, nucleus accumbens; *SNC-SNR*, substantia nigra, pars compacta-substantia nigra, pars reticulata. * significantly different from control patients ($P < 0.02$). (Bokobza et al. 1984)

4.2.1 Hyperactivity of Remaining DA Nerve Terminals in the Striatum

In spite of the 70%–80% reduction in DA concentration, HVA levels are not significantly different from control levels in the nucleus accumbens of parkinsonian patients (Bokobza et al. 1984), due to the increase in DA turnover rate (as indicated by the HVA/DA ratio); this suggests that presynaptic neuronal overactivity is able to compensate for the loss of DA innervation. This might also explain the absence of DA receptor hypersensitivity observed in this structure (Fig. 3). In the putamen, however, where DA depletion reaches 95%, the marked increase in DA turnover does not restore normal DA transmission. DA receptor hypersensitivity in this structure (Fig. 3) may then reflect a second stage of compensation, which becomes operative only when the number of remaining DA neurons is too small to insure normal transmission. In the latter case, despite the large increase in DA turnover, stimulation of hypersensitive DA receptors (due to denervation) is generally accepted to be responsible for the appearance of hyperkinesia: an undertreated akinetic patient (decreased striatal DA transmission) will become abruptly hyperkinetic when treatment is increased (overstimulation of hypersensitive DA receptors). It might be hypothesized that the localization of hypersensitive DA receptors within the striatum may be responsible for the topography of L-dopa-induced AIMs, a result which is in accordance with the development of dyskinesias on the more severely affected part of the patient's body.

4.2.2 Hyperactivity of Remaining DA Neurons in the Substantia Nigra

A large increase in the HVA/DA ratio in the substantia nigra (especially in the pars reticulata) of parkinsonian patients, contrasting with the massively reduced DA concentrations, might indicate adequate compensation for the loss of DA neurons (Bokobza et al. 1984). The 30%–40% reduction in nigral HVA suggests that nigral DA transmission is reduced in patients with Parkinson's disease. Impairment of nigral DA transmission, which probably varies from patient to patient, may modulate L-dopa-induced AIMs in two ways: (a) The metabolism of DA in the striatum in parkinsonian patients may be continuously modified during long-term L-dopa treatment, since nigral DA release is known to influence the activity of ipsilateral DA neurons and that of striatonigral afferents is known to modulate the activity of the mesostriatal DA system (Cheramy et al. 1981); and (b) the output of DA neurons in substantia nigra is not only directed towards the striatum but also to other structures, such as the thalamus and the tectum (Rinvik et al. 1976). The resulting dysfunction may also interfere with the type and distribution of L-dopa-induced AIMs in patients.

4.3 Role of Accumulated Metabolites of L-Dopa?

There is evidence supporting the hypothesis that a deviation in the catabolism of DA towards abnormal metabolites is implicated in the genesis of L-dopa-induced AIMs. Among the various possible compounds the major metabolite O-methyl-dopa is a reasonably good candidate (Ericsson et al. 1971). Increased plasma concentrations of O-methyl-dopa have been found in patients with AIMs and fluctuation disability (Feuerstein et al. 1977; Rivera-Calimlin et al. 1977). Accumulation of O-methyl-dopa is also a possible source of the on-off phenomena observed during chronic L-dopa treatment: (a) its biological half-life is long (approximately 12 hours) (Kuruma et al. 1970); (b) there is an inverse correlation between fasting plasma levels of 3-O-methyl-dopa and the duration of improvement with L-dopa therapy (Muenter et al. 1972); (c) simultaneous injection of L-dopa and O-methyl-dopa into the carotid artery prevents the amino acid from crossing the blood-brain barrier (Wade and Katzman 1975); (d) uptake and utilization of L-dopa in the rat striatum are reduced by the presence of high plasma concentrations of O-methyl-dopa (Reches and Fahn 1981). However, a role of O-methyl-DA synthesized from O-methyl-dopa in inducing L-dopa-induced AIMs remains extremely improbable, since the characteristics of ^{3}H-spiperone binding in the rat striatum are not modified by increasing concentrations of 3- and 4-O-methyl-DA (Ruberg, Agid, unpublished).

4.4 Pathogenesis of Interdose and Onset and End-of-Dose Dyskinesias

Although all L-dopa-induced AIMs are to some extent related to the modification of central DA transmission, the pattern in interdose dyskinesias is opposite to that in onset and end-of-dose dyskinesias, thus suggesting their mechanism is also different (Agid et al. 1979). Current evidence suggests that the former result from maximal stimulation of striatal DA receptors, whereas the latter are related to partial stimulation of the same DA receptors (see above). Since both types of dyskinesias may be observed in the same patients, their development could be mediated through the stimulation of different DA receptors. With the present knowledge concerning the function of DA receptors (Seeman 1980) a precise description of the molecular alterations occurring in the DA synapse would be too speculative.

Pharmacological studies in animals with lesions of the mesostriatal DA pathway (rotating model in the rat, Ungerstedt 1971; ventrotegmental lesions in the monkey, Poirier et al. 1966) may help us to understand the timing of interdose dyskinesias that occur beyond a critical threshold of stimulation of hypersensitive DA receptors in the striatum. In this case, the role of overstimulation of DA receptors in other basal ganglia structures, such as the nucleus accumbens and the globus pallidus, remains unclear. The pathophysiology of onset and end-of-dose dyskinesias is even more difficult to interpret (Agid et al. 1979). The following elements should be taken into consideration: (a) their incidence during the increase and the decrease of plasma dopa concentrations following the administration of one dose of L-dopa strongly suggests that they are triggered by partial stimulation of DA receptors; (b) their biphasic pattern with time resembles the two-peak profile of rotation observed in rats after administration of L-dopa or apomorphine, contrasting with the one-peak pattern of rotation described in animals treated with other DA agonists such as bromocriptine or pergolide (Herrera-Marschitz and Ungerstedt 1984); (c) their predominantly dystonic and ballistic features (in contrast to the more common choreoathetoid interdose dyskinesias) and their preferential occurrence in the trunk, neck, and lower limbs, whereas interdose dyskinesias affect the head, upper and lower limbs, suggest that they result from dysfunction in different topographically organized systems (pallidohypothalamic area?) than interdose dyskinesias (putaminocaudate area?); (d) since both interdose and onset and end-of-dose dyskinesias are frequently observed in the same patient (Lhermitte et al. 1977a), their chronology after L-dopa treatment may possibly be related to stimulation of different types of DA recep-

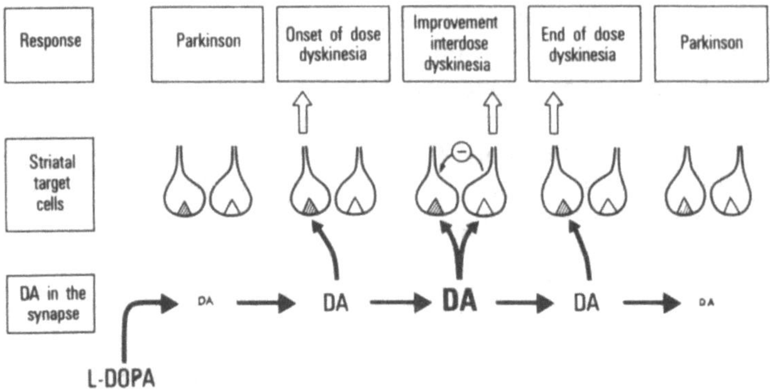

Fig. 5. Hypothetical model of synaptic DA transmission in patients with interdose and onset and end-of-dose dyskinesias

tors; (e) the observed clinical pattern of interdose and of onset and end-of-dose dyskinesias is related to dysfunction of the DA neuronal output, which is itself modulated by impaired activity of other neurotransmitter-containing neurons.

With these ideas in mind, a speculative and oversimplified model of L-dopa-induced interdose and onset and end of dose AIMs is proposed in Fig. 5. After peripheral administration of L-dopa, DA concentrations progressively increase and then decrease in the DA synaptic cleft. When synaptic DA levels are low, the various DA receptor sites located on different striatal target cells are not stimulated and the patient remains akinetic. When synaptic DA levels are high enough, stimulation of one subtype of hypersensitive DA receptors, perhaps because it has a higher affinity for the neurotransmitter, interferes with the DA motor output to give rise to the first set of onset and end-of-dose dyskinesias.

When DA levels are at their maximum in the synapse both DA receptor subtypes are stimulated. Stimulation of the second hypersensitive receptor may be responsible for clinical improvement of parkinsonian signs, and also interdose dyskinesias. To explain why the first burst of AIMs disappears an inhibitory influence on the striatal output of the first overstimulated target cells must be assumed.

When DA levels decrease, the second receptor sites are no longer stimulated, so that end-of-dose dyskinesias recur due to stimulation of the first type of DA receptors, together with the disappearance of interdose dyskinesias. Then parkinsonian disability again becomes manifest because of the reduction in synaptic DA concentrations.

References

Agid Y, Javoy F, Glowinski J (1973) Hyperactivity of remaining dopaminergic neurons after partial destruction of the nigrostriatal dopaminergic system in the rat. Nature 245:150–151

Agid Y, Bonnet AM, Signoret JL, Lhermitte F (1979) Clinical, pharmacological and biochemical approach of "onset and end-of-dose" dyskinesias. In: Poirier LJ, Sourkes TL, Bedard PJ (eds) Advances in neurology, vol 24. Raven, New York, pp 401–409

Barbeau A (1976) Neurological and psychiatric side-effects of L-DOPA. Pharmacol Ther 1:475–494

Barbeau A, Mars H, Gillio-Joffroy L (1971) Adverse clinical side-effects of levodopa therapy. In: McDowell FH, Markham CH (eds) Parkinson's disease. Davis, Philadelphia, pp 203–237

Bernheimer H, Birkmayer W, Hornykiewicz O, Jellinger K, Seitelberger F (1973) Brain dopamine and the syndromes of Parkinson and Huntington: clinical, morphological and neurochemical correlations. J Neurol Sci 20:415–455

Blackwood W, Corsellis JAN (1976) Greenfields neuropathology, 3rd edn. Arnold, London

Bokobza B, Ruberg M, Scatton B, Javoy-Agid F, Agid Y (1984) ^{3}H-spiperone binding, dopamine and HVA concentrations in Parkinson's disease and supranuclear palsy. Eur J Pharmacol 99:167–175

Cheramy A, Laviel V, Glowinski J (1981) Dendritic release of dopamine in the substantia nigra. Nature 289:537

Creese I, Burt DR, Snyder SH (1977) Dopamine receptor binding enhancement accompanies lesion-induced behavioral supersensitivity. Science 197:596–598

Ericsson AD, Wertman BG, Duffy KM (1971) Reversal of the reserpine syndrome with L-DOPA metabolites in reserpinized rats. Neurology 21:1023–1029

Escourolle R, De Recondo J, Gray F (1970) Etude anatomopathologique de syndromes parkinsoniens. In: De Ajuriaguerra J (ed) Monoamines, noyaux gris centraux et syndrome de Parkinson. Symposium Bel Air IV. Masson, Paris, pp 173–229

Fahn S, David E (1972) Oro-facial-lingual dyskinesia due to anticholinergic medication. Trans Am Neurol Assoc 97:277–279

Farley IJ, Hornykiewicz O (1976) Noradrenaline in subcortical brain regions of patients with Parkinson's disease and control subjects. In: Birkmayer W, Hornykiewicz O (eds) Advances in Parkinsonism. Roche, Basel, pp 178–185

Feuerstein C, Serre F, Gavend M, Pellat J, Perret J, Tanche M (1977) Plasma O-Methyldopa in levodopa-induced dyskinesias: a bioclinical investigation. Acta Neurol Scand 56:508–524

Feuerstein C, Demenge P, Barrette G, Silice C, Guerin B, Mouchet P (1981) Long-term effects of nigrostriatal denervation on ^{3}H-haloperidol binding. Eur J Pharmacol 76:457–460

Gershanik O, Heikkila RE, Duvoisin RC (1983) Behavioral correlations of dopamine receptors activation. Neurology 33:1489–1492

Herrera-Marschitz M, Ungerstedt U (1984) Evidence that apomorphine and pergolide induce rotation in rats by different actions on D1 and D2 receptor sites. Eur J Pharmacol 98:165–176

Hornykiewicz O (1966) Dopamine (3-Hydroxytyramine) and brain function. Pharmacol Rev 18:925–964

Javoy-Agid F, Agid Y (1980) Is the mesocortical dopaminergic system involved in Parkinson's disease? Neurology 30:1326–1330

Javoy-Agid F, Ploska A, Agid Y (1982a) Microtopography of TH, CAT, and GAD activity in the substantia nigra and ventral tegmental area of control and parkinsonian human brain. J Neurochem 37:1218–1227

Javoy-Agid F, Ruberg M, Taquet H, Studler JM, Lloyd KG, Garbarg M, Llorens-Cortes C, Grouselle D, Agid Y (1982b) Biochemical neuroanatomy of the human substantia nigra (pas compacta) in normal and parkinsonian subject. In: Friedhoff AJ, Chase TN (eds) Gilles de la Tourette syndrome. Adv Neurol 35:151–163

Javoy-Agid F, Grouselle D, Tixier-Vidal A, Agid Y (1983) Thyrotropin releasing hormone in brain of patients with Parkinson's disease. Neuropeptides 3:405–410

Javoy-Agid F, Ruberg M, Taquet H, Bokobza B, Agid Y, Gaspar P, Berger B, N'Guyen-Legros J, Alvarez C, Gray F, Hauw JJ, Scatton B, Rouquier L (1984a) Biochemical neuropathology of Parkinson disease. In: Hassler RG, Christ JF (eds) Parkinson-specific motor and mental disorders, role of the pallidum: pathophysiological, biochemical, and therapeutic aspects. Adv Neurol 40:189–198

Javoy-Agid F, Taquet H, Cesselin F, Epelbaum J, Grouselle D, Mauborgne A, Studler JM, Agid Y (1984b) Neuropeptides in Parkinson's disease. In: Usdin E (ed) Catecholamines: Neuropharmacology and central nervous system – Therapeutic aspects. Liss, New York, pp 35–42

Javoy-Agid F, Ruberg M, Pique L, Bertagna X, Taquet H, Studler JM, Cesselin F, Epelbaum J, Agid Y (1984C) Biochemistry of the hypothalamus in Parkinson disease. Neurology 34: 672–676

Klawans HL, Weiner WJ (1974) Attempted use of haloperidol in the treatment of L-DOPA induced dyskinesias. J Neurol Neurosurg Psychiatry 37:427–430

Klawans HL, Crossett P, Dana N (1975) Effect of chronic amphetamine exposure on stereotyped behavior: implications for pathogenesis of L-DOPA-induced dyskinesias. In: Calne D, Chase TN, Barbeau A (eds) Dopaminergic mechanisms. Adv Neurol 9:105–112

Kuruma I, Bartholini G, Pletscher A (1970) L-DOPA induced accumulation of 3-O-methyl-DOPA in brain and heart. Eur J Pharmacol 10:189–192

Lee T, Seeman P, Rajput A, Farley IJ, Hornykiewicz O (1978) Receptor basis for dopaminergic supersensitivity in Parkinson's disease. Nature 273:59

Lee T, Seeman P, Hornykiewicz O, Bilbao J, Tourtellotte WW (1981) Parkinson's disease: low density and presynaptic location of D3 receptors. Brain Res 212:494

Lhermitte F, Agid Y, Signoret JL, Studler JM (1977a) Les dyskinesies de "début et fin de dose" provoquées par la L-DOPA. Rev Neurol 133, 5:297–308

Lhermitte F, Agid Y, Feuerstein C, Serre F, Signoret JL, Studler JM, Bonnet AM (1977b) Mouvements anormaux provoquées par la L-DOPA dans la maladie de Parkinson: corrélation avec les concentrations plasmiques de DOPA et de O-méthyl-DOPA. Rev Neurol 133: 445–454

Lhermitte F, Signoret JL, Agid Y (1977c) Etude des effets d'une molécule originale le Tiapride, dans le traitement des mouvements anormaux d'origine extra-pyramidale. Sem Hop Paris 53:9–15

Lhermitte F, Agid Y, Signoret JL (1978) Onset and end-of-dose levodopa-induced dyskinesias, possible treatment by increasing the daily doses of levodopa. Arch Neurol 35:261–263

Marsden CD, Parkes JD, Quinn N (1982) Fluctuations of disability in Parkinson's disease – clinical aspects. In: Marsden CD, Fahn S (eds) Movement disorder. Butterworth Scientific, London, pp 96–122

Mauborgne A, Javoy-Agid F, Legrand JC, Agid Y, Cesselin F (1983) Decrease of substance P-like immunoreactivity in the substantia nigra and pallidum of parkinsonian brains. Brain Res 268:167–170

Mena I, Court J, Fuenzalida S, Papavasiliou PS, Cotzias GC (1970) Modification of chronic manganese poisoning treatment with L-DOPA or 5-OH-tryptophan N Engl J Med 282, 1:5–9

Mones RJ, Elizan TS, Seigel G (1971) Analysis of L-DOPA induced dyskinesias in 51 patients with parkinsonism. J Neurol Neurosurg Psychiatry 34:668–673

Muenter MD, Tyce GM (1971) L-DOPA therapy of Parkinson's disease: plasma L-DOPA concentration, therapeutic response and side effects. Mayo Clin Proc 46:231–239

Muenter MD, Sharpless NS, Tyce GM (1972) Plasma 3-O-methyl-DOPA in L-DOPA therapy in Parkinson's disease. Mayo Clin Proc 47:389–395

Muenter MD, Sharpless NS, Tyce GM, Darley FL (1977) Patterns of dystonia ("I-D-I" and "D-I-D") in response to L-DOPA therapy for Parkinson's disease. Mayo Clin Proc 52:163–174

Nagatsu T, Kanamori T, Kato T, Iikuza R, Narabayashi H (1978) Dopamine stimulated adenylate cyclase activity in the human brain: changes in Parkinsonism. Biochem Med 19:360–365

Ohye C, Bouchard R, Boucher R, Poirier LJ (1970) Spontaneous activity of the putamen after chronic interruption of the dopaminergic pathway: effect of L-DOPA. J Pharm Exp Ther 175:700–708

Peaston MJT, Bianchine JR (1970) Metabolic studies and clinical observations during L-DOPA treatment of Parkinson's disease. Br Med J 1, 5693:400–403

Poirier LJ, Sourkes TL, Bouvier G, Boucher R, Carabin S (1966) Striatal amines, experimental tremor and the effect of harmaline in the monkey. Brain 89:37–52

Quik M, Spokes EG, McKay AVP, Bannister R (1979) Alterations in ^{3}H-spiperone binding in human caudate nucleus, substantia nigra and frontal cortex in Shy-Drager syndrome and Parkinson's disease. J Neurol Sci 43 :429

Reches A, Fahn S (1981) O-methyldopa interferes with striatal utilization of levodopa. Ann Neurol 10:94–95

Reisine TD, Fields JZ, Stern LZ, Johnson PC, Bird ED, Spokes E, Schreiner PS, Enna SJ (1977) Neurotransmitter receptor alterations in Parkinson's disease. Life Sci 21:335

Riederer P, Ransch WD, Birkmayer W, Jellinger K, Danielczyk W (1978) Dopamine sensitive adenylate cyclase activity in the caudate nucleus and metabolic encephalopathies. J Neural Transm [Suppl 14]:153

Rinne UK, Koskinen V, Lonnberg P (1980) Neurotransmitter receptors in the parkinsonian brain. In: Rinne UK, Klinger M, Stamm M (eds) Parkinson's disease. Current Progress, Problems and Management. Elsevier, Amsterdam, pp 93

Rinvik E, Grofova I, Ottersen OP (1976) Demonstration of nigrotectal and nigroreticular projections in the cat by axonal transport of proteins. Brain Res 112:388–394

Rivera-Calimlin L, Tandron D, Anderson F, Joynt R (1977) The clinical picture and plasma levodopa metabolite profile of parkinsonism non responders. Treatment with levodopa and decarboxylase inhibitor. Arch Neurol 34:228–232

Sassin JF, Taub S, Weitzman ED (1972) Hyperkinesia and changes in behavior produced in normal monkeys by L-DOPA. Neurology 22:1122–1125

Scatton B, Javoy-Agid F, Agid Y (1983) Reduction of cortical dopamine, noradrenaline, serotonin and their metabolites in Parkinson's disease. Brain Res 275:321–328

Seeman P (1980) Brain dopamine receptors. Pharm Rev 3:229–313

Shibuya M (1979) Dopamine sensitive adenylate cyclase activity in the striatum of Parkinson's disease. J Neurol Transm 44:287

Sigwald J, Raymondeaud C (1970) Les mouvements anormaux observés au cours du traitement de la maladie de Parkinson par la L-DOPA. Rev Neurol 122, 2:103–112

Taquet H, Javoy-Agid F, Hamon M, Legrand JC, Agid Y, Cesselin F (1983) Parkinson's disease affects differently Met5 and Leu5-enkephalin in the human brain. Brain Res 280:379–382

Tarsy D, Parkes JD, Marsden CD (1975) Metoclopramide and pimozide in Parkinson's disease and levodopa-induced dyskinesias. J Neurol Neurosurg Psychiatry 38:331–335

Tolosa ES, Martin WE, Cohen HP (1975) Dyskinesias during levodopa therapy. Lancet I:1381–1382

Ungerstedt U (1971) Postsynaptic supersensitivity after 6-hydroxydopamine induced-degeneration of the nigrostriatal dopamine system. Acta Physiol Scand [Suppl] 367:69–93

Wade LA, Katzman R (1975) 3-O-methyldopa uptake and inhibition of L-DOPA at the blood brain barrier. Life Sci 17:131–136

Yahr MD (1970) Abnormal involuntary movements induced by dopa: clinical aspects. In: Barbeau A, McDowell FH (eds) L-DOPA and parkinsonism. Davis, Philadelphia, pp 101–108

Discussion Section

Prevalence of Tardive Dyskinesia in a Clinic Population

J. Fleischhauer[1], R. Kocher[2], V. Hobi[2], and U. Gilsdorf[2]

Contents

Abstract 162
1 Introduction 162
2 Methods 164
3 Results 164
4 Discussion 169
References 171

Abstract

The reported prevalence of tardive dyskinesia (TD) widely ranges from 0.5% to 70%. This variability is probably due to many factors, including different patient characteristics, drug treatment exposures, and investigator biases. The aim of this study was to evaluate the prevalence, severity, and symptom type of TD in all 646 patients residing in a psychiatric hospital. Each patient was assessed by a psychiatrist and a neurologist with a special rating scale after drug dose had been stabilized for a minimum of 1 week. The overall prevalence was 32%, with a slightly higher rate and more severe symptoms in women. Age positively correlated with increasing prevalence and severity of TD. Psychiatric diagnosis and duration of neuroleptic therapy were not significantly correlated with TD prevalence. The results are generally consistent with the majority of findings in other studies of the epidemiology of TD.

1 Introduction

We have access in the literature to a large number of reports of studies on the prevalence of tardive dyskinesia (TD). Overall, the prevalence rates recorded vary remarkably widely (0.5%–70%) (Hoff and Hoffmann 1967; Degkwitz et al. 1976), with a number of different intermediate rates (Fleischhauer 1980; Brücher 1983; Wöller and Tegeler 1983). Probably this variability is based on different causes.

Definition of the Syndrome of Tardive Dyskinesia. It is often difficult to differentiate the TD syndrome from similar neurological syndromes, e.g., tardive dystonia, spontaneous hyperkinetic syndromes, or the syndrome caused by nonneuroleptic substances, such as L-dopa (Klawans and McKendall 1971), antihistaminics (Davis 1976), and chronic amphetamine use (Mattson and Calverly 1968).

1 Clinic of Psychiatry of the Canton Lucerne, CH-4915 St. Urban, Switzerland
2 University Clinic of Psychiatry, CH-4000 Basle, Switzerland

Dyskinesia – Research and Treatment
(Psychopharmacology Supplementum 2)
Editors: Casey, Chase, Christensen, Gerlach

Recording of Different Degrees of Severity. It is of importance whether only moderate and severe symptoms of TD are recorded or whether mild and occasional symptoms are included.

Different Patient Populations. Since age and sex seem to be implicated in the etiology of TD, the composition of patient samples in different studies is important for the different rates of prevalence. Observations of geriatric patients only (Bourgeois et al. 1980) yielded a high prevalence of 42%.

Whether only inpatients or only outpatients are observed may also have an influence on the prevalence, since the dose of neuroleptics given may influence the severity of TD symptoms.

In earlier investigations lower prevalence rates were found in outpatients, e.g., 4% (Hippius and Lange 1970), while in later observations showing prevalence rates of 30%–43% there was no difference between outpatients and inpatients (Asnis et al. 1977; Ezrin-Waters et al. 1981).

Dependence of TD Symptoms on Vigilance. The prevalence depends significantly on whether vigilance and affective tension are excluded or included. If the patients are directly observed their vigilance, and therefore the rate of prevalence, is higher. When the information is obtained by the nursing staff by means of a questionnaire the rate of prevalence is lower (as in the study of Hoff and Hoffmann 1967); however, the degree of severity can be higher. This dependence of prevalence on the methodology of the study was shown clearly by Smith et al. (1979).

Influence of Medication. In the opinion of most investigators the chemical construction and the neuroleptic potency of the different neuroleptics have no influence on the prevalence. A few reports allege that TD occurs less frequently with thioridazine (Sayers et al. 1977), clozapine, and also sulpiride. Sulpiride, however, occupies a special position, since the neuroleptic effect is doubtful. The opinion occasionally advanced that cumulative doses of neuroleptics increase the incidence and therewith the prevalence (Crane 1970, Crane 1980; Schmidt 1977) has not been proved by other observations (Chouinard et al. 1979a; Fann et al. 1972; Gardos et al. 1980). Generally the symptoms of TD appear after 1–2 years' therapy with neuroleptics (Crane 1980; Degkwitz et al. 1976), and beyond this the duration of therapy seems to have no additional influence (Degkwitz et al. 1976; Asnis et al. 1977; Schmidt 1977; Perris et al. 1979). We have, however, observed a young schizophrenic patient who developed mild linguo-oral hyperkinesias even after 3 months' therapy with thioridazine, which gradually disappeared after a dose reduction.

Although hyperkinesias can appear during neuroleptic therapy, they often appear after a dose reduction and are then sometimes called masked TD. In young patients this appearance seems to be the rule (Marsden et al. 1975). Since reduction and increase of the neuroleptic dose influence the severity and the existence or nonexistence of TD symptoms, neuroleptic dose seems to be an important factor in the prevalence rate recorded in an investigation.

There are publications positively confirming that an anticholinergic medication has an influence on the prevalence of TD, which seems convincing on a theoretical basis (Crane 1980; Klawans and Rubovits 1974; Jus et al. 1976). On the other hand, there are others that do not confirm such a relationship (Asnis et al. 1977; Gardos et al. 1980).

Although the connection between neuroleptics and TD is obvious and not disputed, there are few directly involved factors; some of them are vague and not precisely comprehensible, so that the possibility of a single factor must also be considered (Hippius and Lange 1970).

The aim of the present study was to record the different variables that might possibly influence the prevalence, the severity and the symptoms of TD (age, sex, diagnosis, duration of illness, neuroleptic medication, kind of neuroleptics, dosage, duration of therapy, other medication, vigilance). The use of a large patient sample, i.e., the total population of inpatients in a large psychiatric clinic should make it possible to see some correlations.

2 Methods

All patients in a psychiatric hospital (total of 646 patients, 272 male and 374 female patients) were seen by a psychiatrist and a neurologist together at the same time on their wards. Each patient was examined a minimum of 1 week after the last change of the dose of neuroleptics and/or anticholinergics. All phenomenological forms of TD were recorded, as were mild, questionable, or occasional forms. The influence of vigilance and of affective tension on TD was investigated by finger-tapping and direct verbal contact. The patients with TD were scored on a special rating scale for hyperkinetic movements (Fig. 1), in which the movements of each muscle group could be quantified from 0 (absent) to 3 (present and marked). The means of the results recorded by the two investigators are the bases of this study.

3 Results

In all, 192 patients (76 men, 116 women) out of 646 inpatients were found to have TD. This was about 32% of the total hospital population (Table 1).

The total scores obtained on the rating scale used ranged from 1 point to a maximum of 18 points. A score of up to 6 points was considered to denote a mild form, and such scores were determined in 64% of the patients; moderate forms were recorded with 7–12 points (29% of the patients); and severe forms of TD, with scores of 13–18 points, were found in 7%.

This numerical classification corresponded rather well with the clinical overall impression of the investigators, with 51% mild, 25% moderate, and 23% severe forms of TD. TD was particularly often observed in the head region and here again it appeared mostly as perioral hyperkinesias. This site was followed by the extremities, primarily by the ankle and toe, then the abdominal muscles and trunk muscles. Rather rarely, TD affecting the muscles of the eyes (rapid and continuous glances) was seen, and occasionally it took the form of involuntary move-

Scale for abnormal hyperkinetic movements

Cantonal Psychiatric Clinic, St. Urban, Lucerne

Name: ....

Date of birth: .... Sex: ....

Diagnosis: 1. ....

2. ....

Parkinsonism Yes ☐ No ☐

	Date of examination:	☐
Head	Ocular and brow musculature	☐
	Perioral musculature	☐
	Tongue	☐
	Jaw	☐
Trunk	Neck area	☐
	Shoulder area	☐
	Abdominal/hip area	☐
Extremities	Elbow joints	☐
	Hand and finger joints	☐
	Knee joint	☐
	Foot and toe joints	☐
	Overall total	☐

Subjective assessment of debility ☐

Exacerbation during consultation No = 0 / Yes = 1 ☐

Severity of abnormal movements ☐

Present medication: 1. .... mg/day

2. .... mg/day

3. .... mg/day

Therapy: .... mg/day

Assessment scale: 0 = none / 1 = slight / 2 = moderate / 3 = pronounced

Fig. 1. Rating scale for abnormal hyperkinetic movements

Table 1. Prevalence of TD symptoms with sex distribution

	Inpatients total	With TD	Percent	Corrected values
Men	255	76	29.8	47.5%
Women	353	116	32.9	52.5%
Total	608	192	31.6	100%

ments of the neck, the shoulders, and the upper arm (Fig. 2). An increase in TD during the study, probably due to raised vigilance, was observed in not less than two-thirds of the patients (66%). Furthermore, it was noticeable that 86% of the patients did not feel debilitated by these rather marked hyperkinesias and only 14% stated a debility. This is an obvious contrast to the feeling of debility with other extrapyramidal movement disorders, e.g., parkinsonism, akathisia. Among the total inpatients observed a rather high prevalence of hyperkinesia was found: 30% in men and 33% in women. The corrected values show a slightly higher value in women (52.5%) than in men (47.5%) (Table 1).

Not all patients were receiving neuroleptics. Of the patients observed 22% did not receive any neuroleptics during the observation period but had had such medication previously, in some cases months before; 48% received neuroleptics

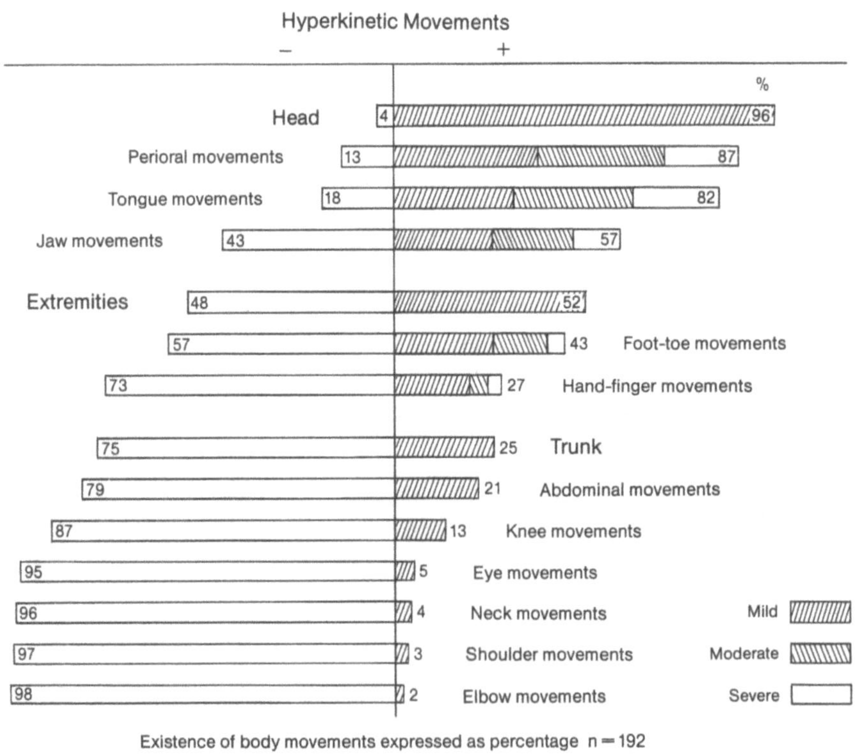

Fig. 2. Distribution of TD symptoms

Table 2. Significant influences of therapy and secondary diagnosis

Feet/toes	Lower values in patients receiving no neuroleptics $P \leq 0.005$ Higher values in patients receiving anticholinergics only $P \leq 0.016$
Shoulder, abdomen trunk	Higher values in patients with organic brain syndrome $P \leq 0.05$

only; and 30% received combinations of neuroleptics and anticholinergics. It is of interest that the factor "Therapy" was shown to have a significant influence on hyperkinesia of toe and ankle (Table 2). Patients with a very long neuroleptic therapy (19–21 years) were in the majority, but a significant difference from other groups was not calculated (Table 3 and Fig. 3).

With reference to the factor "Age distribution" the group of patients aged 66–74 years was oviously the largest, followed by the group aged 75–94 years (Fig. 4 and Table 4). The age now has a remarkable and highly significant influence on the ratio of single TD symptoms, since at higher age the severity of hyperkinetic disorders is obviously increased (Table 5). This increase, however, was not significant for all TD symptoms but only for a few, e.g., perioral and jaw movements and hand and finger movements. The total of head movements and

Table 3. Duration of therapy

Duration	Patients	
	n	%
1– 6 years	53	27.6
7–18 years	52	27.1
19–21 years	87	45.3

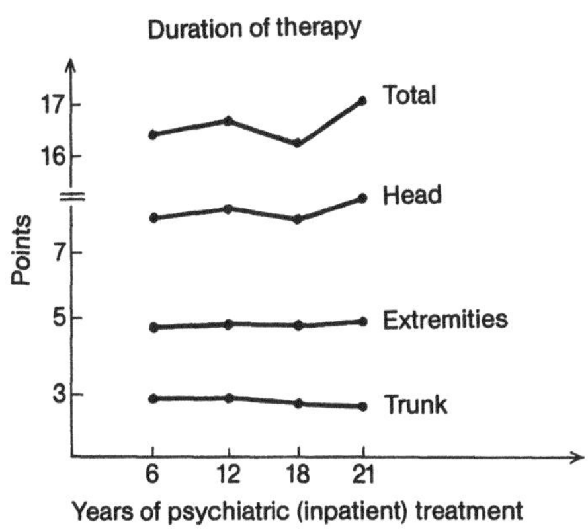

Fig. 3. Influence of duration of therapy on mean total and subgroup scores

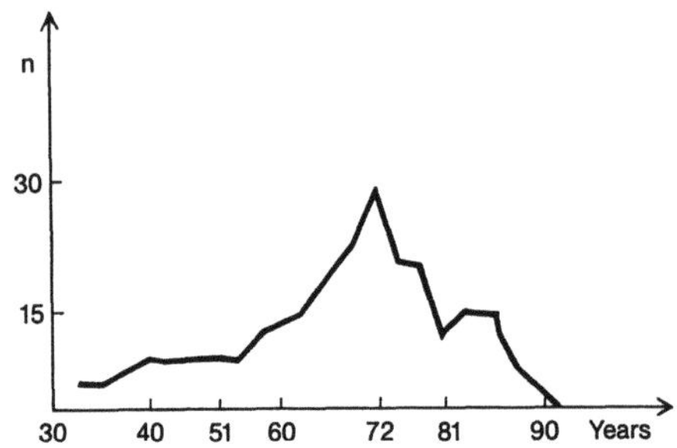

Fig. 4. Age distribution of patients with TD symptoms

Table 4. Age distribution

n	%	Age range
66	34.4	31–65 years
64	33.3	66–74 years
62	32.3	75–94 years

Table 5. Influence of age (mean scores of single significant syndromes)

Symptoms \ Age group	31–65 years ($n = 66$)	66–74 years ($n = 64$)	75–94 years ($n = 62$)	Significance
Perioral hyperkinesias	2.44	2.57	2.79	$P \leq 0.05$
Hyperkinesias of jaw	1.59	1.93	2.19	$P \leq 0.001$
Hyperkinesias of head	7.58	8.12	8.81	$P \leq 0.05$
Hyperkinesias of hands and fingers	1.31	1.34	1.56	T[a]
Total	15.89	16.74	17.77	$P \leq 0.05$

[a] Tendency ($P \leq 0.1$)

the total of all symptoms together is also significantly influenced by age (Table 5).

Sex has a strong influence on TD. In all groups of muscles men have a lower ratio of TD, which is highly significant in some cases. Table 6 shows these groups of muscles, which are significantly different in male and female patients. These are the most frequently recorded symptoms. Only movements of the eye, neck, shoulder, and elbow do not differ significantly between the sexes. These TD symptoms are rare in any case (see Fig. 2).

The influence of the medication was rather small, only the toe and ankle hyperkinesias being less severe in the group without neuroleptics (significant at the 5% level) and more severe in the group receiving anticholinergics only (significant at the 2% level). No influence of the general psychiatric diagnoses on TD was seen, except in patients who had a secondary diagnosis of a psycho-organic brain syndrome. This group had a higher ratio of TD in the area of shoulder,

Table 6. Influence of sex (mean scores of single significant syndromes)

Symptoms	♀ ($n = 116$)	♂ ($n = 76$)	Significance
Perioral hyperkinesias	2.70	2.43	$P \leq 0.05$
Hyperkinesias of tongue	2.68	2.44	T[a]
Movements of jaw	1.99	1.76	T[a]
Movements of head	8.46	7.70	$P \leq 0.05$
Movements of abdomen	1.37	1.12	$P \leq 0.01$
Movements of trunk	3.43	3.17	$P \leq 0.05$
Movements of hands/fingers	1.55	1.17	$P \leq 0.0005$
Movements of knee	1.24	1.08	$P \leq 0.05$
Movements of feet/toes	1.82	1.49	$P \leq 0.01$
Extremities	5.66	4.74	$P \leq 0.0005$
Total	17.55	15.61	$P \leq 0.0005$

[a] Tendency ($P \leq 0.1$)

trunk and abdominal muscles than patients without this diagnosis, and the difference was significant at the 5% level (Table 2).

4 Discussion

In our study sex was seen to have a significant influence, with female patients having a higher prevalence (52%) and more pronounced TD symptoms, i.e., a higher degree of severity, than men (48%). This is confirmed by several other studies (Hippius and Lange 1970; Lehmann et al. 1970; Perris et al. 1979; Jus et al. 1976; Brandon et al. 1971). Crane (1968a), on the other hand, found a higher prevalence in male patients. But there are also other studies where no connection between prevalence and sex could be found (Fann et al. 1972; Asnis et al. 1977; Ezrin-Waters et al. 1981). Since the difference in our study is not so wide, and since at the moment we have no differentiation of the ages in this group between men and women, the possibility cannot be excluded that the apparent sex influence might also be a function of age rather than of sex. On the other hand, the differences are so striking that we tend more to the opinion that there is a genuine sex effect in these data.

The influence of age on TD seems clear enough and confirms other studies. Our study also confirms the findings of other investigators that the TD syndrome rarely occurs in patients under 30 (Crane and Smith 1980).

The discussion as to whether or not medication with anticholinergics leads to a higher degree of severity of TD or even the opposite, is still open. Some studies see a connection between a higher prevalence of TD and anticholinergics (Perris et al. 1979; Itil et al. 1981), but others do not find a relationship (Jus et al. 1976; Chouinard et al. 1979b, c). The experienced clinician can often observe that the initiation of anticholinergic medication can aggravate already existing TD symptoms and also the opposite, that withdrawal of anticholinergics is followed by improvements in TD symptoms. Our material shows an influence insofar as the group of patients receiving no medication but anticholinergics had significantly more severe TD symptoms than the others. Prevalence was not influenced by anticholinergics.

Concerning the psychiatric diagnosis, in our patients we found no influence on the prevalence (Table 7). But we found that the patients with a secondary diagnosis of organic brain syndrome had higher degrees of severity, or a higher ratio of TD symptoms, than the others. This result confirms the findings of Chouinard et al. (1979 a) and of Itil et al. (1981), who found the same in schizophrenic patients. Whether organic brain syndrome also increases the prevalence of TD or not is an open and still controversial question (Perris et al. 1979; Heinrich et al. 1968).

Table 7. Distribution of psychiatric diagnoses[a]

Diagnosis	*n*	%
Schizophrenia	83	43.2
Schizoaffective psychoses	3	1.6
Endogenous depression	12	6.3
Dementias	70	36.5
Oligophrenia (and others)	24	12.5

[a] This factor did not have a significant influence on prevalence

No influence of the length of therapy could be found, if we consider that all our patients had taken neuroleptics for more than 1 year. The three groups, which are fairly roughly divided (1–6, 7–18, 19–21 years of therapy), had equal prevalence rates. Studies with more age-limited groups revealed that long durations of neuroleptic therapy involved a higher risk of TD symptoms (Heinrich et al. 1968; Ezrin-Waters et al. 1981).

In conclusion it can be said that

1. TD can have a relatively high prevalence, 32% in this study.
2. Female subjects have a higher prevalence (52%) than males (48%).
3. Age has a marked influence on the frequency and ratio of TD ($P \leqq 0.05$–0.001).
4. Sex has a similar influence on TD; female patients have more pronounced TD ($P \leqq 0.005$–0.0005).
5. Organic brain syndromes seem to have an influence on the ratio of TD ($P \leqq 0.005$).
6. Absence of neuroleptics is followed by a milder form of TD only in the ankle and toe joints ($P \leqq 0.005$).
7. Medication with anticholinergics alone results in a higher ratio of TD in the ankle and toe joints ($P \leqq 0.016$).
8. Psychiatric diagnosis and duration of therapy had no significant influence on the prevalence of TD.

References

Asnis GM, Leopold MA, Duvoisin RC, Schwartz AH (1977) A survey of tardive dyskinesia in psychiatric outpatients. Am J Psychiatry 134:1367–1370
Bourgeois M, Bouihl P, Tignol J, Yesavage J (1980) Spontaneous dyskinesias. vs. neuroleptic induced dyskinesias in 270 elderly subjects. J Nerv Ment Dis 168:177–178
Brandon S, McClelland MA, Prothero C (1971) A study of facial dyskinesia in a mental hospital population. Br J Psychiatry 118:171–184
Brücher K (1983) Die Spätdyskinesien – eine Übersicht über Klinik, Pathogenese, Prophylaxe und Therapie eines späten neuroleptischen Seiteneffektes. Fortschr Neurol Psychiatry 51:183–199
Chouinard G, Annable L, Ross-Chouinard A, Nestoros JN (1979a) Factors related to tardive dyskinesia. Am J Psychiatry 136:79–83
Chouinard G, Annable L, Ross-Chouinard A, Kropsky MT (1979b) Ethopropazine and benztropine in neuroleptic induced parkinsonism. J Clin Psychiatry 40:73–81
Chouinard G, De Montigny C, Annable L (1979c) Tardive dyskinesia and antiparkinson medication. Am J Psychiatry 136:228–229
Crane G (1968a) Dyskinesia and neuroleptics. Arch Gen Psychiatry 19:700–703
Crane G (1968b) Tardive dyskinesia in patients treated with major neuroleptics: a review. Am J Psychiatry 124:40–47
Crane G (1970) High doses of trifluperazine and tardive dyskinesia. Arch Neurol 22:176–180
Crane G (1980) Neuroleptic drugs and other factors predisposing to TD. In: Fann WE, Smith RC, Davis JM, Domino EF (eds) Tardive dyskinesia, research and treatment. Spectrum, New York
Crane G, Smith RC (1980) The prevalence of tardive dyskinesia. In: Fann WE, Smith RC, Davis JM, Domino EF (eds) Research and treatment. Spectrum, New York
Davis WA (1976) Dyskinesia associated with chronic antihistamine use. N Engl J Med 294:113–116
Degkwitz R, Consbruch U, Haddenbrock S, Neusch B, Oehlert W, Unsöld R (1976) Therapeutische Risiken bei der Langzeitbehandlung mit Neuroleptika und Lithium. Nervenarzt 47:81–87
Ezrin-Waters C, Seeman MV, Seeman P (1981) Tardive dyskinesia in schizophrenic outpatients: Prevalence and significant variables. J Clin Psychiatry 42:16–22
Fann WE, Davis JM, Janowsky DS (1972) The prevalence of tardive dyskinesias in mental hospital patients. Dis Nerv Syst 33:182–186
Fann WE, Smith RC, Davis JM, Domino EF (eds) (1980) Tardive dyskinesia, research and treatment. Spectrum, New York
Fleischhauer J (1980) Späte Hyperkinesien bei neuroleptischer Langzeittherapie. Der Informierte Arzt 8:55–60
Gardos G, Cole JO, La Brie RA (1980) Drug variables in the etiology of TD. In: Fann WE, Smith RC, Davis JM, Domino EF (eds) Tardive dyskinesia research and treatment. Spectrum, New York
Heinrich K, Wegener I, Bender HJ (1968) Späte extrapyramidale Hyperkinesien bei neuroleptischer Langzeittherapie. Pharmacopsychiatry 1:169–195
Hippius H, Lange J (1970) Zur Problematik der späten extrapyramidalen Hyperkinesien nach langfristiger neuroleptischer Therapie. Arzneimittelforsch 20:888–890
Hoff G, Hoffmann G (1967) Das persistierende extrapyramidale Syndrom bei Neuroleptika-Therapie. Wien Med Wochenschr 117:14–17
Itil TM, Reisberg B, Hugue M, Mehta D (1981) Clinical profiles of tardive dyskinesia. Compr Psychiatry 22:282–290
Jus A, Pineau R, Lachance R, Pelchat G, Jus K, Pires P, Villeneuve R (1976) Epidemiology of tardive dyskinesia. Dis Nerv Syst 37:210–214, 257–261
Klawans HL, McKendall R (1971) Observations on the effects of L-DOPA on tardive linguobuccal dyskinesia. J Neurol Sci 14:189–192
Klawans HL, Rubovits R (1974) Effect of cholinergic and anticholinergic agents on tardive dyskinesia. J Neurosurg Psychiatry 37:941–944

Lehmann HE, Ban TA, Saxena BM (1970) A survey of extrapyramidal manifestation in the in-patient population of a psychiatric hospital. Laval Med 41:909–916
Marsden CD, Tarsy D, Baldessarini RJ (1975) Spontaneous and drug induced movement disorders in psychiatric patients. In: Benson DF, Blumer D (eds) Psychiatric aspects of neurologic disease. Grune and Stratton, New York
Mattson RH Calverly JR (1968) Dextroamphetamine-sulphate-induced dyskinesias. JAMA 204:400–402
Perris C, Dimitrijevic P, Jacobsson L, Paulsson P, Rapp W (1979) TD in psychiatric patients treated with neuroleptics. Br J Psychiatry 135:509–514
Sayers AC, Bürki HR, Ruch W, Asper H (1977) Animal models for tardive dyskinesia: Effects of thioridazine. Pharmakopsychiatry 10:291–295
Schmidt P (1977) Verlaufsbeobachtungen an Patienten mit Hyperkinesen. Psychiatr Neurol Med Psychol 29:689–695
Smith JM, Kucharski LT, Oswald WT, Waterman LJ (1979) A systematic investigation of tardive dyskinesia in inpatients. Am J Psychiatry 138:918–922
Wöller W, Tegeler J (1983) Späte extrapyramidale Hyperkinesien Klinik-Prävalenz-Pathophysiologie. Fortschr Neurol Psychiatry 51:131–157

Animal Models

Differential Alteration of Striatal D-1 and D-2 Receptors Induced by the Long-Term Administration of Haloperidol, Sulpiride or Clozapine to Rats [1]

P. Jenner, N. M. J. Rupniak, and C. D. Marsden [2]

Contents

Abstract . . . 174
1 Introduction . . . 174
2 Drug Administration . . . 176
2.1 Alterations in Striatal D-2 Function After 12 Months' Treatment with Haloperidol, Sulpiride or Clozapine . . . 176
2.2 Alterations in Striatal D-1 Function After 12 Months' Treatment with Haloperidol, Sulpiride or Clozapine . . . 177
3 Discussion . . . 179
References . . . 180

Abstract

Rats received haloperidol, sulpiride, or clozapine in their daily drinking water for up to 1 year in clinically equivalent doses. After 12 months' drug intake, and while drug administration continued, striatal dopamine function was assessed. Haloperidol induced D-2 receptor hypersensitivity as shown by enhanced apomorphine-induced stereotypy, elevated B_{max} for specific ^{3}H-spiperone and ^{3}H-NPA binding, and an increase in striatal acetylcholine content. D-1 receptor sites appeared unaffected, since dopamine-stimulated adenylate cyclase and specific ^{3}H-piflutixol binding were not altered. In contrast, neither sulpiride nor clozapine enhanced apomorphine-induced stereotypy or increased B_{max} for ^{3}H-spiperone binding. Sulpiride, but not clozapine, increased B_{max} for ^{3}H-NPA binding; clozapine, but not sulpiride, elevated striatal acetyl choline concentrations. In general, both sulpiride and clozapine enhanced D-1 function as assessed by dopamine-stimulated adenylate cyclase or ^{3}H-piflutixol binding. On acute administration sulpiride and clozapine appear to act at D-2 sites, but continuous chronic administration of these compounds does not result in the development of striatal D-2 receptor hypersensitivity. The absence of change in D-2 function during chronic treatment, coupled with an ability to enhance D-1 function, may contribute to the low incidence of tardive dyskinesia produced by these drugs in man.

1 Introduction

The clinical pharmacology of neuroleptic-induced tardive dyskinesia suggests that an overactivity of brain dopamine function develops during chronic neuroleptic therapy and that this may persist following drug withdrawal (Marsden et al. 1973; Klawans 1973). This hypothesis is complicated by the fact that brain

1 This study was supported by the Wellcome Trust, the Medical Research Council and the Research Funds of the Bethlem Royal and Maudsley Hospitals and King's College Hospital

2 MRC Movement Disorders Research Group, University Department of Neurology and Parkinsons Disease Society Research Centre, Institute of Psychiatry and Kings College Hospital Medical School, Denmark Hill, London SE5, England

Dyskinesia – Research and Treatment
(Psychopharmacology Supplementum 2)
Editors: Casey, Chase, Christensen, Gerlach

dopamine receptors are not a single entity (Seeman 1980). At the simplest level they can be divided into those linked directly to adenylate cyclase (D-1) and those not directly linked to adenylate cyclase (D-2) (Kebabian and Calne 1979). The alterations in motor function produced by the acute administration of neuroleptics are usually attributed to their common action on D-2 sites; the function of D-1 sites in the brain remains unknown (Leysen 1981).

In short-term experiments, the repeated administration of a variety of neuroleptic drugs for some weeks followed by drug withdrawal results in dopamine receptor hypersensitivity, accompanied by consistent increases in D-2 receptor numbers (identified using ^{3}H-spiperone) and in apomorphine-induced behaviours attributed to D-2 receptor effects (Muller and Seeman 1978; Fleminger et al. 1983). In contrast, no consistent changes in D-1 function occur, as judged by changes in dopamine-stimulated adenylate cyclase or by altered ^{3}H-*cis*-flupenthixol or ^{3}H-piflutixol binding. So, the conclusion from this evidence is that it is the alterations in D-2, rather than D-1, receptor function resulting from chronic neuroleptic treatment that are of importance in the development of tardive dyskinesia.

However, in experiments in which animals received trifluoperazine, thioridazine or *cis*-flupenthixol in their drinking water for up to 18 months, alterations in both D-1 and D-2 receptor function occurred (Clow et al. 1979, 1980a; Murugaiah et al. 1983b). Thus, drug treatment enhanced apomorphine-induced stereotypy, elevated B_{max} for ^{3}H-spiperone binding and increased the ability of dopamine to stimulate adenylate cyclase. This last change was of particular interest, since it persisted for 6–12 months following cessation of drug intake; changes in other parameters were only apparent up to 3 months following drug withdrawal (Clow et al. 1980b; Murugaiah et al. 1983a).

Recent evidence has challenged the concept that D-1 and D-2 sites act independently of each other and that only D-2 sites are of functional importance. Thus, Stoof and Kebabian (1981) have shown that selective D-2 antagonists, such as sulpiride, could enhance the efflux of cyclic AMP initiated by agonist stimulation of D-1 receptors. This suggests the existence of a population of D-2 sites which are inhibitory on D-1 function. Recently, the first selective D-1 antagonist drug, SCH 23390, was synthesised; this compound can inhibit apomorphine-induced motor behaviors (Iorio et al. 1983), which are usually attributed to D-2 receptor activation.

This report discusses the role of D-1 receptors in the ability of chronic neuroleptic drug treatment to induce dopamine receptor hypersensitivity in relation to their ability to induce tardive dyskinesia. Three possibilities are evident:

1. Tardive dyskinesia is a result of altered D-2 receptor function alone.
2. Tardive dyskinesia is a result of altered D-1 receptor function alone.
3. Tardive dyskinesia is a result of alterations in both D-1 and D-2 receptor function.

In the present study we have attempted to evaluate the importance of changes of D-1 and D-2 sites during chronic neuroleptic treatment by utilising drugs selective for D-2 sites (haloperidol and sulpiride) and drugs whose use in man is associated with a low incidence of extrapyramidal side-effects (sulpiride and clozapine).

2 Drug Administration

Male Wistar rats (205 ± 14 g at the start of the experiment) were housed initially in groups of eight under standard conditions of lighting (12 h light/dark cycle) and temperature (21 ± 3 °C). Animals were randomly allocated to one of four treatment groups, which received ad libitum as their daily drinking water distilled water alone (controls) *or* haloperidol solution (target intake 2 mg/kg per day) *or* sulpiride solution (target dose 100 mg/kg per day) *or* clozapine (30 mg/kg per day) for a continuous period of up to 12 months. Drug doses were clinically equivalent, being based on the average daily clinical doses used in the control of schizophrenia increased by an arbitrary factor of 5. Doses in our previous studies were calculated in the same manner, so allowing data comparison.

Drinking water containing the drugs was readily acceptable to the animals. The mean daily drug intakes over the 12-month period were haloperidol 1.4–1.6 mg/kg, sulpiride 102–109 mg/kg, and clozapine 24–27 mg/kg. The body weight of the haloperidol group at the end of the 12-month period (477 ± 11 g; $P < 0.05$) was slightly below that of the control group (512 ± 9 g). The body weight of sulpiride-treated rats was normal (501 ± 10 g, $P > 0.05$), whereas that of the clozapine group was reduced (481 ± 6 g; $P < 0.05$). In other respects drug-treated animals did not differ in general health or appearance from control animals. At the end of the 12-month period of drug administration, animals were examined behaviorally and biochemically to assess striatal dopamine function while continuing to receive drug intake.

2.1 Alterations in Striatal D-2 Function After 12 Months' Treatment with Haloperidol, Sulpiride or Clozapine

Stereotyped behavior was assessed following the administration of apomorphine hydrochloride (0.125–1.0 mg/kg SC 15 min previously) (Fig. 1). After 12 months' administration of haloperidol, stereotypy induced by the lowest dose of apomorphine was inhibited but the response to high doses of apomorphine (0.5 and 1.0 mg/kg) was exaggerated. This biphasic effect on stereotypy was observed previously during trifluoperazine treatment, and the apparent inhibition of low dose stereotypy was attributed to a disruption of the stereotypy scoring system caused by an enhancement of locomotor activity (Rupniak et al. 1984).

In contrast to haloperidol, stereotypy induced by apomorphine (0.125–1.0 mg/kg SC) in animals treated for up to 12 months with sulpiride or clozapine did not differ over the time course of the experiment from that observed in age-matched control rats.

Specific ^{3}H-spiperone (0.1–4.0 n*M*; defined by means of (–)-sulpiride 10 μ*M*) binding was used as an index of D-2 sites. The number (B_{max}) of specific ^{3}H-spiperone-binding sites in striatal membranes was increased throughout the 12-month treatment period with haloperidol. In contrast, neither sulpiride nor clozapine treatment altered B_{max} for ^{3}H-spiperone binding, at any time point over this period, from that in tissue from age-matched control animals. None of the drug treatments altered the dissociation constant (K_D) for ^{3}H-spiperone binding.

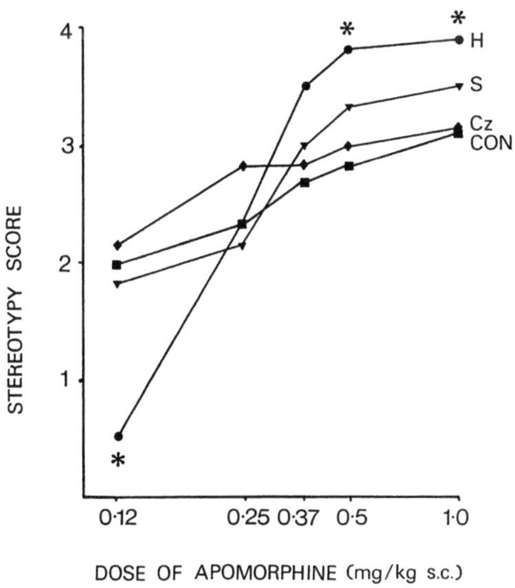

Fig. 1. Stereotyped response to apomorphine hydrochloride (0.125–1.0 mg/kg SC 15 min previously) after 12 months' continuous treatment with haloperidol, sulpiride or clozapine. Results are the mean ± 1 SEM stereotypy scores for between 6 and 11 animals in each dose of apomorphine. Overall group differences were assessed using the Kruskal-Wallis analysis of variance of ratios. Where probabilities associated with H scores were less than 0.05, data were compared by Mann-Whitney U tests. * $P < 0.05$ vs age-matched control rats

Specific ^{3}H-NPA (0.05–2.0 nM; defined by means of ADTN 1 μM) binding was used as an index of agonist-binding sites (presumably the D-3 receptor subpopulation; Grigoriadis and Seeman 1984). B_{max} for specific ^{3}H-NPA binding was increased following 12 months' treatment with either haloperidol or sulpiride compared with values obtained from age-matched control animals. Treatment with clozapine for 12 months, however, had no effect on the number of specific ^{3}H-NPA binding sites. Haloperidol and sulpiride, but not clozapine, elevated K_D for ^{3}H-NPA binding.

As an index of a functional change in striatal D-2 dopamine receptors, striatal acetylcholine concentrations were determined (Scatton 1982). Treatment with both haloperidol and clozapine for 12 months increased the striatal acetylcholine content. Sulpiride treatment had no effect. No changes in choline acetyltransferase, cholinesterase or ^{3}H-QNB binding were found after 12 months' treatment with any drug (data not shown).

So only chronic haloperidol treatment had any consistent effect on striatal D-2 receptor function. The change in acetylcholine content produced by clozapine presumably reflects the marked anticholinergic actions of this drug. Although sulpiride did not alter ^{3}H-spiperone binding, it elevated ^{3}H-NPA binding, so emphasising the difference in the nature of the sites identified by these ligands. It is unclear what effect an elevation of ^{3}H-NPA binding might have, but the recent proposal that the sites labelled by agonist ligands are closely linked to the D-1 site (Grigoriadis and Seeman 1984) is relevant to the present discussion.

2.2 Alterations in Striatal D-1 Function After 12 Months' Treatment with Haloperidol, Sulpiride or Clozapine

The function of D-1 sites was assessed by the ability of dopamine (1–150 μM) to stimulate adenylate cyclase activity in striatal homogenates. The increase in cyclic

Table 1. The effect[a] of continuous chronic administration of haloperidol, sulpiride and clozapine for 12 months on parameters related to striatal D-2 receptor function

Drug treatment	^{3}H-spiperone		^{3}H-NPA		Acetylcholine content (nmol/g)
	B_{max} (pmol/g tissue)	K_D (nM)	B_{max} (pmol/g tissue)	K_D (nM)	
Control	13.8 ± 1.2	0.13 ± 0.03	8.1 ± 0.3	0.8 ± 0.1	19.9 ± 2.1
Haloperidol	26.4 ± 2.2[b]	0.20 ± 0.04	11.0 ± 0.3[b]	1.2 ± 0.1[b]	35.7 ± 3.3[b]
Sulpiride	17.2 ± 1.4	0.13 ± 0.02	13.9 ± 0.4[b]	1.6 ± 0.1[b]	26.5 ± 2.6
Clozapine	15.3 ± 0.9	0.15 ± 0.02	7.2 ± 0.9	0.6 ± 0.1	29.5 ± 3.4[b]

[a] For binding experiments the results are the mean (± 1 SEM) values obtained from Scatchard analysis of three separate tissue pools. The acetylcholine results are expressed as the mean (± 1 SEM) of values obtained from eight individual animals at each time point

[b] $P < 0.05$ vs age-matched control rats

Table 2. The effect[a] of continuous chronic administration of haloperidol, sulpiride or clozapine for 12 months on parameters related to striatal D-1 receptor function

Drug treatment	^{3}H-Piflutixol		Cyclic AMP formation produced by 50 µM dopamine
	B_{max} (pmol/g tissue)	K_D (µM)	(pmol/2.5 min/2 mg tissue)
Controls	88 ± 5	0.32 ± 0.02	38.3 ± 1.9
Haloperidol	83 ± 3	0.31 ± 0.02	25.2 ± 4.7
Sulpiride	102 ± 5	0.38 ± 0.05	54.1 ± 3.1[b]
Clozapine	105 ± 2[b]	0.35 ± 0.02	51.9 ± 6.6

[a] For ^{3}H-piflutixol binding the results are the mean (± 1 SEM) values obtained from Scatchard analysis of three separate tissue pools. For adenylate cyclase activity the values are the means (± 1 SEM) determined from log-lineal regression analysis of assays on tissue from three individual animals examined in duplicate at each of five dopamine concentrations (1–150 µM)

[b] $P < 0.05$ vs control animals (Student's t-test)

AMP formation by 50 µM dopamine was used to express changes in enzyme activity. Administration of haloperidol for 12 months did not enhance cyclic AMP formation; if anything enzyme activity was reduced. In contrast, both sulpiride and clozapine treatment resulted in an increase of approximately 40% in cyclic AMP formation, although this was only significant for the sulpiride group.

Specific ^{3}H-piflutixol [0.08–1.3 nM; defined by *cis*-flupenthixol in the presence of 30 µM (±)-sulpiride] binding was used as an index of D-1 sites. Treatment with haloperidol for 12 months did not alter B_{max} for specific ^{3}H-piflutixol binding to striatal membranes. In contrast, both sulpiride and clozapine treatment increased the number of binding sites by approximately 20%, although this was only significant for the clozapine group.

So, overall only chronic treatment with clozapine and sulpiride induced alterations in striatal D-1 receptor function.

3 Discussion

In this study a comparison has been made of the adaptive changes in striatal dopamine function caused by the chronic administration of neuroleptic drugs with differing abilities to induce extrapyramidal side-effects. Haloperidol, like other typical neuroleptics, induces a high incidence of tardive dyskinesia. In contrast, sulpiride induces a much lower incidence of tardive dyskinesia, while clozapine has a generally low propensity to induce extrapyramidal reactions. These drugs also differ in the nature of their acute interaction with brain dopamine receptors (Hyttel 1980, 1981). Thus, haloperidol is selective for D-2 receptors but can exert a maximal effect on D-1 function, while sulpiride is specific for D-2 sites and exerts little effect on D-1 sites. Clozapine, on the other hand, is weakly active on both D-1 and D-2 sites.

In previous studies we have shown that chronic administration of typical neuroleptic drugs leads to a reversal of initial dopamine receptor blockade in striatum and mesolimbic areas and results in the production of functional D-2 dopamine receptor hypersensitivity in striatum despite continued drug intake (Clow et al. 1979, 1980a; Murugaiah et al. 1983b). If this action is related to the production of tardive dyskinesia in man then it might be expected that drugs such as sulpiride and clozapine would not produce similar effects. Indeed, while chronic haloperidol administration induced all the features of D-2 receptor hypersensitivity previously observed for other typical neuroleptics, this was not observed following sulpiride or clozapine administration. On acute administration both sulpiride and clozapine appear to block D-2 receptors. So, the low incidence of tardive dyskinesia produced by these drugs may be related to their ability to act at D-2 sites without inducing any change in the nature of the receptor population during chronic administration that would result in the development of hypersensitivity.

Of considerable interest, however, was the difference in the ability of the different drugs to induce change in D-1 and D-2 receptor function. Haloperidol administration did not cause an enhancement of D-1 function despite causing an inhibition of adenylate cyclase activity in the early stages of drug administration (data not shown) and despite being present in brain in sufficient amounts to alter D-2 function. This finding suggests that the production of tardive dyskinesia is unrelated to the ability of neuroleptic drugs to enhance D-1 function on chronic administration.

The lack of effect of haloperidol in augmenting D-1 function is perhaps not surprising in view of its predominant effect on D-2 sites. However, sulpiride, which is highly selective for D-2 sites, altered D-1 receptor function without causing adaptive changes in D-2 sites. Since sulpiride has little if any direct effect on D-1 sites it must be presumed that its action is mediated indirectly. Present evidence suggests that at least some D-2 sites have an inhibitory effect on D-1 function (Stoof and Kebabian 1981). It is conceivable that the ability of sulpiride to alter D-1 function is due to a highly selective action on this receptor population, which is unrelated to those D-2 receptors through which hypersensitivity is mediated. Indeed, there are reasons for suggesting that the receptor population acted on by sulpiride differs from that affected by typical neuroleptic drugs (Jenner and Marsden 1984). Interestingly, sulpiride administration did cause a selective adaptation of agonist binding sites. The relationship of these sites to those labelled by ^3H-spiperone remains unclear, but the suggestion that agonist sites may be closely associated with D-1 sites may provide a clue to the actions of sulpiride. Haloperidol administration also led to an up-regulation of agonist binding, so it is still difficult to explain the different effects of these drugs unless the alterations in sites labelled by ^3H-spiperone serve to prevent an action on D-1 function by increasing inhibitory D-2 tone.

The means by which clozapine selectively alters D-1 function appears not to be mediated by a selectivity of action on brain dopamine receptors, as we have suggested for sulpiride. Clozapine is weakly active on dopamine systems, but a much greater proportion of its effect appears to be directed towards cholinergic systems (Hauser and Closse 1978). It is possible, therefore, that the anticholinergic actions of clozapine prevent the drug from inducing any change in the nature of D-2 sites but do not prevent alterations in D-1 function induced by chronic drug administration.

Since adaptations of D-1 receptors to the continued presence of neuroleptic drugs do not appear to be involved in the production of tardive dyskinesia, what is the purpose of alterations in this system? One intriguing possibility is that alterations in D-1 function may serve to reduce the incidence of tardive dyskinesias produced by chronic administration of neuroleptic drugs. Possibly the balance between the degree of functional change induced in D-1 and D-2 sites as a result of chronic drug intake is the critical factor. This would imply that those neuroleptic drugs which can either directly or indirectly enhance D-1 function as a result of chronic therapy are those which are less likely to initiate tardive dyskinesia. Of great interest is the finding that repeated administration of the D-1 antagonist SCH 23390 does not induce dopamine receptor hypersensitivity but prevents the development of supersensitivity caused by repeated administration of haloperidol (Christensen 1983).

At present we cannot explain the role played by alterations of striatal D-1 function during chronic neuroleptic treatment in the aetiology of tardive dyskinesia. It is clear, however, that alterations in D-1 receptor function can no longer be ignored when the functional consequences of chronic neuroleptic treatment are considered.

References

Christensen AV (1983) Animal models for neuroleptic induced neurological dysfunction. In: Usdin E et al. (ed.) Catecholamines: Neuropharmacology and central nervous system – Therapeutic aspects. Liss, New York, pp 99–109

Clow A, Jenner P, Marsden CD (1979) Changes in dopamine mediated behavior during one years neuroleptic administration. Eur J Pharmacol 57:365–375

Clow A, Theodorou A, Jenner P, Marsden CD (1980a) Changes in rat striatal dopamine turnover and receptor activity during one years administration. Eur J Pharmacol 63:135–144

Clow A, Theodorou A, Jenner P, Marsden CD (1980b) Cerebral dopamine function in rats following withdrawal from one year of continuous neuroleptic administration. Eur J Pharmacol 63:145–157

Fleminger S, Rupniak NMJ, Hall MD, Jenner P, Marsden CD (1983) Changes in apomorphine-induced stereotypy, as a result of subacute neuroleptic treatment correlates with increased D-2 receptors but not with increases in D-1 receptors. Biochem Pharmacol 32:2921–2927
Grigoriadis D, Seeman P (1984) The dopamine/neuroleptic receptor. Can J Neurol Sci 11 [Suppl 1]:108–113
Hauser D, Closse A (1978) ^{3}H-Clozapine binding to rat brain membranes. Life Sci 23:557–562
Hyttel J (1980) Further evidence that ^{3}H-*cis*(Z)-flupenthixol binds to adenylate cyclase-associated dopamine receptors (D-1) in rat corpus striatum. Psychopharmacology 67:107–109
Hyttel J (1981) Similarities between the binding of ^{3}H-piflutixol and ^{3}H-flupenthixol to rat striatal dopamine receptors in vitro. Life Sci 28:563–569
Iorio LC, Barnett A, Leitz FH, Hauser VP, Korduba CA (1983) SCH 23390 a potential benzazepine antipsychotic with unique interactions on dopaminergic systems. J Pharmacol Exp Ther 226:462–468
Jenner P, Marsden CD (1984) Multiple dopamine receptors in brain and the pharmacological action of substituted benzamide drugs. Acta Psychiatr Scand 69 [Suppl 311]:109–123
Kebabian JW, Calne DB (1979) Multiple receptors for dopamine. Nature 277:93–96
Klawans HL Jr (1973) The pharmacology of tardive dyskinesia. Am J Psychiatry 130:82–86
Leysen JE (1981) Review on neuroleptic receptors: specificity and multiplicity on in vitro binding related to pharmacological activity. In: Usdin E, Dahl SG, Gram LF, Lingiaerde O (eds) Clinical pharmacology in psychiatry: neuroleptic and antidepressant research. MacMillan, London, pp 35–62
Marsden CD, Tarsy D, Baldessarini RJ (1973) Spontaneous and drug induced movement disorders in psychiatric patients. In: Benson DF, Blummer D (eds) Psychiatric aspects of neurologic disease. Grunne and Stratton, New York, pp 219–266
Muller P, Seeman P (1978) Dopaminergic supersensitivity after neuroleptics: time course and specificity. Psychopharmacology 60:1–11
Murugaiah K, Fleminger S, Theodorou A, Jenner P, Marsden CD (1983a) Persistent increase in striatal dopamine stimulated adenylate cyclase activity persists for more than 6 months but disappears after 1 year following withdrawal from 18 months *cis*-flupenthixol intake. Biochem Pharmacol 32:2495–2499
Murugaiah K, Theodorou A, Jenner P, Marsden CD (1983b) Alteration in cerebral dopamine function caused by administration of *cis*- or *trans*-flupenthixol for up to 18 months. Neuroscience 10:811–819
Rupniak NMJ, Boyce S, Jenner P, Marsden CD (1984) Interpretation of changes in apomorphine-induced stereotyped behavior in rats receiving continuous administration of trifluoperazine for 15 months. Neuropharmacology (to be published)
Scatton B (1982) Effect of dopamine agonists and neuroleptic agents on striatal acetylcholine transmission in the rat: evidence against dopamine receptor multiplicity. J Pharmacol Exp Ther 220:197–202
Seeman P (1980) Brain dopamine receptors. Pharmacol Rev 32:230–313
Stoof JC, Kebabian JW (1981) Opposing roles for D-1 and D-2 dopamine receptors in efflux of cyclic AMP from rat neostriatum. Nature 294:366

Pharmacological Differentiation of Dopamine D-1 and D-2 Antagonists After Single and Repeated Administration

A.V. Christensen, J. Arnt and O. Svendsen [1]

Contents

Abstract 182
1 Introduction 182
2 Effects in Single-Dose Studies 183
3 Interaction Studies 185
4 Effect in Repeated-Dose Studies 186
5 Effect After Combined Long-Term Treatment 188
6 Conclusion 189
References 189

Abstract

In single-dose experiments neuroleptics antagonize dopamine (DA)-agonist-induced stereotypies in animals. The antagonistic potency correlates with their clinical antipsychotic effects.

In a series of experiments where DA-agonist-induced stereotyped gnawing in mice and rats was inhibited by neuroleptics it was shown that the antagonistic effect of butyrophenones was greatly attenuated by concomitant treatment with anticholinergics. The effect of phenothiazines was slightly attenuated and that of thioxanthenes and SCH 23390 remained unchanged. After repeated administration a differentiation is also seen in the ability of the antagonists to suppress DA-agonist-induced stereotypies.

The differentiation in these experiments is similar to that seen in dopamine D-1 and D-2 receptor binding. The compounds can be classified into three pharmacological subgroups: butyrophenones (e.g., haloperidol) with affinity for D-2 receptors; phenothiazines (e.g., fluphenazine and perphenazine) with affinity for both D-2 and D-1 receptors but with preference for the D-2 receptors; and thioxanthenes (e.g., *cis*(Z)-flupentixol and *cis*(Z)-clopenthixol) with equal affinity for D-1 and D-2 receptors, and the selective D-1 antagonist SCH 23390. This compound has the same antistereotypic effect as is seen with the neuroleptics. We have also investigated the effect of the above-mentioned neuroleptics and SCH 23390 after 12 days' treatment and 3–5 days withdrawal. They were given either alone or in combination. When they were given alone a clear differentiation was seen between the groups when mice were tested for methylphenidate antagonism. The thioxanthenes and SCH 23390 retain their ability to antagonize the stereotyped gnawing; the phenothiazines show a reduced effect; and the butyrophenones have almost lost their ability to antagonize the stereotyped behavior.

1 Introduction

Combined chronic treatment with a selective D-2 receptor antagonist (haloperidol) and a mixed D-1/D-2 antagonist [*cis*(Z)-clopenthixol] or a selective D-1 antagonist (SCH 23390) shows that the resulting tolerance/cross-tolerance is not

1 H. Lundbeck A/S, Ottiliavej 7–9, DK-2500 Copenhagen-Valby, Denmark

Dyskinesia – Research and Treatment
(Psychopharmacology Supplementum 2)
Editors: Casey, Chase, Christensen, Gerlach

induced to the same degree. The D-1 component prevents tolerance and hypersensitivity in mice, suggesting that the D-1 and D-2 receptors are closely connected with each other. Since hypersensitivity is postulated to be essential for dyskinesia in man, this syndrome would not be expected to be induced by neuroleptics with a marked D-1 component. Furthermore, the symptoms can possibly also be treated with such compounds as the thioxanthenes and SCH 23390.

2 Effects in Single-Dose Studies

Neuroleptics are a group of divergent chemical structures all used for the treatment of schizophrenia. The most commonly used neuroleptics fall into five chemical groups: thioxanthenes, phenothiazines, butyrophenones, diphenylbutylpiperidines, and benzamides. Table 1 shows a classification of these compounds with respect to their affinity to D-1 and D-2 DA receptors in binding assays. The receptor affinity profile of these compounds has already been described (Hyttel 1978; Kebabian and Calne 1979; Hyttel et al. this volume).

Table 1. Classification of DA-antagonists with respect to D-1 and D-2 DA receptors (Kebabian and Calne 1979)[a]

Selective D-2 antagonists	Mixed D-1 and D-2 antagonists	Selective D-1 antagonist
Butyrophenones	Thioxanthenes	SCH 23390
Haloperidol	*cis*(Z)-Flupentixol	
Spiroperidol	*cis*(Z)-Clopenthixol	
Diphenylbutylpiperidines	Phenothiazines	
Pimozide	Fluphenazine	
	Perphenazine	
Benzamides		
Clebopride		
Sulpiride		

[a] Effects on other neurotransmitter receptors are not considered in terms of selectivity

The only selective D-1 receptor antagonist known is SCH 23390 (Hyttel 1983). The pharmacology of this compound has recently been described (Iorio et al. 1981, 1983; Christensen et al. 1984a, b, c). For our behavioral experiments we have selected one neuroleptic from each of these groups.

In rodent models, where stereotypies are induced by methylphenidate or amphetamine, thioxanthenes, phenothiazines, butyrophenones, diphenylbutylpiperidines, and benzamides antagonize these stereotypies (Table 2). SCH 23390 has a pronounced but very short-lasting effect after systemic administration, but is nearly inactive after oral administration (Christensen et al. 1984a, b).

All neuroleptics and SCH 23390 induce dose-dependent catalepsy in rats (Table 2). This is in contrast to the observations published by Iorio et al. (1983).

However, Iorio's group used oral administration, and we also were unable to demonstrate cataleptogenic activity following administration by this route. Because of the brief action of SCH 23390 it was necessary to shorten the time interval between evaluations of catalepsy, which under standard conditions is 1 h. Since the measurement of full catalepsy in our rat model requires conditioning to

Table 2. Antistereotypic and cataleptic effect of neuroleptics

	Methylphenidate Mouse ED 50		Amphetamine Rat ED 50	Catalepsy Rats ED 50
	IP mg/kg	PO mg/kg	IP mg/kg	SC mg/kg
cis(Z)-Clopenthixol	0.4	0.4	0.5	0.3
Fluphenazine	0.05	0.2	0.05	0.04
Haloperidol	0.2	1.2	0.2	0.1
Pimozide	0.2	0.2	0.5	0.9
Clebopride	0.6	0.5	2.1	0.3
SCH 23390[a]	0.1	5	0.3	0.08

[a] 30 min after administration

Except for SCH23390 the neuroleptics were injected 2 h before testing with the dopamine agonists (methylphenidate 60 mg/kg, SC, or amphetamine 10 mg/kg, SC). The methods have already been described in detail (Pedersen and Christensen 1972; Christensen et al. 1984 a, b, c). In all experiments ED 50 values were calculated by probit analysis, using a log dose scale. Catalepsy was evaluated at the peak effect time. Each rat was placed on a vertical wire grid and catalepsy was defined as being present after at least 15 s immobility. The effect of SCH 23390 was measured every 15 min, the effect of clebopride was measured every 30 min, and for other compounds every hour, 1–6 h after injection. For each dose level at least five rats were used

Table 3. Apomorphine antagonism in dogs

	ED 50 mg/kg SC	
	Vomitus	Stereotypies
cis(Z)-Clopenthixol	0.04	0.6
Fluphenazine	0.005	0.02
Haloperidol	0.01	0.15
Pimozide	0.004	0.03
Clebopride	0.02	0.3
SCH 23390	>10[a]	0.18

[a] Marked sedation

The dogs were pretreated 4 h before testing, except in the case of SCH 23390, which was given 1 h before testing. The antagonism was determined as already described elsewhere (Nymark 1972, Møller Nielsen et al. 1973; Svendsen 1979). Groups of four dogs were given SC doses of test drug. Each drug was given at 3–4 dose levels. The dogs were observed for vomiting after IV injection of 25 μg/kg apomorphine and for stereotypy after IV injection of 1.6 mg/kg apomorphine the test situation during the first three evaluations, the peak response is usually recorded 3–5 h after injection (Arnt 1982). At this time the effect of SCH 23390 is about 10 times weaker than the peak effect seen 30–60 min after injection. Therefore, catalepsy was evaluated every 15 min after SCH 23390. For clebopride an intermediate duration of action is obtained, and for this reason the catalepsy was evaluated every 30 min. Also, 6,7-ADTN-induced hyperactivity and amphetamine-induced circling in unilaterally 6-OHDA-lesioned rats were antagonized both by the neuroleptics and by SCH 23390 (Christensen et al. 1984a, b, c).

In dogs a difference between neuroleptics and SCH 23390 was seen (Table 3). In contrast to the neuroleptics, SCH 23390 has no antagonistic effect against apomorphine-induced vomiting. However, its antistereotypic effect in dogs was comparable to that of the neuroleptics.

3 Interaction Studies

To characterize the neuroleptics further we investigated the effect of the anticholinergic compound scopolamine on the antistereotypic and cataleptic effect of the neuroleptics and SCH 23390. When mice (Table 4) or rats (Table 5) were co-treated with scopolamine, the antistereotypic or cataleptic effects of neuroleptics were not influenced to the same degree. The effects of butyrophenones and diphenylbutylpiperidines were markedly attenuated. The effect of phenothiazines was less attenuated and that of the thioxanthenes and SCH 23390 remained almost unchanged (Scheel-Krüger et al. 1978; Christensen et al. 1979; Arnt and

Table 4. Inhibition by scopolamine of the antistereotypic effect of neuroleptics

Test compound	Saline	Scopolamine 2.5 mg/kg IP
cis(Z)-Clopenthixol	0.4	0.7
Fluphenazine	0.08	0.32[b]
Haloperidol	0.16	> 5[b]
Pimozide	0.32	> 5[b]
Clebopride	0.7	> 5[b]
SCH 23390[a]	0.1	0.1

[a] Pretreatment time 30 min
[b] $P < 0.05$; Parallel line log probit analysis
The methylphenidate antagonistic effect of the neuroleptics is indicated by ED 50 values in mg/kg IP for each dose level. At least five pairs of mice were used. Except for SCH 23390, neuroleptics in various doses were injected IP 90 min before saline or scopolamine. Methylphenidate 60 mg/kg SC was injected 15 min after these compounds. Immediate, after the methylphenidate injection the mice were placed in gnawing cages for 1 h

Table 5. Influence of scopolamine on the antistereotypic and cataleptogenic effects of neuroleptics in rats

	Antiamphetamine		Catalepsy	
	Saline ED 50 mg/kg	Scopolamine IP	Saline ED 50 mg/kg	Scopolamine SC
cis(Z)-Clopenthixol	0.7	1.0	0.3	2.8[a]
Fluphenazine	0.13	> 2.5[a]	0.07	0.29
Haloperidol	0.30	1.2[a]	0.21	20[a]
Clebopride	3	> 20[a]	0.5	> 40[a]
SCH 23390[b]	0.2	0.2	0.1	0.8[a]

[a] $P < 0.05$; Parallel line log probits analysis
[b] Pretreatment time 30 min
In the antistereotypic test neuroleptics except SCH 23390 were injected IP 1.5 h before scopolamine (1.25 mg/kg SC), which was followed 30 min later by IV amphetamine (10 mg/kg, calculated as base). Stereotypies were scored 1 h after amphetamine. In the catalepsy test, scopolamine was injected 3 and 3.5 h after the neuroleptic drug, respectively. Catalepsy was evaluated 2 h after scopolamine. For each dose level 5–10 rats were used

Christensen 1981). In several other behavioral models the same differentiation of thioxanthenes and butyrophenones has been shown when combined with scopolamine: conditioned avoidance response, amphetamine-induced circling in unilaterally 6-OHDA-lesioned rats, and hyperactivity induced by bilateral injection of 6,7-ADTN into rat nucleus accumbens (Arnt et al. 1981; Arnt 1982).

The classifications of the neuroleptics into different groups based on interaction studies are in accordance with the classification given in Table 1.

4 Effect in Repeated-Dose Studies

During long-term treatment with neuroleptics hypersensitivity of DA receptors and tolerance to neuroleptics develop in mice and rats (Christensen et al. 1976; Clow et al. 1979a, b; Christensen and Møller Nielsen 1980; Christensen and Hyttel 1982; Christensen et al. 1984a, b).

In the present experiments this tolerance phenomenon was seen in mice treated daily for 12 days with neuroleptics. Five days after withdrawal there was an increase in the ED50 values of neuroleptics for inhibition of methylphenidate-induced stereotyped gnawing (Table 6), indicating either increased response to the DA agonist or decreased response to the neuroleptics. From the saline column it appears that in acute experiments the four neuroleptics and SCH 23390 are equipotent. After treatment for 12 days with *cis*(Z)-clopenthixol, haloperidol, or SCH 23390 the ED50 value for SCH 23390 was not changed. After 12 days of *cis*(Z)-clopenthixol treatment, the ED50 value for *cis*(Z)-clopenthixol was also unchanged, whereas those for the three other neuroleptics were increased. Repeated administration with fluphenazine, haloperidol, and pimozide induced pronounced tolerance. Thus, it appears that pretreatment with the standard neuroleptics induces tolerance. The tolerance seems to be less pronounced after pre-

Table 6. Methylphenidate antagonistic effect of neuroleptics in mice after repeated administration

Methylphenidate antagonistic effect 5 days after withdrawal by:	Pretreatment for 12 days with					
	Saline	*cis*(Z)-clopenthixol 2.5 mg/kg PO	Fluphenazine 2.5 mg/kg PO	Haloperidol 2.5 mg/kg PO	Pimozide 2.5 mg/kg PO	SCH 23390 2.5 mg/kg SC twice daily
	Methylphenidate antagonistic effect					
cis(Z)-Clopenthixol	0.3	0.4	0.5	0.8[a]	0.8[a]	0.2
Fluphenazine	0.1	0.8[a]	> 5[a]	> 5[a]	> 5[a]	–
Haloperidol	0.2	0.8[a]	> 5[a]	> 5[a]	> 5[a]	0.2
Pimozide	0.2	0.8[2]	> 5[a]	> 5	3.2	–
SCH 23390[b]	0.2	0.2	–	0.2	–	0.2

[a] $P < 0.01$; Parallel line log probit analysis
[b] Pretreatment time 30 min
Except for SCH 23390 the mice were pretreated 2 h before testing with methylphenidate (60 mg/kg SC). The methylphenidate antagonistic effect of the neuroleptics is indicated by ED 50 values in mg/kg IP

treatment with thioxanthenes, which were also the only compounds to which cross-tolerance was not seen. For phenothiazines, butyrophenones, and diphenylbutylpiperidines cross-tolerance was seen. For SCH 23390 neither tolerance nor cross-tolerance was seen.

Besides tolerance to neuroleptics an augmented response to DA agonists was also seen. In mice pretreated as above an increased response to methylphenidate

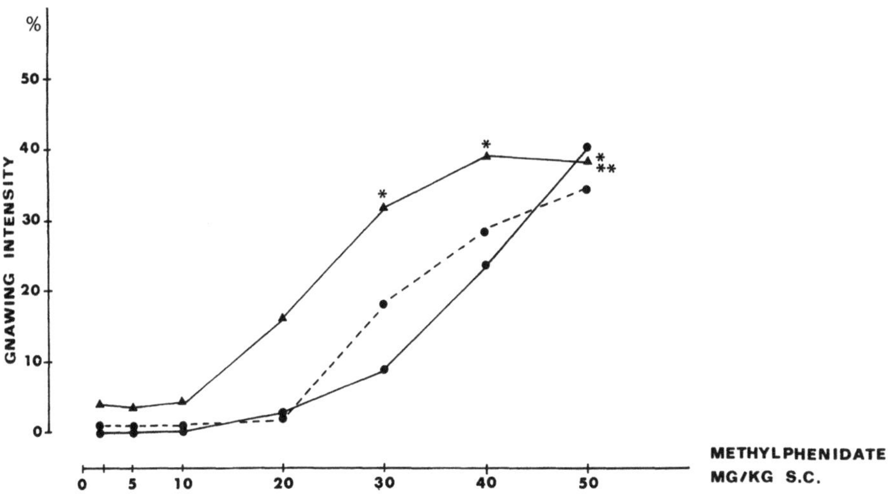

Fig. 1. Dose-response (gnawing) curves for methylphenidate after 12 days pretreatment and 5 days withdrawal of saline (●——●), *cis*(Z)-clopenthixol (●---●), or haloperidol (▲——▲). * Self-mutilation; ** significant difference from the saline- and *cis*(Z)-clopenthixol-pretreated groups

is observed (Fig. 1). The dose-response curve for methylphenidate-induced stereotyped gnawing is shifted significantly to the left after pretreatment with haloperidol. However, after pretreatment with *cis*(Z)-clopenthixol the dose-response curve is very similar to the dose-response curve for the saline group. This is also the case when the mice are pretreated with SCH 23390.

5 Effect After Combined Long-Term Treatment

To measure the effect of D-1 receptor blockade on the development of tolerance and cross-tolerance induced by a D-2 receptor antagonist the following experiments were performed. Mice were treated for 12 days with a D-2 antagonist (haloperidol), combinations of a D-2 and a D-1/D-2 antagonist [haloperidol and *cis*(Z)-clopenthixol, respectively], or a D-2 and a D-1 antagonist (haloperidol and SCH 23390, respectively) and were tested with haloperidol 3 days after withdrawal. Treatment with haloperidol induced tolerance to the effect of haloperidol (Table 7) and cross-tolerance to *cis*(Z)-clopenthixol (Christensen et al. 1984a). Concomitant treatment with either *cis*(Z)-clopenthixol or SCH 23390 induced only slight tolerance (Table 7) and no cross-tolerance to *cis*(Z)-clopenthixol, respectively.

These experiments show that D-1-receptor blockade attenuated the development of tolerance and cross-tolerance induced by D-2-receptor antagonists and may indicate that the D-1-receptor-antagonistic effect of thioxanthenes is probably the explanation for the lack of development of tolerance and cross-tolerance after these neuroleptics.

As shown both in interaction studies and in studies with repeated administration, DA D-1 receptor affinity can now be related to several pharmacological effects exerted via DA (Christensen et al. 1979, 1980; Christensen and Hyttel 1982; Rosengarten et al. 1983; Arnt and Hyttel 1984; Molloy and Waddington 1984). As already mentioned (Hyttel et al., this volume), most neuroleptics also show affinity to other neuron systems, e.g., 5-HT, NA, Ach, and the histaminergic neuron system. Furthermore, many neuron systems are also indirectly

Table 7. Methylphenidate antagonistic effect of haloperidol[a] 3 days after withdrawal of repeated treatment

	Treatment for 12 days with				
	Saline	*cis*(Z)-Clopenthixol 2.5 mg/kg PO	Haloperidol 2.5 mg/kg PO	Haloperidol 2.5 mg/kg PO + SCH 23390 0.8 mg/kg SC x 2	Haloperidol 2.5 mg/kg PO + *cis*(Z)-Clopenthixol 2.5 mg/kg PO
ED 50	0.2	0.8[a]	>5[a]	0.8[a]	0.8[a]

[a] The pretreated mice received haloperidol 2 h before testing with methylphenidate (60 mg/kg SC). The methylphenidate antagonistic effect of the neuroleptics is indicated by ED 50 values in mg/kg IP

[a] $P < 0.05$; Parallel line log probit analysis. ED 50 values are in mg/kg IP

influenced by the neuroleptics (Christensen et al. 1979, 1980; Dunstan and Jackson 1976, 1977; Gerlach 1979; Mogilnicka and Bræstrup 1976; Molander and Randrup 1976; Scheel-Krüger et al. 1977). Therefore, these effects of the neuroleptics can also be relevant to the effect of the compounds in schizophrenia and dyskinesia.

6 Conclusion

In single-dose experiments the behavioral effects of neuroleptics reacting on the DA D-2, D-1 and D-2, or D-1 receptors are very similar.

Anticholinergic drugs attenuate the antistereotypic or cataleptic effects of D-1 and D-2 antagonists but not to the same degree. The effects of butyrophenones, diphenylbutylpiperidines, and benzamides are markedly attenuated. Those of phenothiazines are less attenuated and those of thioxanthenes and SCH 23390 remain essentially unchanged.

After long-term administration the classification of neuroleptics and SCH 23390 in different groups is as mentioned above. The D-2 antagonists (butyrophenones and diphenylbutylpiperidines) induce pronounced tolerance. Phenothiazines induce less and the thioxanthenes and SCH 23390 only slight tolerance. Furthermore, thioxanthenes and SCH 23390 reverse the tolerance development induced by D-2 antagonists.

If hypersensitivity and/or tolerance are related to dyskinesia in man this syndrome would not be expected to be induced or to a lesser degree by thioxanthenes and SCH 23390. Furthermore, the symptoms might possibly be treated with compounds like the thioxanthenes and SCH 23390, since the results in the combined studies indicate induction of less hypersensitivity.

References

Arnt J (1982) Pharmacological specificity of conditioned avoidance response inhibition in rats: inhibition by neuroleptics and correlation to dopamine receptor blockade. Acta Pharmacol Toxicol 51:321–329

Arnt J, Christensen AV (1981) Differential reversal by scopolamine and THIP of the antistereotypic and cataleptic effects of neuroleptics. Eur J Pharmacol 69:107–111

Arnt J, Hyttel J (1984) Differential inhibition by dopamine D-1 and D-2 antagonists of circling behavior induced by dopamine agonists in rats with unilateral 6-hydroxydopamine lesions. Eur J Pharmacol 102:349–354

Arnt J, Christensen AV, Hyttel J (1981) Differential reversal by scopolamine of effects of neuroleptics in rats. Relevance for evaluation of therapeutic and extrapyramidal side-effect potential. Neuropharmacology 20:1331–1334

Christensen AV, Hyttel J (1982) Neuroleptics and the clinical implications of adaptation of dopamine neurons. Pharm Int 3:329–332

Christensen AV, Møller Nielsen I (1980) On the supersensitivity of DA receptors after single and repeated administration of neuroleptics. In: Smith RC (ed) Tardive dyskinesia, research and treatment. Spectrum, New York, pp 35–50

Christensen AV, Fjalland B, Møller Nielsen I (1976) On the supersensitivity of dopamine receptors, induced by neuroleptics. Psychopharmacology 48:1–6

Christensen AV, Arnt J, Scheel-Krüger (1979) Decreased antistereotypic effect of neuroleptics after additional treatment with a benzodiazepine, a GABA agonist or an anticholinergic compound. Life Sci 24:1395–1402
Christensen AV, Arnt J, Scheel-Krüger J (1980) GABA-dopamine/neuroleptic interaction after systemic administration. Brain Res Bull 5 [Suppl 2]:885–890
Christensen AV, Arnt J, Svendsen O (1984a) Animal models for neuroleptic induced neurological dysfunction. In: Usdin E (ed) Catecholamines 3. Liss, New York, pp 316–328
Christensen AV, Arnt J, Hyttel J, Svendsen O (1984b) Behavioral correlates to the dopamine D-1 and D-2 antagonists. Pol J Pharmacol Pharm 36:245–260
Christensen AV, Arnt J, Hyttel J, Larsen J-J, Svendsen O (1984c) Pharmacological effects of a specific dopamine D-1 antagonist SCH 23390 in comparison with neuroleptics. Life Sci 34:1529–1540
Clow A, Jenner P, Marsden CD (1979a) Changes in dopamine-mediated behavior during one year's neuroleptic administration. Eur J Pharmacol 57:365–375
Clow A, Jenner P, Theodorou A, Marsden CD (1979b) Striatal dopamine receptors become supersensitive while rats are given trifluoperazine for six months. Nature 278:59–61
Dunstan R, Jackson DM (1976) The demonstration of a change in adrenergic receptor sensitivity in the central nervous system of mice after withdrawal from long-term treatment with haloperidol. Psychopharmacology 48:105–114
Dunstan R, Jackson DM (1977) The effect of apomorphine and clonidine on locomotor activity in mice after long-term treatment with haloperidol. Clin Exp Pharmacol Physiol 4:131–141
Gerlach J (1979) Tardive dyskinesia. Dan Med Bull 26:209–245
Hyttel J (1978) Effects of neuroleptics on ^{3}H-haloperidol and ^{3}H-*cis*(Z)-flupenthixol binding and on adenylate cyclase activity in vitro. Life Sci 23:551–556
Hyttel J (1983) SCH 23390 – The first selective dopamine D-1 antagonist. Eur J Pharmacol 91:153–154
Iorio LC, Houser V, Korbuda CA, Leitz F, Barnett A (1981) SCH 23390, a benzazepine with atypical effects on dopaminergic systems. Pharmacologist 23:136
Iorio LC, Barnett A, Leitz FH, Houser VP, Korbuda CA (1983) SCH 23390, a potential benzazepine antipsychotic with unique interactions on dopaminergic systems. J Pharm Exp Ther 226:462–468
Kebabian JW, Calne DB (1979) Multiple receptors for dopamine. Nature 277:93–96
Mogilnicka E, Bræstrup C (1976) Noradrenergic influence on the stereotyped behavior induced by amphetamine, phenethylamine and apomorphine. J Pharm Pharmacol 28:253–255
Molander L, Randrup A (1976) Effects of thymoleptics on behavior associated with changes in brain dopamine. II. Modification and potentiation of apomorphine-induced stimulation of mice. Psychopharmacology 49:139–144
Møller Nielsen I, Pedersen V, Nymark M, Franck KF, Boeck V, Fjalland B, Christensen AV (1973) The comparative pharmacology of flupenthixol and some reference neuroleptics. Acta Pharmacol Toxicol 33:353–362
Molloy AG, Waddington JL (1984) Dopaminergic behavior stereospecifically promoted by the D_1 agonist SK&F 38393 and selectively blocked by the D_1 antagonist SCH 23390. Psychopharmacology 82:409–410
Nymark M (1972) Apomorphine provoked stereotypy in the dog. Psychopharmacologia 26:361–368
Pedersen V, Christensen AV (1972) Antagonism of methylphenidate-induced stereotyped gnawing in mice. Acta Pharmacol Toxicol 31:488–496
Rosengarten H, Schweitzer JW, Friedhoff AJ (1983) Induction of oral dyskinesias in naive rats by D-1 stimulation. Life Sci 33:2479–2482
Scheel-Krüger J, Cools AR, Honig W (1977) Muscimol antagonizes the ergometrine-induced locomotor activity in nucleus accumbens: evidence for GABA-dopaminergic interaction. Eur J Pharmacol 42:311–313
Scheel-Krüger J, Christensen AV, Arnt J (1978) Muscimol differentially facilitates stereotypy but antagonizes motility induced by dopaminergic drugs: a complex GABA-dopamine interaction. Life Sci 22:75–84
Svendsen O (1979) Long term effect of teflutixol on apomorphine-induced stereotypy and vomiting in dogs. Eur J Pharm 53:387–390

Pathophysiology of Tardive Dyskinesia [1]

L. M. Gunne and J.-E. Häggström [2]

Contents

Abstract 191
1 Introduction 191
2 Discussion 192
References 193

Abstract

Animal models of persisting tardive dyskinesia have been developed in two species (rats and monkeys). Dyskinetic animals chronically treated with neuroleptics had significant decreases in glutamic acid decarboxylase and GABA in the substantia nigra, the medial globus pallidus, and the subthalamic nucleus, whereas animals without dyskinesias which had been treated similarly had a normal distribution of these biochemical parameters. These changes remained 2 months after neuroleptics were discontinued, and at that point there was a reduced turnover of striatal dopamine in the dyskinetic monkeys. These findings suggest that reduced GABA function in the substantia nigra may play a role in tardive dyskinesia.

1 Introduction

Two animal models for the study of tardive dyskinesia have been developed in our laboratory, one in *Cebus apella* monkeys (Gunne and Bárány 1976) and the other one in rats (Gunne et al. 1982). In both models we have induced long-lasting dyskinetic movements measurable for months after discontinuation of chronic neuroleptic drug administration.

There is now evidence for a regional depression of the GABA-synthesizing enzyme glutamic acid decarboxylase (GAD) and of GABA levels in certain brain areas of animals made dyskinetic by chronic haloperidol or fluphenazine treatment. Changes were observed in the substantia nigra, the medial globus pallidus, and the subthalamic nucleus (Gunne and Häggström 1983; Gunne et al. 1984). Animals which had been chronically treated with neuroleptics for a similar period of time (rats 1 year, monkeys 3–6 years) without developing dyskinesias had a normal distribution of GAD activity (see Table 1) and GABA. In a monkey with unilateral dyskinesia there was a depression of GAD activity only in the opposite nigra (Gunne and Häggström 1984).

1 This study was supported by grant 4546 from the Swedish MRC
2 Psychiatric Research Center, Ulleråker Hospital, S-75017 Uppsala, Sweden

Dyskinesia – Research and Treatment
(Psychopharmacology Supplementum 2)
Editors: Casey, Chase, Christensen, Gerlach

Table 1. Regional brain GAD activity (±SD) in seven untreated controls (UC), and percent deviations in six neuroleptic-treated controls (NC)[a] and six monkeys with neuroleptic-induced persistent dyskinesia (NPD)

Area	nmol/mm³/h GAD UC	Δ% NC	Δ% NPD
Cortex	9.9 ± 1.6	− 7	− 5
Caudate	11.7 ± 2.1	+ 4	0
Putamen	12.2 ± 1.5	− 1	0
Accumbens	19.1 ± 2.6	+ 9	5
Globus pallidus lat.	36.5 ± 7.0	+ 2	−16
Globus pallidus med.	36.9 ± 2.4	+ 4[d]	−26[a]
Amygdala	8.6 ± 0.9	−13	−12
Hypothalamus	21.5 ± 4.4	− 3	− 8
Thalamus	9.8 ± 1.7	− 4	− 4
N. subthalam.	9.7 ± 2.3	+ 5[d]	−32[b]
S. nigra	45.8 ± 6.6	+18[e]	−57[c]
N. ruber	8.9 ± 1.9	+17	+19
Genic. lat.	8.4 ± 1.0	+ 4	−11
Sup. Coll.	13.4 ± 2.9	−18	+10
Form. ret.	18.0 ± 3.9	− 7	− 5
Pons	10.5 ± 5.1	−10	−17

[a] NC did not significantly differ from UC at any brain site
Difference NPD-UC: [a] $P < 0.05$; [b] $P < 0.01$; [c] $P < 0.001$
Difference NPD-NC: [d] $P < 0.01$; [e] $P < 0.001$

2 Discussion

The above findings within the GABA system of dyskinetic animals were still present 2 months after discontinuation of all neuroleptic medication. At this time there was also evidence for a reduced turnover rate of striatal dopamine in dyskinetic monkeys (Fig. 1). The dopamine level was slightly increased, whereas two dopamine metabolites (HVA and DOPAC) were low.

During earlier drug-free periods our monkeys had remained dyskinetic for 1–6 years. Mao and Costa (1978) have shown that chronic neuroleptic treatment reduces the turnover of GABA in the substantia nigra. In such experiments the nigral GABA binding increases (Gale 1980) and nigral injection of GABA ago-

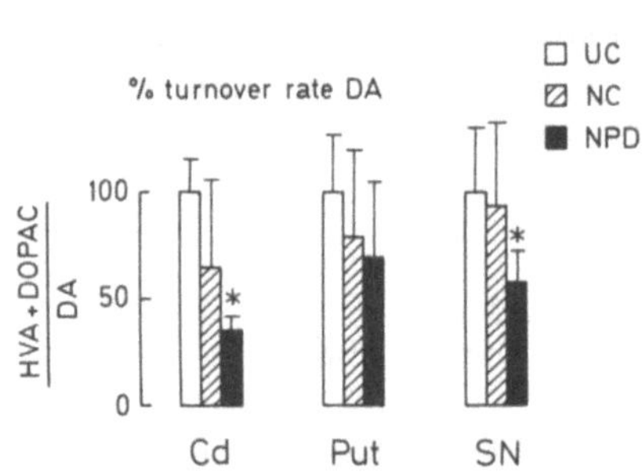

Fig. 1. The ratio (HVA + DOPAC/DA) as a measure of DA turnover in three brain areas: caudate (*Cd*), putamen (*Put*) and substantia nigra (*SN*). Values in neuroleptic-treated controls (*NC*) and monkeys with neuroleptic-induced persistent dyskinesia (*NPD*) are expressed as percentages of values measured in untreated controls (*UC*) for each area (+ SD). The *NPD* group showed a significant depression ($P < 0.05$) in *Cd* and *SN*

nists causes an enhanced behavioral response (Scheel-Krüger et al. 1981). These findings are indicative of a reduced activity in the striatonigral GABA-ergic projection during long-term neuroleptic treatment.

For some unknown reason the striatonigral pathway fails to recover its original function in animals with neuroleptic-induced dyskinesia. Clarification as to whether this dysfunction is due to a regional neuronal cell degeneration or is only a reversible functional depression must await histological evidence. Intranigral injection of the GABA receptor antagonist bicuculline has been reported to induce a particular type of oral dyskinesia in rats without concomitant excitation (Arnt and Scheel-Krüger 1980). It is thus conceivable that a reduced GABA function within the substantia nigra may be an underlying cause of neuroleptic-induced tardive dyskinesia.

References

Arnt J, Scheel-Krüger J (1980) Intranigral GABA antagonists produce dopamine-independent biting in rats. Eur J Pharmacol 62:51–61

Gale K (1980) Chronic blockade of dopamine receptors by antischizophrenic drugs enhances GABA binding in substantia nigra. Nature 283:569

Gunne LM, Bárány S (1976) Haloperidol-induced tardive dyskinesia in monkeys. Psychopharmacology 50:237–240

Gunne LM, Häggström J-E (1983) Reduction of nigral glutamic acid descarboxylase in rats with neuroleptic-induced oral dyskinesia. Psychopharmacology 81:191–194

Gunne LM, Häggström JE (1984) Studies in experimental tardive dyskinesia. In: 5th Catecholamine symposium (to be published)

Gunne LM, Growdon J, Glaeser B (1982) Oral dyskinesia following rat brain lesions and neuroleptic drug administration. Psychopharmacology 77:134–139

Gunne LM, Häggström J-E, Sjöquist B (1984) Association with persistent neuroleptic-induced dyskinesia of regional changes in brain GABA synthesis. Nature 309:347–349

Mao C, Costa E (1978) Biochemical pharmacology of GABA transmission. In: Lipton MA, DiMascio A, Killam KF (eds) Psychopharmacology: a generation of progress. Raven, New York, pp 307–318

Scheel-Krüger J, Magelund G, Olianas MC (1981) Role of GABA in the striatal output system, globus pallidus, nucleus subthalamicus. In: DiChiara G, Gessa GL (eds) GABA and the basal ganglia. Raven, New York, pp 165

Intermittent Treatment with Droperidol, a Short-Acting Neuroleptic, Increases Behavioral Dopamine Receptor Sensitivity

R. H. Belmaker, A. Elami, and J. Bannet [1]

Contents

Abstract . . . 194
1 Introduction . . . 194
2 Methods . . . 197
3 Results . . . 198
4 Discussion . . . 198
References . . . 198

Abstract

Drug holidays have been proposed as a preventive strategy against the development of tardive dyskinesia. Three animal studies in which dopamine receptor hypersensitivity after chronic neuroleptic treatment was used as a model for tardive dyskinesia failed to find any reduction in dopamine receptor hypersensitivity with intermittent, as opposed to continuous, treatment. Since most neuroleptics have a long half-life in vivo, we hypothesized that truly drug-free periods may not have been achieved in previous studies. Droperidol, an ultrashort-acting butyrophenone neuroleptic, was administered to rats for 22 days in twice-daily injections or one injection every 48 hours. At 60 hours after the last dose there was no difference in apomorphine-induced stereotypy between continuously treated and intermittently treated animals. Thus, even totally drug-free periods do not reduce the development of dopamine receptor hypersensitivity.

1 Introduction

Drug holidays have been advocated for patients maintained on long-term neuroleptic treatment as a possible strategy for reducing the incidence of tardive dyskinesia (Editorial 1979). However, a retrospective clinical study has suggested that drug holidays or interruptions of neuroleptic treatment may not reduce and may even increase the incidence of tardive dyskinesia (Jeste et al. 1979). Since prospective studies are extremely difficult in this area and could take years to yield a definitive answer, a study of drug holidays in an animal model of tardive dyskinesia seems relevant. Dopamine (DA) receptor binding increases with chronic neuroleptic treatment in animals and has been considered a molecular model for human tardive dyskinesia (Klawans et al. 1977). Evidence for the similarity of this model to human tardive dyskinesia includes the following facts: (a) human tardive dyskinesia, like increased caudate DA receptor binding, occurs after chronic,

1 Jerusalem Mental Health Center – Ezrath Nashim, P.O.B. 140, Jerusalem, Israel

Dyskinesia – Research and Treatment
(Psychopharmacology Supplementum 2)
Editors: Casey, Chase, Christensen, Gerlach

but not after acute neuroleptic treatment; (b) DA agonists exacerbate and DA blockers, at least temporarily, improve human tardive dyskinesia, as might be expected if DA receptor numbers were increased; and (c) enhanced stereotypy after DA agonists, a behavioral tardive dyskinesia model in animals (Tarsy and Baldessarini 1974), parallels the development of increased caudate DA receptor number (Clow et al. 1979).

We therefore decided to study the effect of drug holidays on the development of increased DA receptor binding in mouse caudate after chronic haloperidol feeding (Bannet et al. 1980).

Sabra wild-type mice were divided into four groups and fed as follows: (a) Drug-free food for 10 weeks; (b) food containing 0.0025% haloperidol for 10 weeks; (c) food containing 0.0025% haloperidol for 1 week alternating with drug-free food for 1 week, for a total of 10 weeks (the last week being haloperidol feeding); and (d) food containing 0.0025% haloperidol for 5 weeks. At the end of the feeding periods the animals were all given a 4-day washout period with drug-free food, after which they were killed and the caudate nucleus of each was dissected. The brain specimens were stored at − 70 °C until assay in randomized batches. The assay for DA receptor binding using ^{3}H-spiroperidol was done as previously described (Ebstein et al. 1979; Burt et al. 1976).

Table 1. The effect (mean + SD) of chronic haloperidol on ^{3}H-spiroperidol[a] binding in mouse striatum (pmol/g tissue)

Control ($n = 15$)	4 Weeks ($n = 16$)	10 Weeks ($n = 18$)	Drug holidays ($n = 20$)
16.56 + 1.94	21 + 5.03[b]	23.3 + 3.6[c]	22 + 5.38[c]

[a] Concentration of ^{3}H-spiroperidol in reaction mixture was 1 n*M*
[b] $P < 0.01$
[c] $P < 0.001$

Table 1 presents the DA receptor binding in each of the four groups. Binding is significantly increased after 5 or 10 weeks of haloperidol treatment, but 10 weeks of drug holiday treatment yielded no different results from 5 or 10 weeks of continuous treatment.

This study (Bannet et al. 1980) contained several methodological flaws. (a) A single concentration of spiroperidol was used instead of the construction of a full Scatchard plot. This was done to obtain individual data on each mouse caudate, but may have obscured a difference between the drug holiday-treated group and the continuous haloperidol group. (b) No difference was found between five continuous weeks of haloperidol feeding and 10 continuous weeks of haloperidol feeding. In such a system with a flat dose-response curve, it is unlikely to be possible to detect differences due to the drug-holiday regimen.

Two recent studies have been completed that add information to that provided by Bannet et al. (1980). Murugaiah et al. (to be published) treated rats for 6 or 12 months with trifluoperazine or *cis*-flupenthixol in the drinking water. Such long periods of treatment might be expected to model the human disorder of tardive dyskinesia more closely. Moreover, Ebstein et al. (1979) found that the percentage increase in caudate-spiperone binding was more pronounced after 3 months of chronic haloperidol treatment than after 3 weeks of haloperidol medication. It might thus be expected that longer periods of treatment would yield larger, more clinically relevant effects, and thereby provide a clearer answer to the question of drug holidays. Murugaiah et al. (to be published) planned a drug holiday group that was withdrawn from trifluoperazine or *cis*-flupenthixol for 1 full month after each 2 months of neuroleptic treatment. Unfortunately, Murugaiah et al. (to be published) did not use an in vivo washout period before testing for apomorphine-induced stereotypy and caudate spiperone binding. Perhaps because of the continued presence of drug in the brain, neither continuous nor discontinuous trifluoperazine treatment had the expected consistent effect of increasing apomorphine-induced stereotypy.

Perhaps because of pharmacokinetic differences between trifluoperazine and *cis*-flupenthixol, continuous and discontinuous *cis*-flupenthixol treatments both increased apomorphine-induced stereotypy, but there was no difference between continuous and drug holiday treatment. Measurement of spiperone binding in caudate was done of course after thorough washing of membranes, but this in vitro washout is known to be incomplete compared with in vivo washout. Thus inconsistent results were reported: continuous *cis*-flupenthixol did not increase spiperone binding after 6 or 12 months; the drug holiday regimen increased spiperone binding after 6 but not after 12 months. Both continuous and discontinuous trifluoperazine increased spiperone binding after 6 months but the increase was less pronounced in the drug holiday group. This study, while commendable for the long duration of treatment, appears comparable to a human epidemiologic study of tardive dyskinesia carried out with patients all receiving continuing neuroleptic treatment. No estimate of the incidence of underlying masked tardive dyskinesia could be made. Moreover, the study of Murugaiah et al. (to be published) uses inordinately long "holidays." A month in a rat is long enough to induce increases in spiperone binding and in this model must be considered equivalent to at least several months in the human. No clinical situation contemplates such a prolonged drug holiday.

Koller (to be published) also studied drug holidays in an animal model. Guinea-pigs were treated with continuous haloperidol for 14 days, haloperidol every other day for 14 injections, or haloperidol every fifth day for 14 injections. The dose was 0.5 mg/kg for each injection. After a final 3-day in vivo washout apomorphine-induced stereotypy was measured and 48 hours later striata were dissected and spiperone binding was determined. All the haloperidol-treated groups showed increased DA receptor sensitivity behaviorally and increased spiperone binding biochemically; none of the treatment regimens gave different results from any other. These consistent results agree closely with those of Bannet et al. (1980); it should be noted, however, that guinea-pigs often differ from other animal models in neuropharmacology, and that 14 days is a short treatment period for the demonstration of increases in spiperone binding.

An issue not previously raised in animal studies of neuroleptic drug holidays is the long half-life of haloperidol. In humans the half-life of haloperidol is at least

24 hours (Soudijn et al. 1967). Moreover, it is a highly lipophilic drug and in vivo receptor binding in brain could continue for several days after the drug is undetectable in blood (Goldman et al. 1981). A 1-week drug holiday, as used by Bannet et al. (1980), or a 5-day drug holiday, as used by Koller (to be published), may not be a drug holiday at all. We decided to study this question using droperidol, a butyrophenone neuroleptic with a distribution half-life of 10 minutes and an elimination half-life of 134 minutes in humans (Cressman et al. 1973). Droperidol is a typical DA receptor antagonist, and clinical studies have demonstrated its neuroleptic properties in human psychosis (Burns 1980; Granacher and Ruth 1979; Neff et al. 1972; VanLeevman et al. 1977). However, it is most widely used in preanesthesia, where it can induce a rapidly reversible neuroleptic sedation (Morrison 1969).

2 Methods

We hypothesized that the use of droperidol might allow short but truly total drug holidays and that this technique might achieve a reduction in long-term neuroleptic effects on DA receptors. We divided 49 Sabra strain rats into three groups: (a) Control rats received twice-daily injections of saline, every 12 hours, for 22 days; (b) continuous treatment rats received twice-daily injections of 2.5 mg/kg droperidol at each injection for 22 days; and (c) drug holiday rats received 10 mg/kg droperidol once every 48 hours and saline for each of the three remaining injection times per 48 hours. After 22 days all injections were stopped. At 60 hours from the last injection rats were evaluated for apomorphine-induced stereotypy according to the method of Kelly and Iversen (1976). In brief, each rat was observed for 1 minute every 3 minutes for a total of 30 minutes (ten observations).

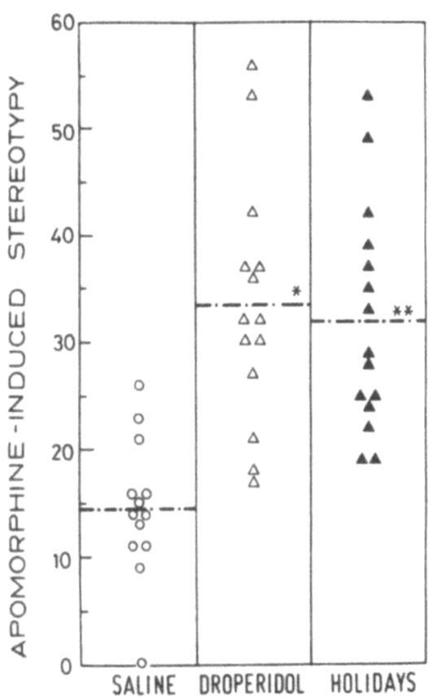

Fig. 1. The effect of continuous (DROPERIDOL) or intermittent (HOLIDAYS) treatment on the development of behavioral DA receptor supersensitivity. * Saline vs droperidol, $P < 0.001$, Student's t-test; ** saline vs holidays, $P < 0.001$, Student's t-test: droperidol vs holidays, NS

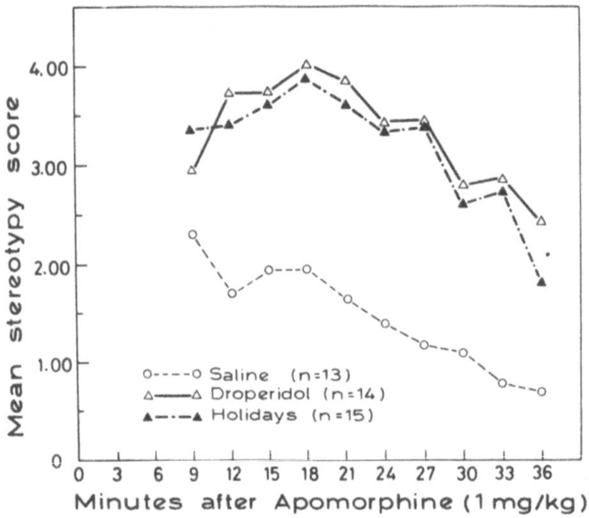

Fig. 2. Time course of stereotypy response to apomorphine in rats pretreated with saline, continuous droperidol (*Droperidol*) or intermittent droperidol (*Holidays*)

Apomorphine-induced stereotypy was rated using the following scale: 0 = sleep or stationary; 1 = active without stereotypy; 2 = bursts of stereotyped sniffing (S), head movements (HM) or rearing (R); 3 = intense stereotyped S-R-HM or confined to one area; 4 = stereotyped S-R-HM accompanied by bursts of licking or gnawing including self-licking or biting; 5 = stereotyped licking or gnawing; 6 = stereotyped licking or gnawing confined to a small area. Scores in Fig. 1 are the sum of ten ratings over 30 minutes after IP apomorphine (1 mg/kg).

3 Results

Figure 1 illustrates the results. There is no difference between the total stereotypy scores of the continuous treatment and drug holiday groups.

Figure 2 illustrates the time course of apomorphine-induced stereotypy in the three groups. No reduction in the duration of apomorphine-induced stereotypy is observed in the drug holiday group.

4 Discussion

These results imply that continued presence of drug is not the explanation for the failure of drug holidays to reduce the intensity of DA receptor supersensitivity induced by neuroleptics. Intermittent treatment, even with an ultrashort-acting neuroleptic, is quite capable of inducing marked increases in apomorphine-induced stereotypy. It would be interesting to speculate whether a parallel phenomenon occurs with regard to the antipsychotic effect of neuroleptics: clear antipsychotic effects require about 3 weeks to develop. Would droperidol every other day induce an equivalent antipsychotic effect at the end of 3 weeks, or must DA receptors be continuously blocked to induce antipsychotic effects? Such questions may lead to knowledge about the basic relationship between DA blockade, psychosis, and tardive dyskinesia; however, they seem unable to lead to a simple technique for preventing tardive dyskinesia.

References

Bannet J, Belmaker RH, Ebstein RP (1980) The effect of drug holidays in an animal model of tardive dyskinesia. Psychopharmacology 69:223–224

Burns ME (1980) Droperidol in the management of hyperactivity, self-mutilation and aggression in mentally handicapped patients. J Int Med Res 8:31–33

Burt DR, Creese I, Snyder SH (1976) Properties of ^{3}H-haloperidol and ^{3}H-dopamine binding associated with dopamine receptors in calf brain membranes. Mol Pharmacol 12:800–812

Clow A, Jenner P, Theodorou A, Marsden CD (1979) Striatal dopamine receptors become supersensitive while rats are given trifluoperazine for six months. Nature 278:59–61

Cressman WA, Plostnieks J, Johnson PC (1973) Absorption, metabolism and excretion of droperidol by human subjects following intramuscular and intravenous administration. Anesthesiology 38:363–369

Ebstein RP, Pickholz D, Belmaker RH (1979) Dopamine receptor changes after long-term haloperidol treatment in rats. J Pharm Pharmacol 31:558–559

Editorial (1979) Tardive dyskinesia. Lancet II:447–448

Goldman Z, Ebstein RP, Lerer B, Zohar J, Hermoni M, Belmaker RH (1981) Haloperidol blood levels during dosage reduction in chronic schizophrenic patients. Neuropsychobiology 7:281–284

Granacher RP, Ruth DD (1979) Droperidol in acute agitation. Curr Ther Res 25:361–365

Jeste DV, Potkin SG, Sinha S, Feder S, Wyatt RJ (1979) Tardive dyskinesia: reversible and persistent. Arch Gen Psychiatry 36:585–590

Kelly PH, Iversen SD (1976) Selective 6-OHDA-induced destruction of mesolimbic dopamine neurons: abolition of psychostimulant-induced locomotor activity in rats. Eur J Pharmacol 40:45–56

Klawans HL, Hitri A, Nausieda PA, Weiner WL (1977) Animal models of dyskinesia. In: Hanin I, Usdin E (eds) Animal models in psychiatry and neurology. Pergamon, Oxford, pp 351–363

Koller WC (to be published) Intermittent haloperidol treatment in animal models of tardive dyskinesia.

Morrison JD (1969) Drugs used in neuroleptanalgesia. Int Anesthesiol Clin 7:41

Murugaiah K, Theodorou A, Clow A, Jenner P, Marsden CD (to be published) Effects of drug-holiday regimes on the development of dopamine receptor supersensitivity during continuous chronic trifluoperazine or *cis*-flupenthixol administration to rats.

Neff KE, Denney D, Blachly PH (1972) Control of severe agitation with droperidol. Dis Nerv Syst 33:594–597

Soudijn W, Van Wijngaarden I, Allewijn F (1967) Distribution, excretion and metabolism of neuroleptics of butyrophenone type. Eur J Pharmacol 1:47–57

Tarsy D, Baldessarini RJ (1974) Behavioral supersensitivity to apomorphine following chronic treatment with drugs which interfere with the synaptic function of catecholamines. Neuropharmacology 13:927–940

VanLeevman AMH, Molders J, Sterkmans P (1977) Droperidol in acutely agitated patients. J Nerv Ment Dis 164:280–283

Induction and Reversal of Dopamine Dyskinesia in Rat, Cat, and Monkey

K. G. Lloyd [1], M. T. Willigens [1], and M. Goldstein [2]

Contents

Abstract 200
1 Introduction 201
2 Methods 201
3 Results and Discussion 202
3.1 Dopamine Mimetic-Induced Stereotypies in the Rat 202
3.2 Dyskinetic and Stereotypic Movements in the Cat 206
3.3 Dyskinetic Movements in the Monkey 206
4 Summary and Conclusions 208
References 208

Abstract

Abnormal involuntary movements (AIMs, stereotyped or dyskinetic movements) were induced with different dopamine mimetics in rat, cat, and monkey. In the rat only stereotyped movements were observed, whereas in the cat dopamine agonists (apomorphine) preferentially induced dyskinesia but dopamine/noradrenaline uptake inhibitors (*d*-amphetamine, nomifensine) induced predominantly stereotypies; L-dopa induced an equal, low, number of both kinds of movements in the cat. In the monkey with bilateral lesions of the nigrostriatal dopamine pathways the AIMs could be divided into type 1 dyskinesia (behavioral), type 2 dyskinesia (oral and psychomotor), and chorea. GABA agonists (progabide, muscimol) had a biphasic action on apomorphine stereotypies in the rat, slightly (10%–20%) augmenting these movements at low doses and antagonizing (> 50%) them at higher doses. As these latter doses of progabide also antagonize apomorphine-induced circling in rats with a unilateral lesion of the substantia nigra, it is likely that this action is exerted at or beyond the dopamine target cell. In cats the dyskinetic movements induced by apomorphine were abolished by progabide. In contrast, L-dopa-induced stereotypies were resistant to the antidyskinetic action of progabide, and at low doses of L-dopa an increased incidence of stereotypies was noted. In the monkey, the type 1 dyskinesia following L-dopa and piribedil were also relatively resistant to progabide administration, whereas the type 2 dyskinesia and chorea were abolished by progabide. These studies are parallel to and support the clinical observations that dyskinetic movements following a direct action at the dopamine receptor (tardive dyskinesia) may be reversed by progabide whereas those associated with dopamine neuron activity, perhaps together with noradrenergic activation (L-dopa dyskinesia), are resistant to the antidyskinetic action of progabide.

1 L.E.R.S. – Synthélabo, 31 Av. P.V. Couturier, F-92220 Bagneux, France
2 Department of Psychiatry, New York University Medical Center, 550 First Ave, New York, NY 10016, USA

Dyskinesia – Research and Treatment
(Psychopharmacology Supplementum 2)
Editors: Casey, Chase, Christensen, Gerlach

1 Introduction

The treatment of Parkinson's disease with L-dopa, and subsequently with dopamine agonists, has been viewed as a milestone in rational medical research and therapy. It is undisputed that these patients benefit from the treatment and that their quality of life is greatly improved. However, although these treatments effectively overcome the dopamine deficiency that is the major neurochemical observation in Parkinson's disease (Hornykiewicz 1966; Lloyd et al. 1975), such treatment with L-dopa or dopamine mimetics is accompanied, in a disturbingly high number of cases, by dyskinetic movement disorders, which seem to be inherent to the treatment itself (Barbeau 1978). Thus, stimulation of dopamine receptors is essential for the amelioration of the parkinsonian symptoms but also leads to dyskinesia.

A relevant series of questions may be asked, however, in an effort to overcome this apparent dilemma: (a) are there different dopamine receptor subtypes involved in the relief of parkinsonian symptoms versus the induction of dyskinesia? (b) are the dopamine receptors responsible for the antiparkinsonian effects located on different cell bodies or in different brain regions than those responsible for the dyskinetic movements?

If the latter is true, then it should be possible to manipulate the system by pharmacological means in such a way that the dyskinetic movements are antagonized or prevented without modification of the antiparkinsonian effect of the dopamine mimetic.

The present study has attempted to test this hypothesis in different laboratory models. Dyskinetic movements in cats and monkeys or stereotyped behavior in rats have been induced by either L-dopa or different dopamine agonists. Subsequently the GABA agonists progabide and muscimol have been assessed for their effects on these abnormal movements. The results indicate that the action of GABA mimetics on AIMs is dependent on several factors: the type of dopamine mimetic (direct versus indirect); the parameter studied (dyskinetic movements or stereotyped behavior; the state of the test animal (intact or lesioned nigrostriatal dopamine system); and the relative affinity of the GABA agonist for GABA A and GABA B receptors.

2 Methods

The induction of stereotyped behavior was assessed in rats (CD, COBS male rats, Charles River France, 150–200 g body weight) as described by Worms and Lloyd (1979) using either an "all-or-none" technique where each observation is negative or positive according to the respective absence or presence of stereotyped movements (repetitive licking, sniffing, gnawing and biting) or a five-point rating scale. Compounds were injected either SC (apomorphine, nomifensine) or IP (L-dopa, *d*-amphetamine, piribedil). In cats (male mongrel cats, 1.5–3 kg weight) stereotypies (purposeless patterned elements from the pre-existing behavioral repertoire) were differentiated from dyskinetic movements (limb flicks, shaking, athetosis, not normally observed in cats) by means of a remote television camera (Lloyd et al. 1981). Tongue protrusions and other oral movements were not assessed due to the large variation in salivation seen between individual cats.

In monkeys with bilateral lesions of the nigrostriatal dopamine pathway, the AIMs induced by L-dopa or piribedil were grouped as follows (Lloyd et al. 1981): Type 1 dyskinesia, comprising restlessness, chattering increased irritability, aggressivity; type 2 dyskinesia, including repetitive oral and facial movements, hyperkinesia, swaying and stereotypies; chorea.

3 Results and Discussion

3.1 Dopamine Mimetic-Induced Stereotypies in the Rat

As shown in Fig. 1, stereotypic movements can be induced in the rat by different mechanisms of dopamine receptor activation, by direct agonists (apomorphine, piribedil), by uptake inhibitors (*d*-amphetamine, nomifensine), or by the dopamine precursor, L-dopa. Although the doses vary widely for the different compounds, the stereotypies elicited are very similar. However, other behavioral components (e.g., locomotor activation and emesis) vary greatly between these dopamine mimetics (see also Lloyd at al. 1981, 1983a). This is probably due to the involvement of other neurotransmitters (e.g., noradrenaline) in the action of some compounds (e.g., amphetamine and nomifensine) (Delina-Stula 1983; Iversen 1975).

Studies were then performed with the actions of GABA-mimetic drugs on the stereotypies induced by the dopamine agonist apomorphine and the dopamine precursor L-dopa. Three GABA agonists – progabide, SL 75.102 and muscimol – produced similar biphasic actions on the apomorphine-induced stereotypies in the rat. Thus, at very low doses, a small (10%–20%) but significant ($P < 0.05$) increase in the stereotypies was noted (Fig. 2). At higher doses, all three GABA agonists diminished (by at least 50% for progabide and SL 75.102) the stereotypies.

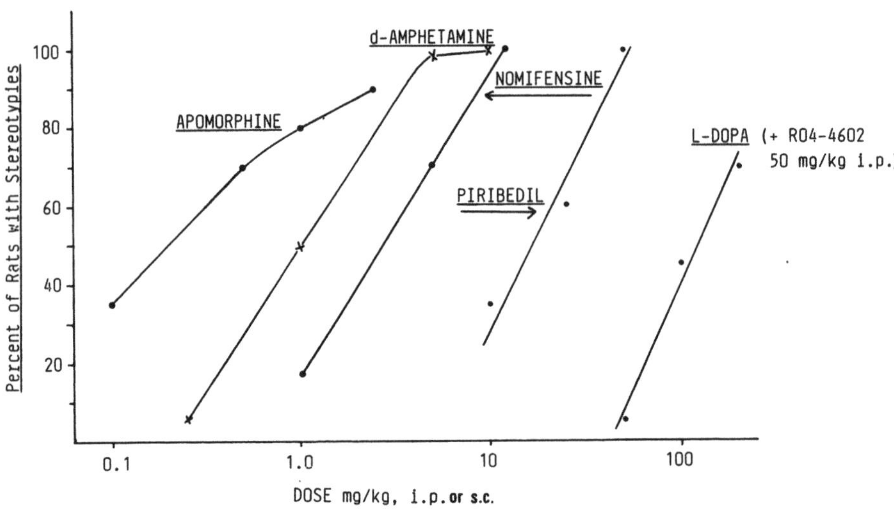

Fig. 1. Induction of stereotypies by dopamine mimetics in the rat. Animals received drugs either SC (apomorphine, nomifensine) or IP, and the presence or absence of stereotyped behavior (repetitive licking, sniffing, gnawing, and biting) was noted every 30 min for 4 h

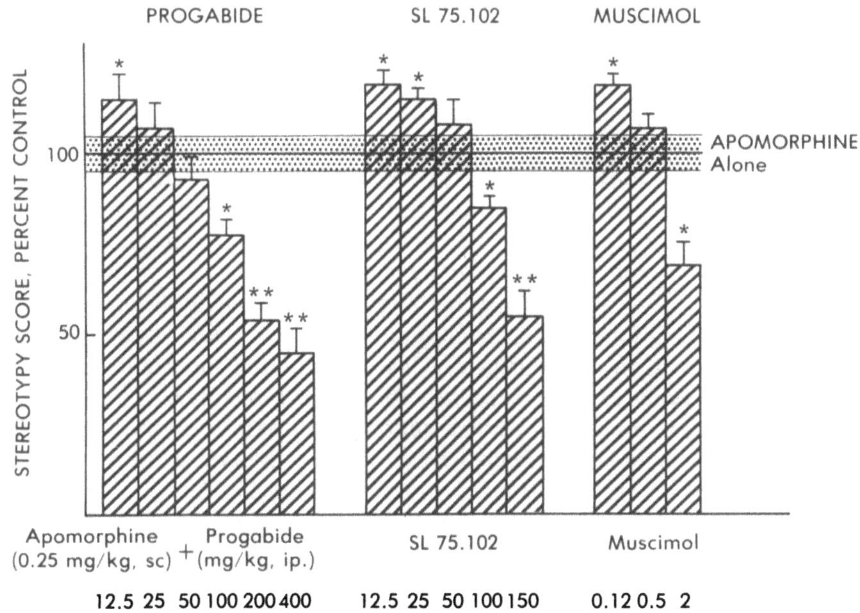

Fig. 2. The action of different GABA agonists on apomorphine-induced stereotyped behavior in the rat. Rats received injections of apomorphine and immediately afterwards of the GABA agonist. Stereotyped behavior was scored on five-point rating scale and was noted every 10 min for 1 h. $n = 20$ rats per group. * $P < 0.05$; ** $P < 0.01$ vs apomorphine alone. (Data from Worms et al. 1979, 1982)

It is likely that both these biphasic actions are mediated by GABA A receptors, as all three compounds have a similar profile for GABA A receptors, but muscimol has at best a very low affinity for the GABA B site (Table 1). Furthermore, baclofen, the specific GABA B agonist (Hill and Bowery 1981), neither potentiates nor inhibits apomorphine-induced stereotypies at nonmyorelaxant doses (Lloyd, unpublished results).

It is likely that these effects are exerted on different receptive cells which have GABA A receptors. In this regard, GABA mimetics inhibit striatal cholinergic neurons at the same dose range presently observed to potentiate apomorphine-induced stereotypies (Scatton and Bartholini 1982). The higher dose range that antagonizes the apomorphine stereotypies is within the dose range that decreases

Table 1. Profile of SL 75.102 and muscimol on the binding of ligands to GABA receptors (Calculated from Lloyd et al. 1982)

	Ratio of IC_{50} to that for the GABA A site			
	^{3}H-GABA A	^{3}H-GABA B	^{3}H-Isoguvacine	^{3}H-Muscimol
Progabide	1	3.0	0.2	0.2
SL 75.102	1	1.4	0.4	0.6
Muscimol	1	> 10000	1.1	0.9

dopaminergic synaptic activity in the striatum (Scatton et al. 1982). These observations are in parallel with the effect on stereotyped behavior as anticholinergic compounds exacerbate stereotypies and dyskinesia (cf. Lloyd 1978, for references) and dopamine receptor blockade effectively antagonizes the stereotypies (Worms and Lloyd 1979).

The above actions are observed in rats with an intact nigrostriatal dopamine system. In rats with a unilateral lesion of the nigrostriatal dopamine system, GABA agonists such as progabide appear to have only a monophasic action in decreasing the rotation induced by apomorphine in this model. For progabide the dose producing 50% reduction in the circling provoked by apomorphine (1 mg/kg IP) is 200 mg/kg IP, i.e., the same dose as decreases apomorphine-stereotyped behavior to the same degree. This suggests that the same synapses may be involved in both antiapomorphine activities of progabide.

In contrast to the homogeneity of their actions on dopamine agonist-induced stereotypies, GABA agonists exhibit different profiles vis-à-vis L-dopa-induced stereotypies in the intact rat. Progabide at doses of 100 and 200 mg/kg IP together with a low dose of L-dopa (50 mg/kg IP plus RO4-4602 50 mg/kg IP) provoked the appearance of stereotyped movements (Fig. 3A). However, at higher doses of L-dopa (100 and 200 mg/kg IP), which per se induced stereotypic movements, progabide had no effect. In contrast, muscimol (2 mg/kg IP) (Fig. 3B) only inhibited L-dopa stereotypies. These doses of muscimol and progabide are those that inhibit apomorphine-induced stereotypies. Thus, although the difference between the two GABA agonists is not evident when the dopamine receptor is stimulated by a direct agonist, if the receptor activation depends on presynaptic dopamine neuron activity there is a clear differentiation between progabide and muscimol.

Such a difference is paralleled by the clinical effects of GABA agonists. Thus both progabide (Lloyd et al. 1983b; Morselli et al. 1984) and muscimol (Tamminga et al. 1979) are effective in reducing neuroleptic-induced tardive dyskinesia, a phenomenon that directly involves the dopamine receptor. In contrast to this, and in parallel with the present experimental results, progabide is inactive in reducing L-dopa dyskinetic movements in parkinsonian patients and causes an exacerbation in some cases, whereas the parkinsonian condition is actually improved (Morselli et al. 1984).

The neurochemical basis for such an action on L-dopa-mediated events is not clear. It is unlikely that it is a direct action on dopamine neurons, as these doses of progabide (100–200 mg/kg IP) or muscimol (2 mg/kg IP) decrease indices of dopamine turnover and release, in both the resting and the activated states (Scatton et al. 1982; Lloyd et al. 1980). One possibility is that the GABA B action of progabide is important for the interaction of the compound with L-dopa in both dyskinesia and parkinsonian symptoms. This could be related to the control of noradrenergic neuron activity by GABA B receptors (Karbon et al. 1983; Hill and Bowery 1981), as noradrenaline is also a metabolite of L-dopa and has been implicated both in behavioral (Lloyd 1977) and in motor (Lloyd and Hornykiewicz 1975) actions of L-dopa. The involvement of the GABA B receptor is supported by the observation that the stereotyped behavior induced by the L-dopa-progabide combination is not reversed by bicuculline (unpublished results).

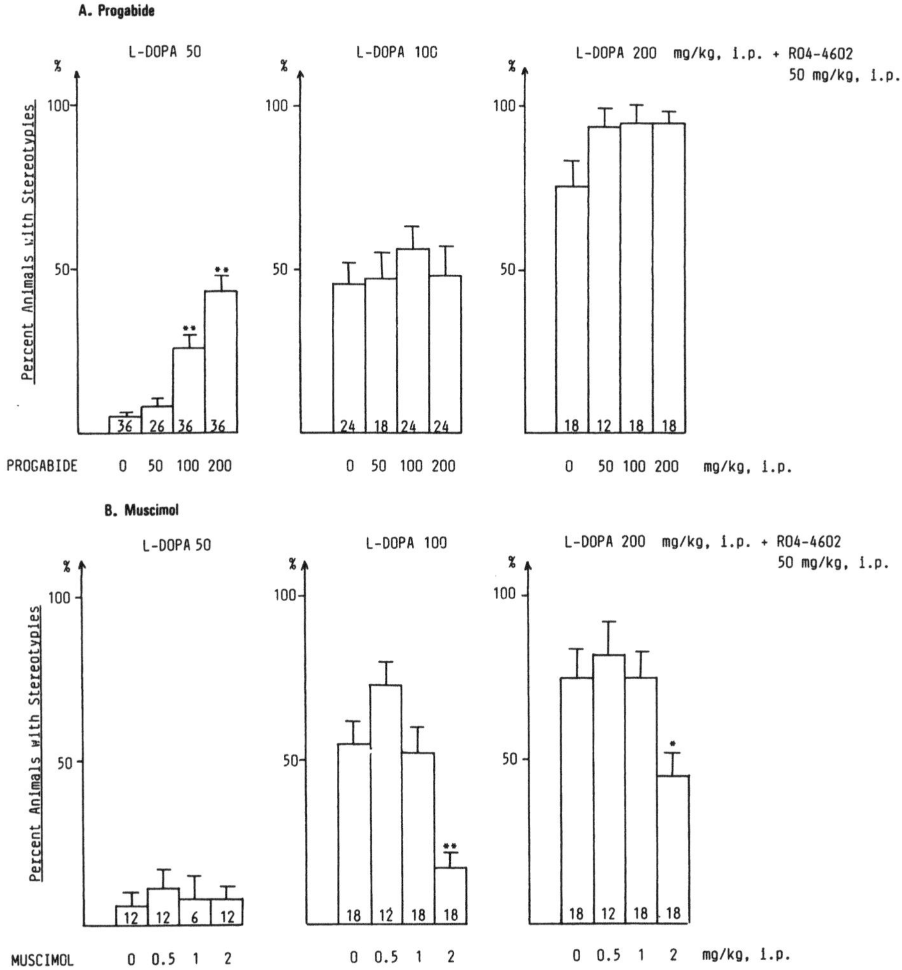

Fig. 3 A, B. The actions of progabide (A) and muscimol (B) on L-dopa-induced stereotypies in the rat. Progabide or muscimol was administered immediately after L-dopa and the presence or absence of stereotypies noted every 30 min for 4 h. The number of rats is indicated within each histogram. * $P < 0.05$; ** $P < 0.01$ vs L-dopa alone

The low-dose GABA-mimetic accentuation of apomorphine stereotypies and the provocation of stereotypies by the progabide-low dose L-dopa combination are supported by certain observations in the literature. Thus, Scheel-Krüger et al. (1979) have reported that in the rat injections of GABA mimetics in the substantia nigra pars reticulata induce stereotyped behavior, whereas when injected into the pars compacta these compounds have an antistereotypic action. When injected systemically, muscimol and THIP are reported to augment methylphenidate-induced stereotypies (Scheel-Krüger et al. 1979). This effect is qualitatively greater than the small potentiation of apomorphine stereotypies presently observed with low doses of muscimol and progabide. Furthermore, in both experimental settings, the GABA agonists potentiate neuroleptic catalepsy (Lloyd et al. 1979, 1980; Scheel-Krüger et al. 1979; Worms et al. 1982).

3.2 Dyskinetic and Stereotypic Movements in the Cat

As previously demonstrated (Lloyd et al. 1981), dopamine mimetics provoke both stereotypic and dyskinetic movements, which can be readily distinguished from each other. The proportion of dyskinetic to stereotypic movements varies between dopamine mimetics, with uptake inhibitors (nomifensine, *d*-amphetamine) inducing a much greater proportion of stereotypies than dyskinesia (almost no dyskinetic movements). L-Dopa produces a similar (rather low) occurrence of each type of abnormal movement, whereas with apomorphine at a dose of 3 mg/kg (PO) dyskinesia is exclusively induced; at high doses (10 mg/kg PO) both stereotypic and dyskinetic movements are observed (Lloyd et al. 1981). It is tempting to suggest that the stereotypies are related to an activation of both dopaminergic and noradrenergic synapses, as both nomifensine and *d*-amphetamine inhibit noradrenaline in addition to dopamine uptake (Delina-Stula 1983; Iversen 1975), and noradrenaline and dopamine are both L-dopa metabolites.

Further studies were performed to assess the action of the GABA agonist progabide on apomorphine-induced dyskinesia (Lloyd et al. 1983a). At doses of 50 and 100 mg/kg IP, progabide caused a dose-dependent reduction in dyskinetic movements ($P < 0.01$ for both doses vs apomorphine alone). At 100 mg/kg the dyskinetic movements were almost completely abolished.

Thus, in the cat progabide exerts an antiapomorphine action qualitatively and quantitatively similar to that seen in the rat.

3.3 Dyskinetic Movements in the Monkey

The animal model closest to the parkinsonian state is that induced by bilateral lesion of the substantia nigra in the monkey (Poirier et al. 1966; Battista et al. 1969). When dopamine mimetics are administered to such animals, not only are the parkinsonian signs (e.g., tremor) reduced, but a series of abnormal involuntary movements are also induced (Goldstein et al. 1973). These have been grouped into dyskinesia type 1 (behavioral), dyskinesia type 2 (psychomotor), and chorea.

The effect of progabide on the different abnormal involuntary movements induced by piribedil or L-dopa (plus RO4-4602) have been investigated in this monkey model for Parkinson's disease (Fig. 4). For both piribedil- and L-dopa-induced AIMs, the type 1 dyskinesia (behavioral) was the least sensitive to progabide. Even at the maximum dose of progabide tested (100 mg/kg PO for piribedil and 50 mg/kg PO for L-dopa) these movements were still present. Such, or even lower, doses completely abolished the psychomotor and oral dyskinesia and the chorea. The action of progabide on these latter AIMs (type 2 dyskinesia and chorea) was similar for both piribedil and L-dopa. In the presence of progabide the antitremor activity of L-dopa was unaltered.

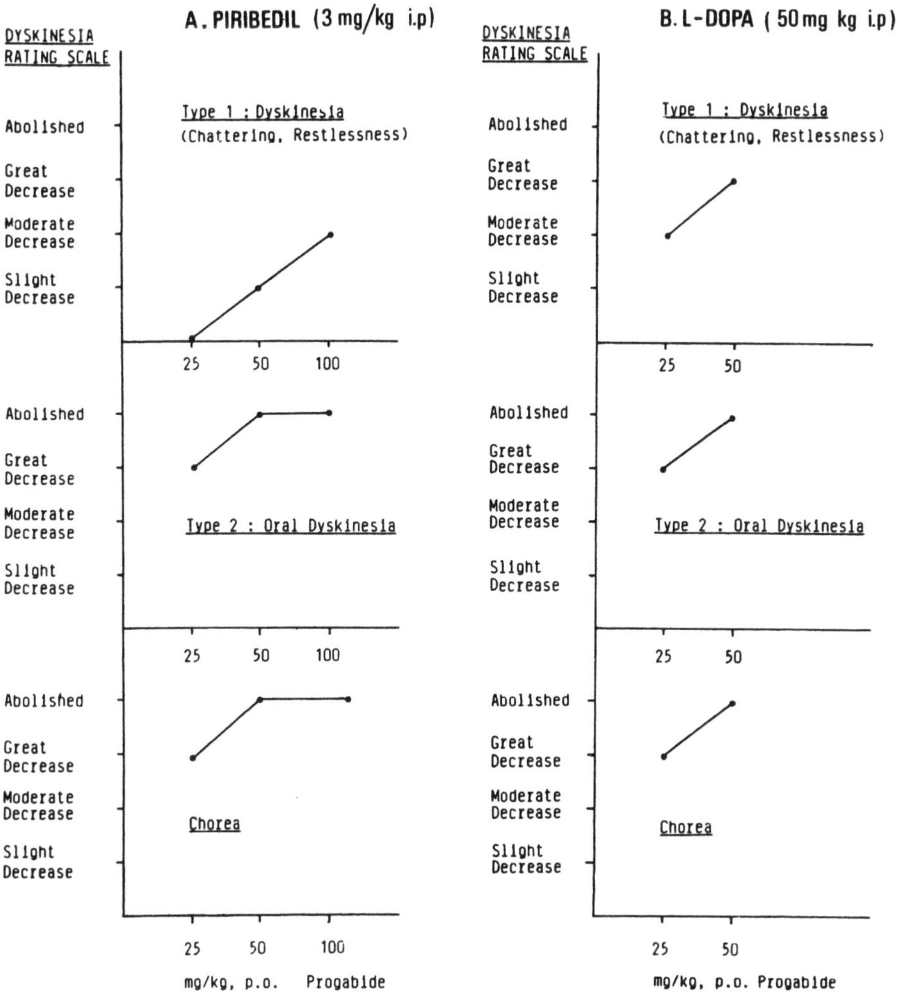

Fig. 4 A, B. Effect of progabide on **A** piribedil- and **B** L-dopa-induced dyskinesia and chorea in the lesioned monkey. In monkeys bearing a bilateral ventromedial tegmental lesion resulting in hypokinesia and tremor, progabide was administered immediately after L-dopa or piribedil and the different dyskinetic movements, chorea, and tremor assessed over 2 h

These results, when taken together with the clinical observations with progabide given for L-dopa dyskinesia in parkinsonian patients (Morselli et al. 1984), suggest that the type 1 dyskinesia in this monkey model is the best reflection of the L-dopa-induced dyskinesia in man. Thus, both these types of AIMs are resistant to progabide. Furthermore, in parallel with the clinical observation that progabide does not exacerbate Parkinson's disease, and actually increases the "on" time in those patients with "on-off" episodes (Morselli et al. 1984), progabide does not diminish the antitremor effect of L-dopa at all in the monkey model of Parkinson's disease.

4 Summary and Conclusions

The AIMs induced by dopamine mimetics (agonists or L-dopa) vary markedly in different animal models. In the rat, stereotyped behaviors are routinely observed with very few clear "dyskinetic" movements; in the cat dyskinetic movements can clearly be dissociated from stereotyped behavior; and in a monkey model of Parkinson's disease, dyskinetic movements predominate with few stereotypies being observed.

The action of GABA agonists on these abnormal movements also varies markedly in different models. The diminution by progabide or muscimol of apomorphine-induced stereotypies in intact rats, or of rotation in unilaterally lesioned rats, correlates well with the actions of these compounds in tardive dyskinesia. In addition, both these GABA agonists have a low-dose stimulatory effect on apomorphine stereotypies in the rat, and progabide has a similar action in combination with low doses of L-dopa. These actions parallel the lack of effect of progabide on L-dopa dyskinesia in Parkinson's disease patients. These results suggest that dyskinesia related to a direct action on dopamine receptors (e.g., apomorphine, neuroleptics) may be blocked by GABA agonists but that those related to presynaptic dopamine neuron activity, perhaps with the involvement of noradrenergic neurons (e.g., L-dopa), are less susceptible to such intervention.

This hypothesis receives support from the observation that the apomorphine-induced dyskinetic movements in the cat are completely antagonized by progabide.

In the model of Parkinson's disease produced by a bilateral lesion of the nigrostriatal dopaminergic paths, the behavioral dyskinesia (chattering, restlessness induced by piribedil or L-dopa) is relatively resistant to the antidyskinetic action of progabide, whereas the psychomotor and oral dyskinetic movements and the chorea induced by these dopamine mimetics can be completely abolished by the GABA agonist. In this manner, the behavioral dyskinesia seems to be the most similar pharmacologically to the L-dopa-induced dyskinesia in the parkinsonian patient.

References

Barbeau A (1978) The last ten years of progress in the clinical pharmacology of extrapyramidal symptoms. In: Lipton MA, DiMascio A, Killam KF (eds) Psychopharmacology: a generation of progress. Raven, New York, pp 771–776

Battista AF, Goldstein M, Nakatani S, Anagnoste B (1969) The effect of ventrolateral thalamic lesions on tremor and the biosynthesis of dopamine in monkeys with lesions of the ventromedial tegmentum. J Neurosurg 31:164–171

Delina-Stula A (1983) Mode of action of antidepressant drugs – primary effects. In: Angst J (ed) The origins of depression: current concepts and approaches. Springer, Berlin Heidelberg New York, pp 351–366

Goldstein M, Battista AF, Ohmoto T, Anagnoste B, Fuxe K (1973) Tremor and involuntary movements in monkeys: effect of L-dopa and of a dopamine receptor stimulating agent. Science 179:816–817
Hill DR, Bowery NG (1981) ^{3}H-Baclofen and ^{3}H-GABA bind to bicuculline insensitive $GABA_B$ sites in rat brain. Nature 210:149–152
Hornykiewicz O (1966) Dopamine (3-hydroxytyramine) and brain function. Pharmacol Rev 18:925–964
Iversen LL (1975) Uptake processes for biogenic amines. In: Iversen LL, Iversen SD, Snyder SH (eds) Biochemistry of biogenic amines. Plenum, New York, pp 381–432 (Handbook of psychopharmacology, vol. 3)
Karbon EW, Duman R, Enna SJ (1983) Biochemical identification of multiple $GABA_B$ binding sites: associations with noradrenergic terminals in rat forebrain. Brain Res 274:393–396
Lloyd KG (1977) Psychiatric disturbances occurring during levodopa therapy of Parkinson's disease. Primary Care 4:561–575
Lloyd KG (1978) Neurotransmitter interactions related to central dopamine neurons. In: Youdim MBH, Lovenberg W, Sharman DF, Lagnado JR (eds) Essays in neurochemistry and neuropharmacology, vol 3. Wiley, New York, pp 129–208
Lloyd KG, Hornykiewicz O (1975) Catecholamines in regulation of motor function. In: Friedhoff AJ (ed) Catecholamines and behavior. Plenum, New York, pp 41–57
Lloyd KG, Davidson L, Hornykiewicz O (1975) The neurochemistry of Parkinson's disease: effect of L-dopa therapy. J Pharmacol Exp Ther 195–453–464
Lloyd KG, Worms P, Depoortere H, Bartholini G (1979) Pharmacological profile of SL 76.002, a new GABA-mimetic drug. In: Krogsgaard-Larsen P, Scheel-Krüger J, Kofod H (eds) GABA-neurotransmitters. Munksgaard, Copenhagen, pp 308–325
Lloyd KG, Worms P, Zivkovic B, Scatton B, Bartholini G (1980) Interaction of GABA mimetics with nigro-striatal dopamine neurons. Brain Res Bull 5 [Suppl 2]:439–445
Lloyd KG, Broekkamp CLE, Cathala F, Worms P, Goldstein M, Asano T (1981) Animal models for the prediction and prevention of dyskinesia induced by dopaminergic drugs. In: Corsini GU, Gessa GL (eds) Apomorphine and other dopaminomimetics, vol. 2. Raven, New York, pp 123–133
Lloyd KG, Arbilla S, Beaumont K, Briley M, DeMontis G, Scatton B, Langer SZ, Bartholini G (1982) γ-Aminobutyric acid (GABA) receptor stimulation II. Specificity of progabide (SL 76.002) and SL 75.102 for the GABA receptor. J Pharmacol Exp Ther 220:672–677
Lloyd KG, Broekkamp CLE, Worms P (1983a) Involvement of GABA neurons in the induction and reversal of dopamine receptor related dyskinesia. In: Zbinden G, Cuomo V, Racagni G, Weiss B (eds) Application of behavioral pharmacology in toxicology. Raven, New York, pp 203–215
Lloyd KG, Morselli PL, Depoortere H, Fournier V, Zivkovic B, Scatton B, Broekkamp CLE, Worms P, Bartholini G (1983b) The potential use of GABA agonists in psychiatric disorders: evidence from studies with progabide in animal models and clinical trials. Pharmacol Biochem Behav 18:957–966
Morselli PL, Fournier V, Bossi L, Musch B (1984) Clinical activity of GABA agonists in neuroleptic and L-dopa induced dyskinesia. In: Casey D, Chase TN, Christensen AV, Gerlach J (eds) Dyskinesia, research and treatment. Psychopharmacology [Suppl] (this volume, p 128)
Poirier LJ, Sourkes TL, Bouvier G, Boucher R, Carabin S (1966) Striatal amines, experimental tremor and the effect of harmaline in the monkey. Brain 89:37–52
Scatton B, Bartholini G (1982) γ-Aminobutyric acid (GABA) receptor stimulation IV. Effect of progabide (SL 76.002) and other GABAergic agents on acetylcholine turnover in rat brain areas. J Pharmacol Exp Ther 220:689–695
Scatton B, Zivkovic B, Dedek J, Lloyd KG, Constantinidis J, Tissot R, Bartholini G (1982) γ-Aminobutyric acid (GABA) receptor stimulation III. Effect of progabide (SL 76.002) on norepinephrine, dopamine and 5-hydroxytryptamine turnover in rat brain areas. J Pharmacol Exp Ther 220:678–688
Scheel-Krüger J, Arnt J, Braestrup C, Christensen AV, Magelund G (1979) Development of new animal models for GABAergic actions using muscimol as a tool. In: Krogsgaard-Larsen P, Scheel-Krüger J, Kofod H (eds) GABA-neurotransmitters. Munksgaard, Copenhagen, pp 447–464

Tamminga C, Crayton TW, Chase TN (1979) Improvement in tardive dyskinesia after muscimol therapy. Arch Gen Psychiatry 36:595–598

Worms P, Lloyd KG (1979) Predictability and specificity of behavioral screening tests for neuroleptics. Pharmacol Ther 5:445–450

Worms P, Depoortere H, Durand A, Morselli PL, Lloyd KG, Bartholini G (1982) γ-Aminobutyric acid receptor stimulation I. Neuropharmacological profiles of progabide (SL 76.002) and SL 75.102, with emphasis on their anticonvulsant spectra. J Pharmacol Exp Ther 220:660–671

Behavioral Effects of Long-Term Neuroleptic Treatment in Cebus Monkeys [1]

D. E. Casey [2]

Contents

Abstract 211
1 Introduction 211
2 Materials and Methods 213
3 Results 213
4 Discussion 214
References 216

Abstract

Tardive dyskinesia (TD) occurs in predisposed individuals receiving neuroleptic treatment, but prior to the onset of symptoms it is not possible to predict who is at risk for this disorder. If the time course for evolving symptoms, perhaps mediated through dopamine hypersensitivity, could be identified, treatment interventions could be initiated. Eight male Cebus monkeys (15–18 years old) were tested with the dopamine agonists apomorphine, *d*-amphetamine, bromocriptine, and pergolide before, during, and after 3 months of treatment with haloperidol 0.25 mg/kg daily PO. This treatment cycle was repeated four times. Apomorphine and amphetamine produced moderate buccolinguo-masticatory (BLM) signs. Bromocriptine and pergolide produced very few BLMs. Initially haloperidol suppressed dopamine agonist-induced BLMs, but tolerance to the effect developed and was replaced by a potentiation of apomorphine-induced BLMs. Markedly increased apomorphine- and amphetamine-induced BLMs were seen following the first 3 months of haloperidol medication (behavioral hypersensitivity), but this gradually decreased to near-baseline levels, even with re-exposure to neuroleptics in the four treatment cycles. Bromocriptine and pergolide produced no signs of BLM behavioral hypersensitivity. These findings suggest that long-term neuroleptic treatment in nonhuman primates induces dynamic compensatory CNS changes, which may not fully explain the pathogenesis of TD on the basis of dopamine hypersensitivity.

1 Introduction

Tardive dyskinesia (TD) occurs as a late complication of prolonged neuroleptic treatment in predisposed individuals (Casey and Gerlach 1984). The syndrome classically involves involuntary repetitive movements in the orofacial region, with tongue protrusions and chewing motions, although limb and truncal choreoathetosis may also develop. Increasing age and possibly female sex are risk factors

1 This work was supported in part by funds from the Veterans Administration Career Development Award and Merit Review Program and by grant no. 36657 from NIMH

2 Psychiatry Service, VA Medical Center, Portland, OR 97207, USA

Dyskinesia – Research and Treatment
(Psychopharmacology Supplementum 2)
Editors: Casey, Chase, Christensen, Gerlach

associated with TD, but it is not possible prior to the onset of the disorder to predict who is likely to develop this syndrome. The concept of individual vulnerability is also indirectly supported by the lack of a correlation between TD and either total dose or duration of neuroleptic treatment (Kane and Smith 1982). One recent study of TD in the elderly treated for varying lengths of time over a 20-year span found that the prevalence of TD primarily increased during the first 3 years of treatment (Toenniessen et al. 1985). Thereafter, no significant increase in TD prevalence occurred. These data suggest that vulnerability to TD includes critical time aspects as well as individual patient characteristics. Unfortunately, no clinical laboratory techniques are currently available for reliable assessment of the potential susceptibility of each patient to develop TD.

Although the exact pathophysiology of this syndrome is unclear, dopamine receptor hypersensitivity is thought to play a primary role (Schelkunov 1967; Klawans 1973; Tarsy and Baldessarini 1973; Baldessarini et al. 1980).Animal models of neuroleptic-induced hypersensitivity show both behavioral and biochemical changes following acute (Christensen et al. 1976), short-term (Klawans and Rubovits 1972; Tarsy and Baldessarini 1973), and long-term (Clow et al. 1979, 1980 a, b) neuroleptic treatment, and in central nervous system (CNS) lesion studies (Ungerstedt 1971) in rodents. During the acute and short-term neuroleptic treatment studies evaluating the interaction between dopamine agonists and antagonists, each class of compounds counteracted the opposing drug effects in a dose-dependent relationship. However, with longer-term neuroleptic treatment of 6 months or more, antagonists lost the ability to suppress dopamine agonist-induced behavior. With even longer treatment, behavioral hypersensitivity provoked by dopamine agonist challenge doses of apomorphine was present both during and after neuroleptics (Clow et al. 1979). Though these rodent models have provided valuable insights, the relationship between TD in humans and the dopamine agonist-provoked abnormal behaviors is as yet unclear.

Models closer to the human syndrome have been produced in monkeys (Gunne and Barany 1976; Kovacic and Domino 1982). Though reversible and irreversible TD in Cebus monkeys (Gunne and Barany 1976; Kovacic and Domino 1982; Domino, this volume) and short-lasting behavioral hypersensitivity in *Cercopithecus aethiops* monkeys (Casey et al. 1980) following haloperidol have been shown, the evolution of neuroleptic-induced behavioral alterations in nonhuman primates has not been sufficiently studied. Furthermore, the individual vulnerability of monkeys to provocative challenges with dopamine agonists and antagonists prior to neuroleptic treatment has not been evaluated. This may provide a fruitful line of investigation to identify individual differences prior to treatment that correlate with the eventual development of TD.

The aim of this study was to assess the responses in aged Cebus monkeys to provocative challenges with dopamine agonists and antagonists before, during, and after prolonged haloperidol treatment. The possible tolerance to dopamine antagonist effects and the evolution of behavioral hypersensitivity in the presence of continued haloperidol treatment were also evaluated.

2 Materials and Methods

Subjects. Eight male Cebus albifrons monkeys, 15–18 years old, were tested.

Drugs. The dopamine agonists were apomorphine 0.5 mg/kg, *d*-amphetamine 1.0 mg/kg, and the ergots bromocriptine 5.0 mg/kg and pergolide 0.5 mg/kg, each given SC. The dopamine antagonist haloperidol was given SC in doses of 0.01 mg/kg, 0.05 mg/kg, and 0.25 mg/kg. Oral haloperidol 0.25 mg/kg was given in a 30-ml aliquot of apple juice 7 days per week. Placebo was sterile saline, 0.25 mg/kg SC.

Design. The dopamine agonists and placebo were evaluated in the above order with 7 days between tests. Haloperidol challenges were then given, with an additional 7 days between tests, followed by oral haloperidol for 3 months. During the last month of haloperidol, the dopamine agonists were retested on the same schedule noted above. Five days after haloperidol was discontinued the dopamine agonists were again retested with 7 days between each trial. Then no medications were administered for 1 month. The next treatment cycle was initiated with once-weekly challenge doses of haloperidol prior to initiation of the 3-month period of oral haloperidol medication. This cycle was repeated four times.

Rating. Drug-induced buccolinguo-masticatory (BLM) movements, consisting of chewing, tongue choreoathetosis and protrusion, and compulsive licking or gnawing were scored. The rating scale was 0 = normal; 1 = occasionally present; 2 = regularly present; and 3 = continually present. Behaviors were scored prior to and at regular intervals after drug injections for 6 hours. Apomorphine was scored for only 2 hours. All scoring was done by a rater who was blind to drug dosage. Group mean scores are used for data analysis.

3 Results

Prior to haloperidol treatment, apomorphine and amphetamine produced low to moderate signs of BLM. Bromocriptine and pergolide produced very few BLM dyskinesias. Apomorphine-induced BLMs were reduced during the first treatment cycle with concomitant haloperidol, but increased above the baseline scores after haloperidol was discontinued for 1 week (Fig. 1). At the end of the second 3-month treatment cycle, concomitant haloperidol no longer suppressed the apomorphine-induced BLMs. Rather, the BLM score during this combination treatment was equal to the elevated apomorphine only score 1 week after haloperidol had been discontinued in the previous cycle. By 1 week after haloperidol was discontinued in the second cycle, the apomorphine score was still above the original baseline, but lower than the score at the end of the first cycle (Fig. 1). The third and fourth cycles showed similar responses with higher scores for haloperidol plus apomorphine than for apomorphine alone. Furthermore, the trend of decreasing BLM scores over the second, third, and fourth treatment cycles continued, so that at the end of the fourth cycle scores had returned to almost the pretreatment baseline level (Fig. 1).

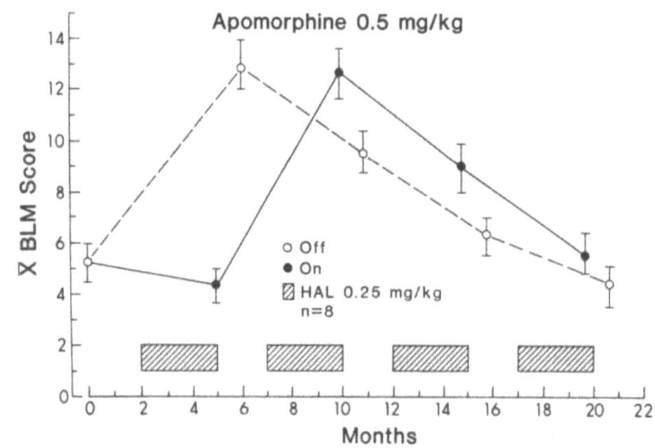

Fig. 1. Mean buccolinguo-masticatory (BLM) score induced by apomorphine 0.5 mg/kg before, at the end of, and 1 week after each 3-month treatment with haloperidol 0.25 mg/kg PO

Similar patterns of posthaloperidol hypersensitivity responses were seen with the amphetamine challenge. This response was most pronounced after the first 3-month cycle, and slowly returned to the baseline score over the second, third, and fourth treatment cycles. However, with amphetamine there was no increase above the baseline score when haloperidol and amphetamine were given in combination during each of the 3-month haloperidol treatment periods.

Bromocriptine and pergolide did not cause increase in BLM signs either during or following any of the four haloperidol treatment cycles. Though there was complete suppression of the bromocriptine-induced BLM signs at the end of the first 3-month haloperidol treatment period, this suppressive effect resolved, so that the scores in the second, third, and fourth treatment periods remained at the pretreatment baseline level.

4 Discussion

Different dopamine agonists have widely varying capacities for production of BLM behavior. Whereas apomorphine, a partial agonist, and amphetamine, an indirect agonist, consistently produced moderate BLM signs of tongue protrusion and chewing, the ergot agonists bromocriptine and pergolide, even at very high doses, were much less effective in producing these behaviors in monkeys. Similar behavioral differences among these classes of dopamine agonists have also been seen in rodents (Gianutsos and Moore 1980).

The initial differences seen in the preneuroleptic phase continued throughout the four cycles of haloperidol treatment. Apomorphine and amphetamine, but not the ergots, showed typical behavioral hypersensitivity, with exaggerated responses to agonists following the cessation of antagonist treatment. The inability of bromocriptine and pergolide to produce BLM dyskinesias questions the validity of these behaviors as models of iatrogenic movement disorders, because these drugs produce obvious hyperkinetic dyskinesias in parkinsonian patients. The absence of bromocriptine- or pergolide-induced BLMs as a hypersensitivity response may be explained by a desensitization process initiated by the doses of apomorphine and amphetamine given in the previous 2 weeks. However, this seems unlikely to be the sole explanation, because the striking behavioral hypersensitivity seen with amphetamine (scores nearly twice those of the original baseline) would not be expected to resolve completely in only 7 days. Furthermore, this desensitization process could not explain why the ergots were generally ineffective in producing BLM dyskinesias prior to any neuroleptic treatment. Rather, it is more likely that the ergot agonists function in mechanisms that are, at least in part, different from apomorphine or amphetamine.

The behavioral hypersensitivity of increased BLM responses seen after extended neuroleptic treatment is discontinued are consistent with many earlier observations of postneuroleptic behavioral hypersensitivity in rodents and monkeys (Schelkunov 1967; Klawans and Rubovits 1972; Tarsy and Baldessarini 1973; Christensen et al. 1976; Casey et al. 1980). However, the observations that this apomorphine- and amphetamine-provoked behavioral hypersensitivity gradually decreases toward the initial pretreatment baseline level with repeated treatment over 1–2 years raises many questions. Perhaps the BLM syndrome is not correlated with parameters of long-term neuroleptic treatment which eventually lead to TD. The tendency to focus on behavioral changes seen during or after relatively short treatment durations may have incorrectly led to the assumption that these changes were related to TD. Indeed, they may only reflect an intermediate phase in CNS compensating processes set in motion by neuroleptics, or they may be related to something else entirely.

The ability of haloperidol to suppress apomorphine-induced BLMs conforms to the classic model of counteracting antagonist-agonist effects. However, the antagonist not only lost its suppressive effects (tolerance), but also eventually enhanced (potentiation) the apomorphine influences during the second, third, and fourth 3-month treatment periods. This may be interpreted as evidence for behavioral hypersensitivity in the presence of chronic dopamine antagonist treatment. This observation, previously noted in rodents (Clow et al. 1979), has now been shown in nonhuman primates. The tolerance phase of this response may be a model for the gradual resolution of neuroleptic-induced parkinsonism seen in the clinic.

The potentiation phase implies that during long-term treatment the neuroleptic effects switch from classic antagonist influences early in drug exposure to paradoxical enhancement of apomorphine agonist effects in later phases of treatment. Though the reversal of the classic antagonist-agonist effect continued after the first treatment phase, the gradual decrease toward pretreatment baseline levels during extended treatment illustrates the dynamic alterations in function seen with long-term neuroleptic exposure. The clinical relevance of this paradoxical response is unknown, since it was seen with apomorphine but not amphetamine, bromocriptine, or pergolide. It may or may not be a model of evolving TD.

Though these results are preliminary and need to be replicated in other laboratories, they stimulate provocative questions. The validity of dopamine agonist-induced BLM behavior as a model for TD is challenged. The gradual evolution of antagonist-agonist effects from suppression to tolerance to potentiation of agonist-induced behaviors reflects incompletely understood adaptive processes. The eventual resolution of hypersensitivity responses, even with continued re-exposure to neuroleptics, illustrates the dynamic quality of CNS adaptive processes. These observations may be early clues that the traditional explanation that neuroleptics have their therapeutic effects via dopamine receptor blockade needs revision. The induction of hypersensitivity or other compensatory CNS events in response to neuroleptic treatment may be the mechanism of beneficial antipsychotic effects rather than of undesirable side-effects.

Acknowledgments. Haloperidol was supplied by McNeil Laboratories, bromocriptine by Sandoz, Inc., and pergolide by Eli Lilly Company.

References

Baldessarini RJ, Cole JO, Davis JM, Gardos G, Preskorn SH, Simpson GM, Tarsy D (1980) Tardive dyskinesia: a task force report. American Psychiatric Association, Washington DC

Casey DE, Gerlach J (1984) Tardive dyskinesia: management and new treatment. In: Stancer HC, Garfinkel PE, Rakoff VM (eds) Guidelines for the use of psychotropic drugs. Spectrum, New York, pp 183–203

Casey DE, Gerlach J, Christensson E (1980) Behavioral aspects of dopamine receptor hypersensitivity in primates. Prog Neuropsychopharmacol [Suppl] 110:101

Christensen AV, Fjalland B, Møller Nielsen I (1976) On the supersensitivity of dopamine receptors induced by neuroleptics. Psychopharmacology 48:1–6

Clow A, Jenner P, Marsden CD (1979) Changes in dopamine-mediated behavior during one year's neuroleptic administration. Eur J Pharmacol 57:365–375

Clow A, Theodorou A, Jenner P, Marsden CD (1980a) Changes in rat striatal dopamine turnover and receptor activity during one year's neuroleptic administration. Eur J Pharmacol 63:135–144

Clow A, Theodorou A, Jenner P, Marsden CD (1980b) Cerebral dopamine function in rats following withdrawal from one year of continuous neuroleptic administration. Eur J Pharmacol 63:145–157

Gianutsos G, Moore KE (1980) Differential behavioral and biochemical effects of four dopaminergic agonists. Psychopharmacology 68:139–146

Gunne LM, Barany S (1976) Haloperidol-induced tardive dyskinesia in monkeys. Psychopharmacology 50:237–240

Kane JM, Smith JM (1982) Tardive dyskinesia: prevalence and risk factors, 1959 to 1979. Arch Gen Psychiatry 39:473–481

Klawans HL (1973) The pharmacology of tardive dyskinesia. Am J Psychiatry 130:82–86

Klawans HL, Rubovits R (1972) An experimental model of tardive dyskinesia. J Neural Transm 33:235–246

Kovacic B, Domino EF (1982) A monkey model of tardive dyskinesia (TD): evidence that reversible TD may turn into irreversible TD. J Clin Psychopharmacol 2:305–307

Schelkunov EL (1967) Adrenergic effect of chronic administration of neuroleptics. Nature 214:1210–1212

Tarsy D, Baldessarini RJ (1973) Pharmacologically induced behavioral supersensitivity to apomorphine. Nature 245:262–263

Toenniessen LM, Casey DE, McFarland BH (1985) Tardive dyskinesia in the aged. Arch Gen Psychiatry (to be published)

Ungerstedt U (1971) Stereotaxic mapping of the monoamine pathways in the rat brain. Acta Physiol Scand [Suppl] 367:1–48

Induction of Tardive Dyskinesia in *Cebus apella* and *Macaca speciosa* Monkeys: A Review

E. F. Domino [1]

Contents

Abstract 217
1 Introduction 217
2 Methods 218
3 Results 219
4 Discussion 221
References 223

Abstract

Two different studies were performed in subhuman primates in an attempt to induce symptoms of tardive dyskinesia. The first study lasted for over 5 years. This involved elderly *Macaca speciosa.* The animals were given first 25 mg of fluphenazine decanoate and later the enanthate IM (3.2 mg/kg) every 2 weeks and on 5 days a week, haloperidol, first IM and later PO. Haloperidol was given first in doses of 1.0 mg/kg and ultimately after years of therapy, in doses of 6.4 mg/kg per day. Those animals who survived gained weight to over 10 kg. After neuroleptic withdrawal, tardive dyskinesia became evident in 1 month. The symptoms of tardive dyskinesia following cessation of medication lasted a maximum of 1 year. This animal model produced very impressive symptoms in one of the three animals treated who survived. This is not a very practical animal model from the aspects of economics (costly), time (5 years), and animal availability (rare and endangered species). However, the symptoms of tardive dyskinesia are very striking and identical with human tardive dyskinesia in a susceptible animal.

A more practical experimental animal model involved *Cebus apella.* Depot fluphenazine (0.1 to 3.2 mg/kg) was given continuously every 2 weeks for 1 year. In this species the symptoms of tardive dyskinesia became progressively prolonged and intense with each course of fluphenazine therapy and withdrawal, suggesting that reversible tardive dyskinesia may turn into irreversible tardive dyskinesia. With each succeeding course of fluphenazine therapy (1 month) and withdrawal (1–3 months), the animals appeared to be sensitized to both the acute extrapyramidal and the tardive dyskinesia symptoms. These animals were also given various experimental drug treatments including biperiden lactate, benztropine mesylate, and *d*-amphetamine after they developed signs of tardive dyskinesia.

1 Introduction

It is well known that elderly humans given chronic neuroleptic medication are more likely to develop tardive dyskinesia than young adults (Jeste and Wyatt 1981). While there are many possible reasons for this, it is highly probable that

1 Department of Pharmacology, University of Michigan, M6414 Medical Science Building I, Ann Arbor, MI 48109-0010, USA

Dyskinesia – Research and Treatment
(Psychopharmacology Supplementum 2)
Editors: Casey, Chase, Christensen, Gerlach

pre-existing age-related alterations in neurotransmitter function account for the increased susceptibility of the elderly. Neurotransmitter changes in old age are very numerous and involve most neurotransmitter systems (Domino et al. 1978). It occurred to us that the use of elderly subhuman primates might facilitate symptoms of tardive dyskinesia more readily than the use of younger animals. It proved to be difficult to obtain only geriatric animals for this study and instead middle-aged to geriatric animals were used. The results of these studies have been described in detail elsewhere (Kovacic and Domino 1982; Domino and Kovacic 1983; Domino and Kovacic 1984; Kovacic and Domino 1984). These reports have not emphasized the fact that many of the animals were geriatric, and that this may be an important factor in the success achieved in inducing tardive dyskinesia in two species of subhuman primates, *Macaca speciosa* and *Cebus apella.*

2 Methods

Macaca speciosa. Eight adult animals, three males and five females, weighing 3.2 kg or more, were started on this study. All were sexually mature and had previously been used in reproductive research. They were near middle age to geriatric and were not good breeders. Some were used experimentally for chronic electroencephalographic studies with a large variety of centrally acting drugs including hallucinogens, anesthetics, and convulsants. Those monkeys with chronic indwelling brain electrodes lost their implants over a period of months to years and were then entered into this study as their scalps healed. All animals were in excellent physical condition prior to neuroleptic treatment. Three of the monkeys completed 3–5 years of uninterrupted neuroleptic treatment. Another three were found dead after 1–3 weeks of neuroleptic treatment (37% incidence of unexpected death). Two animals, after several months of neuroleptic therapy, developed self-mutilation syndromes that were so destructive (eating off fingers, chewing on testicles, etc.) that treatment was discontinued for humane reasons (see Domino 1983). The animals were housed in separate cages in a room controlled for temperature and humidity. Food and water were allowed ad libitum. The diet consisted of Purina Monkey Chow pellets and fresh fruit.

Cebus apella. Five feral-born females, each weighing approximately 2 kg, were started on this study. None of these animals had been used previously in research. Three of the monkeys completed a full year of neuroleptic treatment. One monkey dislocated her knee after only 6 months of treatment, developed gangrene (dry), and was sacrificed. Except for the leg, no gross pathologic lesions were found on necropsy. The fifth monkey died after 9 months of neuroleptic treatment from undetermined causes (20% incidence of unexpected death). These animals were housed in smaller individual cages in a separate room with conditions similar to those for the *Macaca speciosa.* The diet consisted of Purina Monkey Chow pellets, Marmoset Science Diet, and fresh fruit. Except for one animal, the monkeys maintained stable body weights throughout the study. One was estimated by veterinarians to be geriatric, and one was found to be carrying a dead infant in utero during the quarantine period just before the start of the study; the other monkeys were estimated to be middle-aged to geriatric.

Drugs. The *Macaca speciosa* were given first 25 mg total IM fluphenazine decanoate and later the enanthate (3.2 mg/kg) IM every 2 weeks, and 5 days a week haloperidol first IM and later PO. Haloperidol was given first in doses of 1.0 mg/kg and ended after years of therapy with 6.4 mg/kg. Those animals who survived gained weight to over 10 kg. The drugs used were fluphenazine decanoate and enanthate and haloperidol pure substance.

The most systemic study was done in *Cebus apella.* Depot fluphenazine (0.1–3.2 mg/kg, IM) as the enanthate ester was selected because, in patients, the incidence of neurologic reactions to this agent appears to be somewhat greater than that caused by the decanoate. The species *Cebus apella* was selected because *Cebus apella* had shown more tardive dyskinesia than other species of subhuman primates that had been given neuroleptics on a long-term basis, as recorded by Gunne and his colleagues (Barany et al. 1979; Barany and Gunne 1979; Gunne and Barany 1976, 1979, 1980).

Assessment of Behavior. Videotapes of the animals' behavior were obtained before the start of drug treatment and at various times throughout the study. The animals were observed at least once a day, 5 days/week. A log was kept of each animal's behavior.

3 Results

Macaca speciosa. These animals were first given fluphenazine decanoate in a dose of 25 mg IM every 2 weeks. Haloperidol was added as a daily dose of 1.0 mg/kg IM Monday through Friday. This regimen produced marked reductions in motor activity and behavior, giving rise to terms like "zombies." Sudden death (3 animals) and self-mutilation (2 animals) syndromes were observed in some of the monkeys (Domino 1983). Three of the animals tolerated chronic neuroleptic therapy very well. These three *Macaca speciosa* showed relatively few signs of dyskinetic and dystonic reactions, but more signs of parkinsonism, especially bradykinesia. Tremor was not prominent, although years later one developed an intention tremor as well as a tremor at rest. Considerable tolerance was observed to the effects of these neuroleptics; so, over a course of months and years, the dose of haloperidol was gradually increased to 6.4 mg/kg and the route of administration changed from IM to PO. In addition, fluphenazine enanthate (3.2 mg/kg) was given. Throughout the period of 3–5 years of continuous combined neuroleptic therapy, these three monkeys continued to gain weight. They showed mostly bradykinesia, and no significant dyskinetic or dystonic reactions. Tardive dyskinesia-like symptoms were never seen while the monkeys received neuroleptics. Because of financial constraints, neuroleptic treatment of these animals was discontinued abruptly. Within a few weeks all showed an increase in alertness and loss of the bradykinesia. The hand tremors that one had disappeared. Within one month after drug withdrawal another animal showed a slight increase in mouthing and chewing movements, which disappeared in about 2 weeks. The third animal showed no tardive dyskinesia-like movements whatsoever. In contrast, the first animal started to have prominent mouthing movements within 1 month, which remained prominent for about 9 months after abrupt withdrawal of the fluphenazine and haloperidol. Akathisia of the hands and feet was also evident. This first animal showed the most characteristic human-like tardive dyskinesia ever produced in any of our monkeys. However, after about 9 months the symptoms of tardive dyskinesia gradually disappeared, and 1 year later they were totally absent.

Cebus apella. The monkeys were treated with fluphenazine enanthate given IM every other week. During the first 2 months of treatment the dose was raised in half-log increments from 0.1 to 3.2 mg/kg. At the high dose the animals stopped eating and drinking, so the dose was dropped back to 1 mg/kg for 4 months and then raised again to 3.2 mg/kg and held there for the last half of the year. From the 4th to the 8th month of fluphenazine treatment, attempts were made to add haloperidol to the treatment regimen by adding 0.5 mg/kg to food (fruit or juice) daily. However, the animals would not reliably eat the drugged food. Decreased food and water intake became a problem so the attempt was abandoned.

During the first month of treatment, the predominant effects seen in all monkeys were sedation, slowing of movements, akinesia, tremor of the extremities, trembling of the entire body, and decreased water intake. During the following months, parkinsonian symptoms (evident for the entire 2-week period after injection) intensified and a variety of dystonic postures, dyskinesias, and akathisia-like symptoms appeared. These occurred in episodes which had their peak occurrence from 3 hours to 2 1/2 days after each injection. Usually, monkeys had one episode lasting several hours on the day of injection and another lasting several hours on the second or third day after injection. During these episodes, any or many of the various dystonic, dyskinetic, and akathisia-like reactions could occur. As the year of treatment progressed, such symptoms increased in type, frequency, and severity. The number of episodes of reactions increased and during the later months occurred sporadically throughout the entire 2-week period after each injection. Stress, especially the stress of eye contact with the investigator, appeared to precipitate episodes of drug reactions.

The following signs were displayed by all monkeys. The animals circled in a well-coordinated, quadrupedal manner, or they thrashed about the cage in a poorly coordinated manner, assuming bizarre postures. An abnormal posture commonly seen was with the feet on the floor, head close to the feet, legs extended and rump high. A dystonic posture often displayed was with arms and/or legs widespread and extremities clinging to the walls or ceiling (often resembling a horizontal crucifixion posture); at such times the animals were rigid and trembling and unresponsive to verbal or tactile stimuli. Retrocollis was very common; sometimes the monkeys would sit immobile for hours with the face parallel to the ceiling. At times the monkeys would fling themselves violently (crash) into the walls or ceiling of the cage. Parts of the cages were padded to prevent the animals from injuring themselves. Crashing spells occurred sporadically and usually lasted only a minute or so. A spell could be terminated by pulling the squeeze wall of the cage forward to within about 6 in. from the front wall. The animals often appeared glassy-eyed and unresponsive to stimuli just before a crash.

In addition to the above, effects characteristic of the individuals were observed. One had oral dyskinesias which first appeared during the 8th month of treatment. The animal would hold her mouth wide open and protrude her tongue far to the side, holding it out for many seconds at a time, sometimes moving her jaw up and down rhythmically. Sometimes she would gnaw on the cage wall, ceiling, or floor, protruding her tongue far through the cage mesh, either straight out or curved downward to the side, moving it irregularly.

Another animal often held her right arm in a characteristic posture. She held the arm straight up with the wrist flexed so that the palm of her hand was parallel to the top of her head. Often when in this position, she made bicycling movements with her legs while either staying in one location or prancing around the cage. Sometimes she was quite graceful about this, giving the appearance of dancing. During the later months she was not graceful and this characteristic behavior became a signal that crashing was imminent if not prevented by pulling the squeeze wall forward. Two other animals would lie on the floor on their backs and circle constantly for hours. Their elbows were scraped raw from this activity. Medicated ointment had to be applied to the elbows, and bulky bandages to prevent further injury and permit healing. During circling, the animals' arms and legs often thrashed about or flexed and extended rhythmically.

Effect of Benztropine on Acute Reactions to Fluphenazine. The ability of benztropine to affect the monkeys' abnormal movements was examined during the 2 weeks following the last injection of the year of fluphenazine treatment. Shortly after an animal went into an episode of acute reaction to fluphenazine, she was given benztropine (0.2–0.5 mg/kg, IM). The drug very effectively terminated the episode.

Symptoms Reminiscent of Tardive Dyskinesia. Within a few months after abrupt cessation of chronic treatment with fluphenazine three of the animals displayed symptoms similar to tardive dyskinesia. Such symptoms worsened under stress.

4 Discussion

Centrally acting dopamine antagonists (neuroleptic drugs) induce in various subhuman and human primates at least two different extrapyramidal syndromes, which respond to pharmacological challenges in totally different ways. The first constellation of signs and symptoms is the acute dyskinetic, dystonic, parkinsonism syndrome. This syndrome can occur early or late after chronic neuroleptic treatment. It is made worse by single doses of neuroleptics and is relieved by centrally acting, predominantly muscarinic anticholinergic drugs. The second constellation of signs and symptoms is tardive dyskinesia. This syndrome occurred in our monkeys after chronic neuroleptic medication given continuously for 0.25–5 years. It is sometimes manifest while the animals are still receiving neuroleptic medication and becomes prominent within about 1 month after neuroleptic withdrawal. Generally, but not always, the tardive dyskinesia syndrome subsides after a period of months without medication. Repeated intermittent neuroleptic medication regimens prolong the tardive dyskinesia syndrome. Single doses of neuroleptics relieve this syndrome temporarily. Many motor movements and effects of various drug treatments are similar to those in humans with tardive dyskinesia.

This study shows that *Macaca speciosa* and *Cebus apella* monkeys given long-term treatment with neuroleptics develop two distinct motor syndromes, one corresponding to the early extrapyramidal symptoms of neuroleptic-treated patients, the other corresponding to tardive dyskinesia. The first syndrome consisted initially of parkinsonian symptoms and, as the year progressed, in *Cebus apella* a variety of dystonic, dyskinetic, and akathisia-like reactions appeared, which worsened after each injection, were not exacerbated by drug withdrawal, and could be treated very effectively with benztropine mesylate. The second syndrome made its first appearance after cessation of neuroleptic treatment, consisted of abnormal movements very similar in appearance to those of patients with tardive dyskinesia, and could be abolished completely by resumption of neuroleptic treatment.

The results of this study using Cebus confirm the studies of Bárány's group (Bárány et al. 1979; Bárány and Gunne 1979) and others (see Domino and Kovacic 1983), which show that monkeys given long-term treatment with a neuroleptic show progressive changes in overt motor behavior. The neuroleptic elicits dramatic dystonia and dyskinesia in these animals, which resemble the acute dyskinetic or dystonic syndrome observed in humans at the beginning of neuroleptic treatment. Although not all monkeys given long-term treatment with a neuroleptic develop the dystonic and dyskinetic effects (Gunné and Bárány 1976, 1979, 1980; Paulson 1972, 1973), once established in an animal they can be reliably elicited with a single injection of the neuroleptic. This has been reported to occur even after a drug-free hiatus of as long as 508 days (Weiss et al. 1977). In such "primed" animals the effects can also be elicited by single injections of many neuroleptics (Liebman and Neale 1980; Neale et al. 1981; Porsolt and Jalfre 1981). The ability of various neuroleptics to precipitate dystonias and dyskinesias in primed monkeys appears to correspond with their propensity to produce acute dystonic-dyskinetic reactions in patients.

The present study provides evidence that *Cebus apella* also can be primed for tardive dyskinesia, since when tardive dyskinesia symptoms were fading they could be restored to full force with a short (4-week) course of fluphenazine treatment. In the one monkey that received three courses of fluphenazine the duration of display of pronounced symptoms of tardive dyskinesia was longer after the second course of treatment than after the first, and longer after the third course than after the second. This suggests that spontaneously remitting tardive dyskinesia might eventually turn into irreversible tardive dyskinesia with continued neuroleptic treatment.

Of special interest is the marked tolerance over the months and years that the *Macaca speciosa* showed to neuroleptic medication, which allowed very large doses to be given. Perhaps the best animal model of tardive dyskinesia was that produced in one of the geriatric male *Macaca speciosa* treated with neuroleptics continuously for 5 years after which they were abruptly withdrawn. Unfortunately, this species of monkey is relatively rare, expensive, and difficult to handle because of the large size, which makes special caging and related animal facilities necessary. This species is also somewhat more susceptible than others to sudden death and self-mutilation syndromes induced by neuroleptics (Domino 1983). Although this species showed the most characteristic form of "human"-like tardive dyskinesia, it is not practical or efficient to study these animals unless excellent long-term facilities are available. *Cebus apella* is a much more practical animal to study as a model of tardive dyskinesia, although the animals require much more care and attention during neuroleptic treatment because of their severe dyskinetic and dystonic symptoms.

Acknowledgements. The author would like to acknowledge the research efforts of B. Kovacic, B. Mathews, D. Ruffing, and S. Tart in these studies.

References

Bárány S, Ingvast A, Gunne LM (1979) Development of acute dystonia and tardive dyskinesia in cebus monkeys. Res Commun Chem Pathol Pharmacol 25:269–279

Bárány S, Gunne LM (1979) Pharmacological modification of experimental tardive dyskinesia. Acta Pharmacol Toxicol 45:107–111

Domino EF (1983) Sudden death, acute and chronic extrapyramidal syndromes including tardive dyskinesia and self-mutilation induced by fluphenazine and haloperidol in monkeys. Abst Soc for Neurosci 13th Annual Meeting, Boston, MA Abst 893:9

Domino EF, Dren AT, Giardina WJ (1978) Biochemical and neurotransmitter changes in the aging brain. In: Lipton MA, DiMascio A, Killam KF (eds) Psychopharmacology: a generation of progress. Raven, New York, pp 1507–1515

Domino EF, Kovacic B (1983) Monkey models of tardive dyskinesia. In: Bannet J, Belmaker RH (eds) New directions in tardive dyskinesia Research. Karger, Basel, pp 21–33

Domino EF, Kovacic B (1984) Monkey models of tardive dyskinesia. In: Catecholamines. Liss, New York (to be published)

Gunne LM, Bárány S (1976) Haloperidol-induced tardive dyskinesia in monkeys. Psychopharmacology 50:237–240

Gunne LM, Bárány S (1979) A monitoring test for the liability of neuroleptic drugs to induce tardive dyskinesia. Psychopharmacology 63:195–198

Gunne LM, Bárány S (1980) A primate model for tardive dyskinesia. In: Fann WE, Smith RC, Davis JM, Domino EF (eds) Tardive dyskinesia research and treatment. Medical and Scientific Books, New York, pp 1–12

Jeste DV, Wyatt RJ (1981) Changing epidemiology of tardive dyskinesia – an overview. Am J Psychiatry 138:297–309

Kovacic B, Domino EF (1982) A monkey (Cebus apella) model of tardive dyskinesia (TD): Evidence that reversible TD may turn into irreversible TD. J Clin Psychopharmacol 2:305–307

Kovacic B, Domino EF (1984) Fluphenazine-induced acute and tardive dyskinesias in monkeys. Psychopharmacology (to be published)

Liebman J, Neale R (1980) Neuroleptic-induced dyskinesias in squirrel monkeys. Correlation with propensity to cause extrapyramidal side effects. Psychopharmacology 68:25–29

Neale R, Fallon S, Gerhardt S, Liebman JM (1981) Acute dyskinesias in monkeys elicited by halopemide, mezilamine, and the "antidyskinetic" drugs, oxiperomide and tiapride. Psychopharmacology 75:254–257

Paulson GW (1972) Dyskinesias in rhesus monkeys. Am Neurol Assoc Trans 97:109–110

Paulson GW (1973) Dyskinesias in monkeys. Adv Neurol 1:647–650

Porsolt RD, Jalfre M (1981) Neuroleptic-induced acute dyskinesias in rhesus monkeys. Psychopharmacology 75:16–21

Weiss B, Santelli S, Lusink G (1977) Movement disorders induced in monkeys by chronic haloperidol treatment. Psychopharmacology 53:289–293

List of Contributors

Agid, Y. 145
Arbilla, S. 39
Arnt, J. 9, 46, 60, 182

Bannet, J. 194
Bartholini, G. 39
Belmaker, R. H. 194
Bonnet, A.-M. 145
Bossi, L. 128

Carlsson, A. 31
Casey, D. E. 88, 137, 211
Chase, T. N. 122
Christensen, A. V. 9, 182
Cunningham Owens, D. G. 79
Cross, A. J. 104
Crow, T. J. 104
Domino, E. F. 217

Elami, A. 194

Fage, D. 39
Ferrier, I. N. 104
Fleischhauer, J. 162
Fog, R. 118
Fournier, V. 128

Gerlach, J. 98
Gilsdorf, U. 162
Goldstein, M. 200
Gunne, L. M. 191

Häggström, J. E. 191
Herrera-Marschitz, M. 19
Hobi, V. 162
Hyttel, J. 9

Javoy-Agid, F. 145
Jenner, P. 174
Johnson, J. A. 104
Johnstone, E. C. 104

Kane, J. M. 72
Kocher, R. 162

Langer, S. Z. 39
Larsen, J.-J. 9
Lieberman, J. 72
Lloyd, K. G. 200

Marsden, C. D. 64, 174
Morselli, P. L. 128
Musch, B. 128

Oblin, A. 39
Owen, F. 104
Owens, D. G. C. 104

Pakkenberg, H. 111
Pedersen, B. 111
Poulter, M. 104

Ruberg, M. 145
Rupniak, N. M. J. 174

Scatton, B. 39
Scheel-Krüger, J. 46
Seeman, P. 2
Ståhle, L. 19
Svendsen, O. 182

Tamminga, C. A. 122
Thaker, G. K. 122
Tossman, U. 19

Ungerstedt, U. 19

Willigens, M. T. 200
Woerner, M. 72

Zetterström, T. 19
Zivkovic, B. 39

Subject Index

Page numbers in *italics* indicate pages where the subject is discussed in detail

Abnormal involuntary movement scale (AIMS) 74, 81, 92, 104, *145–159*, *200*
Acetylcholine 28, 29, 42, 43, *46–57*, 101, 120, *137*, *174*
^{3}H-Acetylcholine 14, 101
γ-Acetylenic GABA 39, 139
Adenylate cyclase 2, 3, 10, 13, 20, *174*
Adrenergics *137*
α-Adrenoceptors (α_1) *9*, 14
Age *64*, *72*, *79*, *98*, 118, *162*, 218
AIMS 81
Akathisia 129, 140, 220
  tardive *98*
Akinesia 147, 149
Amantadine 129
Amphetamine-induced stereotyped behaviour 60, 129, 183, *211*, *217*
Amygdala 49
Anhedonia 120
Anticholinergics 100, *111*, *137*, 163, 170, *182*, 221
Apomorphine 13, *19*, 32, 33, 35, 41, 47, 48, 124, *200*, *211*
Apomorphine antagonism vomiting 184
Arecoline 138
Association areas *46–57*
  prefrontal *46–57*
Associative cortex *46–57*
  parietal area *46–57*
Autoreceptors *2–6*, 26, *31–45*

Baclofen 139, 203
Ballistic movements i11
Barbiturates 141
Basal ganglia *39*, 51, *104*, 114, 118–120, *122*, 138, *145*
Behaviour, spatial aspects *128*, 219
Benzamides *9*, 183
Benzodiazepines 100, *111*, 139, 141, 149
Benztropine *217*
BHT 920 34
Bicuculline 193, 204
Biperiden lactate *217*
Bleuler 80
BLM (bucco-linguo-masticatory) syndrome 65, 67, 69, 71, 75, 83, 118, *211*
Bradykinesia 219
Bromocriptine 133, *211*
Brueghel's syndrome 114
Butyrophenones *9*, *182*, *194*
Butaclamol 15
γ-Butyrolactone 33

Carbachol 52, 53
Carbamazepine 113
Catalepsy 33, 37, 50, 54, 183, 206
Caudate nucleus *2*, 13, 36, 40, 46, 48, 106, 150, 152, 195
CCK 8 147
Cebus apella monkeys 102, 191, *211–216*, *217–223*
Cerebellar afferents
  cortex 19–30
  cortex interneurones 19–30
  input-output systems 19–30
  stimulation 19–30
Cerebello-thalamo-cortical pathway *19–30*, *46–57*
Cerebro-cerebellar-motor cortex pathways 19–30
Cerebro-striato-premotor cortex pathways 19–30
Chewing movements 98–103, *211–216*
Chlorpromazine 14, 64
Chlorprothixene *9–18*
Choline 138
  acetyltransferase (CAT) 105, 108, 151, 177
Cholinergic 134, *137*, 149
  interneurones 51, 52
Chorea *200*
Chronic treatment *64–71*, *79–87*, *104–110*, *182–190*, *194–199*
Circling 186, *200*
cis(Z)-Flupentixol 10, 13, 14, 21, 26, 28, 47, 60, 100, 175, *182*
cis(Z)-Clopenthixol 14, 60, *182*
Clebopride 184
Clonazepam 125

Clonidine 140
Clothiapine 15
Clozapine 15, 101, 119, 163, *174–181*
Combined treatment stereotypy *182–190*
Cortex
  association 46–57
  orbitofrontal 46–57
  parietal 46–57
  precentral motor 50
  prefrontal 49–51
  sulcal 50
  visual 46–57
Cortico-striatal pathways 43
Cortico-striatate projections *46–57*
Cross-tolerance *182–190*
CT scans 85
Cyclic AMP 175

Deanol 134
Denervation hypersensitivity 21
Dentato-thalamo-cortical circuit 46-57
^{14}C-2-Deoxyglucose
Des-tyrosine-gamma-endorphin 140
Diazepam 101
Differentiation of DA antagonists *9–18*, *182–190*
Dihydroxyphenylacetic acid (DOPAC) 105, 109, 192
Diphneylbutylpiperidines 183, 186
Dogs 184–185
Dopa accumulation 113
L-Dopa 44, 48, 101, 120, *128–136*, *145–159*, *200*
L-Dopa therapy *141–162*
Dopamine (DA) 2, 28, 31, 32, 39, *46–57*, *98*, 119, *122*, 138, *145*, *182–190*
  autoreceptors *32*, 43
  receptor
    agonists *32–38*, *60*, *61*, 101, *145*, *211*
    antagonists 47, 51, *60*, *61*, *118–121*, *145*
    D-1 antagonists 35, *182–190*
    D-1 and D-2 antagonists, mixed *9–18*
    D-2 antagonists 35, *182–190*
    blockade *9*, *137*, 198
    hypersensitivity *194*, *211*
    sensitivity 101, 119, 120, *194–199*
    stimulation *145*
  receptors *2–8*, *19–30*, 32, 36, 37, 43, 101
    D-1 receptors 2, *9*, *19*, *60*, *61*, *104*, *174–181*
    D-2 receptors *2*, *9*, *19*, *60*, *61*, *104*, *174–181*
    D-3 receptors 3, 10
    D-4 receptors 2, 10
  release 40, 44
Dopaminergic innervation *1–30*
Dopaminergic neurons of substantia nigra *1–30*
Dopaminergic nigro-neostriatal pathway *1–30*
Droperidol *194–199*
Drug holidays *194*
Dysfunction in agonist-antagonist coordination *182–190*
Dyskinesia (D) *9*, *38*, *64*, *72–78*, *122–127*, *200*
  anatomical substrates *64–70*, *79–87*, *104–110*
  and interactions of mesocortical/mesolimbic/striatal dopamine *79*–87, *104–110*, *174–181*
  and the nigral cholinergic system *182–190*
  and the nucleus basalis magno cellularis (NBM) cholinergic system 51
  and the role of striatal acetylcholine *182–190*
  behavioral *200*
  D-1/D-2 dopamine receptors, role of *9–18*, *182–190*
  differential role of
    dopamine in dorsal/ventral striatum 46, 53
    dorsal/ventral striatal acetylcholine 174–181
    pallidal and nigral GABA systems 200–210
  /distinct GABA systems 122–127, 206–210
  dopamine-induced *200–210*
  L-dopa-induced *128–136*, *145–159*, *200*
  dynamic interactions of the GABA systems in series 39–57, *200–210*
  dysfunction of the efferent GABA systems 39–57, 200–210
  /GABA, a mediator and moderator of dopamine functions 39–57, 200–210
  /GABA in striatal and limbic output systems 39–57, 200–210
  /GABA in non-dopaminergic nigral output systems 39–57, 200–210
  /GABA in zona reticulata of substantia nigra (SNR) 39–57, 200–210
  /GABA. SNR stereotyped gnawing/licking activities 39–57, 200–210
  neuroleptic-induced *128–136*
  oral 193, *200*
  orofacial 82, 84, 114, 131
    prevalence 81, 84
  psychomotor *200*
  spontaneous *118–121*
    orofacial 114

Dyskinesia (D) (continued)
tardive 2–8, *32*, 39, 44, *46–57*, *64–71*, 79, 85, *89–103*, *118–121*, *128*, *137–144*, *162–171*, 175, *191–194*, *217–223*
incidence *72–78*, *174*, 194, *200*
irreversible *88–97*, 120, *217*
prevalence *72–79*, 81, 90, 124, *162–171*
reversible 70, *88–97*, *137*, *217*
risk factors *72–78*
vulnerability, individual *72*, 82, 84
Dyskinetic movements *128*
Dysphonia *111*
Dystonia *64*, *98*, *111–117*
focal *111*
segmental *111*
Dystonia musculorum deformans 65, *111*, 129
tardive 65, *111*, 129

Emetic trigger zone 34
EMG test *128*
Enanthate *217*
Enkephalin peptidergic nerve terminals 151
Epidemiology 72, *162*
Estrogen 134, 141
Ethybenztropine 149
Extrapyramidal symptoms *32*, 77, *98*, 166, 175, *217*
Extrapyramidal system 76
Eye movements 164

Feedback 41, 55
compensated 41, 55
position 41, 55
Fluperlapine *9–18*
Fluphenazine 14, 47, *182*
decanoate *217*
Fluspiriline *9–18*
Fusaric acid 141

GABA *19*, 40, 43, *46–57*, *98*, 102, *104*, 105, *122–127*, *137*, 139, *191*
agonists *128–136*, *200*
GABA mimetics *39–45*, 201
Gamma-acetylenic GABA 39, 139
Gamma-vinyl GABA 125, 139
Geriatric animals 218
Geriatric patients *74*, 163
Gilles de la Tourette syndrome 118–121
Globus pallidus 29, 47, 150, *191*
Glutamate decarboxylase 151, *191*

^{3}H-piflutixol (^{3}H-PIF) *9–18*, *104–110*
^{3}H-spiroperidol (^{3}H-SPI) *9–18*, *39–45*, *104–110*

Haloperidol 10, 34, 37, 40–43, 47, 54, 119, *174–181*, *182*, 195, *211*
Histamine receptors (H–1) *9*
Homovanillic acid (HVA) *104*, 192
Huntington's chorea 51, 65, 106, *118*
6-Hydroxydopamine (6-OHDA) lesions 10, 12, 13, 20, 28, 29, 36, 41, 46, *60*, *61*, 124
5-Hydroxyindacetic acid (5-HIAA) 109
3-(3-Hydroxyphenyl)-*N*-*n*-propylpiperidine (3-PPP) *31–45*
Hyperactivity 186
Hyperkinetic dyskinesia 94, *98*, *118*, 163
Hypersensitivity 20, 36, 37, *39–45*, 49, *98*, *104*, *122*, *145*, *174*
Hypothalamus 3

Immobility 54
Inhibitory nigro-striatal pathways 39–57
Involuntary movements *72*, *79–87*

Kainic acid 48
Kraepelin 80

Lactotroph receptor 35
L-Dopa 44, 48, 101, 120, *128–136*, *145–159*, *200*
L-Dopa therapy *141–162*
Leu-enkephalin 147
Lecithin 138
Levomepromazine 14, 100
Lithium *39–45*, 91, 93, 134, *137*

Macaca speciosa *217–223*
Mania *39*
MAO-inhibitors 109, 129
Medial thalamus 46–57
Mesencephalic locomotor area
Met-enkephalin 147
Methyl-dopa 133
Meige syndrome *111*
Methakvalon 100
3-Methoxytyramine 40
Methylphenidate antagonism 12, 15, 16, *182*
Methylscopolamine 54
Metoclopramide 13, 129
Monkey models of TD *191*
Movement accuracy
disorder *104–110*
initiation 104–116
onset 212
parameters 111–121
reaction time 111–121
related neuronal discharge 111–121
Muscarinic cholinergic receptors *9*, 109
Muscarinic presynaptic receptors 14
Muscimol 29, 41, 50, 54, 124, *128*, 139, *200*

Neuroleptics *9–18*, 51, *64*, *72*, *104*, *118*, *125*, *162*, *194–199*
combination treatment 119
withdrawal 120, 169, 175, 192, *217*
Neuropeptides 105, *137*, *145*
Nigro-neostriatal complex 19–30, 46–57, 60, 61
Nigro-neostriatal-pallidal complex 19–30, 46–57, 60, 61
Nigro-striatal bundle 19–30, 60, 61
damage 19–30, 60, 61
dopamine system 19–30, 60, 61
impulses 19–30, 60, 61
Nigro-striatal dopaminergic system 41, 42, *200*
Nigro-thalamic pathway 47–56
Non-dopaminergic nigral efferents 47–56
Non-human primates 211–223
Noradrenaline 17, 151
3-H-NPA *174*
Nomifensine 202
Nucleus accumbens *2*, 33, 46, 49–51, *104*, 152
subthalamic 150, *191*

Onset of movement 74, *145*
Opiate receptors *19–30*, 137
Oxotremorine 54
Oxypertine 133

Pallido-thalamic afferents *46–57*
Pallidum 50
Parkinsonism 37, 49, 55, 69, *98*, 119, 129, 139, 140, 201, 219
agonist burst 141–162
bradykinesia 141–162
movements 141–162
Pathogenesis *211*
Pathophysiology *89–103*, *122–127*, *145–159*, *191–193*, 212
Penfluridol 15
Peptides 109, 120, 151
Pergolide 13, *19*, *211*
Perphenazine 14, 101, *182*
Phenothiazines *8*, 66, *182*
Phenytoin 141
Physostigmine 134, 138
Picrotoxin 23, 24, 29, 30
^{3}H-Piflutixol 10, 105, *174*
Pimozide 15, 119, 186
Pipamperone 15
Piribedil 19–30, *200*
Pituitary *2*, 36
Post-mortem brain 103, *104*, *145*
Postsynaptic supersensitivity 174–190
3-PPP (– and +) *31–45*
Presynaptic supersensitivity 31–45
Progabide 39, 125, *128*, *200*
Prolactin 4
Prognosis (in TD) 88–103
Propranolol 140
n-Propylapomorphine 123
Psychosis *64*, 66, 198
PSE criteria 80
Putamen *2*, 17, *104*, 150, 152
Pyridoxine (vit. B_6) 134, 140, 141

Repeated administration 174–190, 194–199
Reserpine 33, 35, 36, 54, 119, 123
Response, conditioned avoidance 186
Reticular formation 124
Reticulo-spinal pathway 46–57
Rigid 149
Rigidity 149

Sadness 120
Schizoaffective disorders 77
SCH 23390 10, 13, 15, *19*, 47, 48, 53, 60, 175, *182*
Schizophrenia *2–8*, 13, 16, 37, *64*, 74, 77, *79–87*, *104*, 125, 176
Schizophrenic involuntary movements, neuroleptic *64*, *72*, *98*
Scopolamine 12, 185, 186
Sedation 184
Self-mutilation 218, 219
Senile dementia 84, 106
Serotonin 9, 14, 16, *137*
Serotonin (S-2) receptors *9*, 17, 139
Sex 74, 76, 163, 170
Simpson dyskinesia scale 75, 131
SK&F 38393 13, 60
SL 75102 203
Slowing of movements 65, 98, 111
Sodium valproate 44, 139
Spiperone *2*
^{3}H-Spiperone 4, 36, 105–107, 152, *174*
^{3}H-Spiroperidol 9, 10, 40, 47, 195
St. Louis criteria 80
Stereotype *128*, *174*, 176, *182*, *194*, *200*
Striatal cholinergic interneurones 41
complex 151
dopamine depletion (40?), 151, 152
system 37, 42
Striatonigral pathway 193
Striatum/striatal structure 4, 20, 23, 24, 29, 30, 40, 42, 43, *46*, 102, *122*, 153
Substance P 42, 52, 109, 151
Substantia innominata 51
Substantia nigra 29, 33, 42, 49, 51, 52, 54, 107, 120, 124, *145*, *191*, *200*
lesion *19–30*, 60
pars compacta (SNC) 49

Substantia nigra (continued)
  pars reticulata (SNR) 49, 54, 124, 125, 134, 205
Subthalamic neurons *46–57*
Sulpiride 3, *19*, 47, 48, 53, 163
Superior colliculus *46–57*
Supersensitivity 35, 41, 43, *182–190*

Tectum 124
Tefludazine 9–18
Tetrabenazine 101
Thalamic relay stations *46–57*
Thalamo-cortical projections *46–57*
Thalamus 51, 124
Thioridazine 14, 100, 119, 163, 175
Thioxanthenes *9*, *182*
THIP 50, 124, 125, *128*, 139
Thyrotropin releasing hormone (TRH) 151
Tolerance 13, 41, 42, 51, 102, 182, 219, 222
Tonus 65, 111
Torticollis 66, *111*
Tourette's (Gilles de la) syndrome *64*, 111, *118*
Tremor 114, 219
Treatment
  acute *182–190*
  subacute *182–190*
  chronic *182–190*
Trifluoperazine 14
Trihexyphenidyl 113
Tyrosine hydroxylase activity 41

Vasopressin 140
Ventral forebrain *46–57*
Ventral striatum *46–57*
Ventral-lateral thalamus *46–57*
Ventricular enlargement 86
Ventrolaterial thalamic nucleus *46–57*
Vigilance 163
γ-Vinyl-GABA 125, 139
VIP 147

Withdrawal 49, 70, *98*, *182*

MIX
Papier aus verantwortungsvollen Quellen
Paper from responsible sources
FSC® C105338

If you have any concerns about our products,
you can contact us on
ProductSafety@springernature.com

In case Publisher is established outside the EU,
the EU authorized representative is:
Springer Nature Customer Service Center GmbH
Europaplatz 3, 69115 Heidelberg, Germany

Printed by Libri Plureos GmbH
in Hamburg, Germany